Liver Ultrasound

From Basics to Advanced Applications

Edited by

Adrian K.P. Lim, MD, FRCP, FRCR
Professor and Consultant Radiologist
Department of Imaging, Imperial College Healthcare NHS Trust, London, UK;
Department of Metabolism, Digestion and Reproduction,
Imperial College London, UK

Matteo Rosselli, MD, PhD, FRCP
Consultant in Internal Medicine and Honorary Associate Professor
Department of Internal Medicine, San Giuseppe Hospital, USL Toscana Centro, Empoli, Italy;
Division of Medicine, Institute for Liver and Digestive Health, University College London,
Royal Free Hospital, London, UK

WILEY Blackwell

This edition first published 2024

© 2024 John Wiley & Sons Ltd

Registered Offices

John Wiley & Sons, Inc., 111 River Street, Hoboken, NJ 07030, USA

John Wiley & Sons Ltd, The Atrium, Southern Gate, Chichester, West Sussex, PO19 8SQ, UK

For details of our global editorial offices, customer services, and more information about Wiley products visit us at www.wiley.com.

Wiley also publishes its books in a variety of electronic formats and by print-on-demand. Some content that appears in standard print versions of this book may not be available in other formats.

Library of Congress Cataloging-in-Publication Data

Names: Lim, Adrian, editor. | Rosselli, Matteo, editor.

Title: Liver ultrasound : from basics to advanced applications / edited by Adrian K.P. Lim, Matteo Rosselli.

Description: First edition. | Hoboken, NJ : Wiley-Blackwell, 2024. | Includes bibliographical references and index.

Identifiers: LCCN 2022017515 (print) | LCCN 2022017516 (ebook) | ISBN 9781119612599 (cloth) | ISBN 9781119612605 (adobe pdf) | ISBN 9781119612636 (epub)

Subjects: MESH: Liver Diseases–diagnostic imaging | Liver–diagnostic imaging | Ultrasonography

Classification: LCC RC847.5.I42 (print) | LCC RC847.5.I42 (ebook) | NLM WI 710 | DDC 616.3/620754–dc23/eng/20220610

LC record available at https://lccn.loc.gov/2022017515

LC ebook record available at https://lccn.loc.gov/2022017516

Cover Design by Wiley

Cover Image: Courtesy of Matteo Rosselli

Set in 9.5/12.5pt STIXTwoText by Straive, Pondicherry, India

Printed in Singapore

M100222_020124

Contents

List of Contributors

Ali Alsafi
Department of Imaging
Imperial College Healthcare NHS Trust
London, UK

Annalisa Berzigotti
Department of Visceral Surgery and Medicine,
Inselspital, Bern University Hospital
University of Bern
Bern, Switzerland

James P.F. Burn
Department of Imaging
Imperial College Healthcare NHS Trust
London, UK

Annamaria Deganello
Department of Radiology, King's College Hospital;
Division of Imaging Sciences, King's College London
London, UK

Caroline Ewertsen
Department of Radiology
Rigshospitalet
Copenhagen, Denmark

Giovanna Ferraioli
Department of Clinical, Surgical, Diagnostic and
Pediatric Sciences, University of Pavia
Pavia, Italy

M. Ángeles García-Criado
Radiology Department, Hospital Clínic i Provincial
University of Barcelona
Barcelona, Spain

Ivica Grgurevic
University Hospital Dubrava
Department of Gastroenterology, Hepatology and Clinical
Nutrition,
University of Zagreb School of Medicine and Faculty of
Pharmacy and Biochemistry
Zagreb, Croatia

Sevan Harput
Division of Electrical and Electronic Engineering
London South Bank University
London, UK

Chris J. Harvey
Department of Imaging
Imperial College NHS Healthcare Trust
London, UK

Tom Heller
Lighthouse Trust, Lilongwe, Malawi;
International Training and Education Center for Health,
University of Washington, Seattle, WA, United States

Michaëla A.M. Huson
Radboud University Medical Center, Department of
Internal Medicine and Radboud Center of Infectious
Diseases (RCI), Nijmegen, The Netherlands

Robert de Knegt
Department of Gastroenterology and Hepatology
Erasmus MC University Medical Centre
Rotterdam, The Netherlands

Adrian K.P. Lim
Department of Imaging, Imperial College Healthcare NHS
Trust, London, UK;
Department of Metabolism, Digestion and Reproduction,
Imperial College London, UK

Andreas Panayiotou
Department of Radiology
King's College Hospital
London, UK

Neeral R. Patel
Department of Imaging
Imperial College Healthcare NHS Trust
London, UK

Thomas Puttick
Department of Radiology
King's College Hospital
London, UK

Maija Radzina
Radiology Research laboratory, Riga Stradins University;
Diagnostic Radiology Institute, Paula Stradins University
Hospital; Medical Faculty, University of Latvia,
Riga, Latvia

Matteo Rosselli
Department of Internal Medicine, San Giuseppe Hospital,
USL Toscana Centro, Empoli, Italy;
Division of Medicine, Institute for Liver and Digestive
Health, University College London, Royal Free Hospital,
London, UK

Davide Roccarina
Department of Internal Medicine and Hepatology,
Azienda Ospedaliero-Universitaria di Careggi,
Florence, Italy;
Division of Medicine, Institute for Liver and Digestive
Health, University College London, Royal Free Hospital,
London, UK

Maria E. Sellars
Department of Radiology
King's College Hospital
London, UK

Paul S. Sidhu
Department of Radiology
King's College Hospital
London, UK

Ioan Sporea
Department of Gastroenterology and Hepatology
Victor Babes University of Medicine and Pharmacy
Timisoara, Romania

Francesca Tamarozzi
Department of Infectious Tropical Diseases and
Microbiology, WHO Collaborating Centre on
Strongyloidiasis and other Neglected Tropical Diseases,
IRCCS Sacro Cuore Don Calabria Hospital,
Negrar di Valpolicella, Verona, Italy

Meng-Xing Tang
Department of Bioengineering
Imperial College London
UK

Xiaowei Zhou
State Key Laboratory of Ultrasound Engineering in
Medicine, College of Biomedical Engineering, Chongqing
Medical University, Chongqing, China

Forewords

It gives me great pleasure to write the foreword for this very exciting book. Every practical aspect of the discipline has been covered by an energetic team of experts, providing an easily accessible manual for a branch of medical imaging that for some non-experts has been seen as highly specialised and difficult to unlock.

Professor Adrian K.P. Lim is a Professor of Medical Imaging at Imperial College London who, over the years, has majored on new ultrasound techniques, improving visualisation and discrimination of malignant from non-malignant lesions. Dr Matteo Rosselli has worked at the Institute for Liver and Digestive Health at University College London for many years. Together with Professor Adrian K.P. Lim, he has organised the International Hepatology Ultrasound Course at the Royal Free Hospital in London with an active opportunity for 'hands-on' experience for each delegate.

It was this practical approach to teaching and problem solving that has informed this easily digestible book. As a hepatologist who has relied on the expertise of Professor Adrian K.P. Lim and Dr Matteo Rosselli for important diagnostic advice on a tidal wave of patients over the years, it is gratifying to see their knowledge opened up to a wider audience.

Professor Simon Taylor-Robinson
Professor of Translational Medicine
Imperial College London

Undoubtedly, Adrian K.P. Lim and Matteo Rosselli are genuine experts in the field of liver ultrasonography. Together they combine the skills and knowledge of the clinical radiologist with the domain expertise of the practicing hepatologist to address an aspect of patient care which is crucial in the day-to-day management of patients with liver disease. Not only are they experts in the art and science of liver ultrasound but, as illustrated in this book, they are also world class teachers of liver ultrasound.

As a clinical hepatologist at St Marys Hospital London for over 30 years and a professor of hepatology at Imperial College, I have witnessed and appreciated the evolution of liver ultrasound and the increasing dependence on this diagnostic technology in hepatology. Whilst most hepatologists, usually with a gastroenterology training, understand the strengths and limitations of endoscopy, the same cannot be said of ultrasonography. Unfortunately, relatively few hepatologists have mastered ultrasound and consequently fail to fully comprehend the full versatility of this crucial diagnostic tool. Within this book lies an opportunity to correct this deficiency.

Whilst no one can be expected to master a sophisticated skill such as ultrasound without the guidance and training provided by an expert, Adrian K.P. Lim and Matteo Rosselli's 'Liver Ultrasound' goes a long way in providing the information required to get started in this field. The first few chapters provide the novice with the essentials of ultrasound physics, liver anatomy and indeed the anatomy of the ultrasound machine, appropriately termed 'knobology'. Subsequent chapters deal with the common and, in some cases less common, causes of liver disease with focus on focal liver lesions, biliary tract disease, vascular disease and ultrasound in chronic liver disease. This book also deals with relatively new developments in ultrasound including the use of shearwave elastography for assessment of liver fibrosis and microbubble ultrasound for characterisation of space-occupying lesions. The practical nature of this book is illustrated by the chapter on interventional radiology techniques which includes a guide to managing patients with coagulopathy requiring invasive procedures - frequently a source of tension between radiologist and hepatologist.

This is a book which I would strongly recommend to all trainee hepatologists and gastroenterologists. It really should be considered as essential reading for those hepatologists planning to undertake training in liver ultrasound and should definitely be included in the induction pack for radiology trainees. I would like to see an era when all hepatologists undertook their own liver ultrasounds. This book may be one of the catalysts which help to make this happen.

Professor Mark Thursz
Professor of Hepatology and Head of Department
Faculty of Medicine, Department of Metabolism
Digestion and Reproduction
Imperial College London, UK

It is with great pleasure that I introduce to you this book on Liver Ultrasound conceived and led by Adrian K.P. Lim and Matteo Rosselli. The book includes chapters ranging from very basic physical concepts of medical ultrasound to the most updated guidelines for the use of ultrasonography in the clinical management of patients with liver diseases. Since my early training as a clinical hepatologist, I have witnessed the progressive technical development of this field and how ultrasonography has become an essential instrument in everyday clinical practice. The latest developments, including the use of elastography for the assessment of liver tissue fibrosis and contrast agents for the characterization of liver lesions, have made ultrasonography a solid omni-comprehensive asset in Hepatology.

The concept of the book derives from the success of the series of International Liver Ultrasound workshops organized at the Royal Free Hospital in London in the past ten years and is directed at providing a written and illustrated basis to everybody who is interested in developing skills in liver ultrasonography and relative clinical applications. The book is obviously directed to radiologists and sonographers but, most importantly, to trainees in Hepatology and hepatologists, who will have the highest professional advantage by becoming independent users of ultrasonography.

In conclusion, I am truly enthusiastic about this book, and I wish huge success to all those who wish to become expert users of this technology.

Professor Massimo Pinzani
MD, PhD, FRCP, FAASLD, MAE
Sheila Sherlock Chair of Hepatology
University College London, Royal Free Hospital

Preface

The origins of this book stemmed from a series of workshops that we put together and the realisation that there was an appetite for most clinicians and allied health professionals to learn how to scan a liver. While most of us learn via mentors and on the job, rarely are the basics, the 'tips and tricks', put into words. Instead, these nuggets of information tend to be passed on from generation to generation by word of mouth.

With ultrasound becoming the modern-day 'stethoscope', the initial aim of this book was to provide an 'all you need to know' about liver ultrasound, from the basics to advanced practice. As the chapters developed, it progressed from a relatively basic to intermediate-level book into one that encompasses a wide range of diseases. Our esteemed co-authors also provided in-depth knowledge on the multifaceted aspects of liver pathology, its clinical background, and how to apply the latest and advancing technologies.

Overall, it has turned into a book for the beginner to take with them through their journey and medical career, offering a pictorial review of both common and uncommon diseases. We hope this will serve the current and future generations of multidisciplinary liver ultrasound imagers well.

To our past, present, and future colleagues and students – thank you for teaching, helping, and inspiring us to write this book!

Adrian K.P. Lim and Matteo Rosselli

About the Companion Website

This book is accompanied by a companion website.

www.wiley.com/go/LiverUltrasound

This website includes:

- Video clips

1

Getting Started
Ultrasound Physics and Image Formation
Sevan Harput[1], Xiaowei Zhou[2], and Meng-Xing Tang[3]

[1] Division of Electrical and Electronic Engineering, London South Bank University, London, UK
[2] State Key Laboratory of Ultrasound Engineering in Medicine, College of Biomedical Engineering, Chongqing Medical University, Chongqing, China
[3] Department of Bioengineering, Imperial College London, UK

What Is Ultrasound?

Ultrasound refers to an acoustic wave whose frequency is greater than the upper limit of human hearing, which is usually considered to be 20 kHz. Medical ultrasound operates at a much higher frequency range (generally 1–15 MHz) and it is inaudible. Medical ultrasound images are produced based on the interaction between the ultrasound waves with the human body. For this reason, producing and interpreting an ultrasound image require an understanding of the ultrasound waves, their transmission and reception by sensors, and the mechanisms by which they interact with biological tissues.

Ultrasound Waves

Unlike electromagnetic waves used in optical imaging, X-ray, and computed tomography (CT), ultrasound waves are mechanical waves that require a physical medium to propagate through. For example, ultrasound waves can travel in water or human tissue, but not in a vacuum. Ultrasound waves transport mechanical energy through the local vibration of particles. In other terms, an ultrasound wave propagates by the backwards and forwards movement of the particles in the medium. It is important to note that while the wave travels, the particles themselves are merely displaced locally, with no net transport of the particles themselves. For example, if a lighted candle is placed in front of a loudspeaker, the flame may flicker due to local vibrations, but the flame would not be extinguished since there is no net flow of air, even though the sound can travel far away from the speaker [1]. While propagating in a medium, both the physical characteristics of the ultrasound wave and the medium are important for understanding the wave behaviour. Therefore, this section will first introduce the relevant physical processes and parameters that affect ultrasound wave propagation.

Ultrasound Wave Propagation

There are many types of acoustic waves, such as longitudinal, shear, torsional, and surface waves. The mechanical energy contained in one form of an acoustic wave can be converted to another, so most of the time these waves do not exist in isolation. However, for the sake of simplicity we will only describe the longitudinal or compressional waves, which are most commonly used in B-mode and Doppler imaging.

The propagation of longitudinal ultrasound waves is illustrated in Figure 1.1 using discrete particles. As we know, human tissue is not made up of discrete particles, but rather a continuous medium with a more complicated structure. This is merely a simplified physical model to explain wave propagation. During the wave propagation, particles are displaced due to the acoustic pressure in parallel to the direction of motion of the longitudinal wave, as illustrated in Figure 1.1a–c. When the pressure of the medium is increased by the wave, which is called the compression phase, particles in adjacent regions move towards each other. During the reduced pressure phase (rarefaction), particles move apart from each other. During these two phases, the change in the concentration of particles changes the local density, shown in Figure 1.1d as the higher-density regions with darker colours. This change in local density can be related to the change in acoustic pressure, which is also proportional to the velocity of the particles, Figure 1.1e.

Liver Ultrasound: From Basics to Advanced Applications, First Edition. Edited by Adrian K.P. Lim and Matteo Rosselli.
© 2024 John Wiley & Sons Ltd. Published 2024 by John Wiley & Sons Ltd.
Companion website: www.wiley.com/go/LiverUltrasound

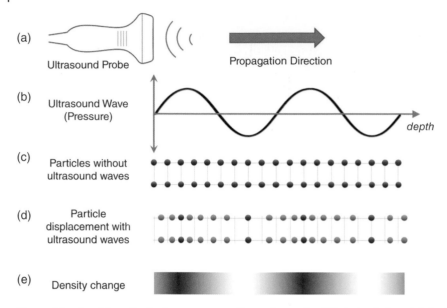

(a) Ultrasound Probe — Propagation Direction

(b) Ultrasound Wave (Pressure) — depth

(c) Particles without ultrasound waves

(d) Particle displacement with ultrasound waves

(e) Density change

Figure 1.1 (a–e) Longitudinal wave propagation using a simplified physical model depicted graphically. A detailed explanation is in the text above.

Particle velocity should not be confused with the speed of sound. The ultrasound wave travels, while the particles oscillate around their original position. The particle velocity is relatively small in comparison to the speed of sound in the medium.

Speed of Sound, Frequency, and Wavelength

A propagating ultrasound wave can be characterised by its speed, frequency, and wavelength. Similar to other types of waves, the speed of propagation of an ultrasound wave is determined by the medium it is travelling in. Propagation speed is usually referred to as the speed of sound, denoted by 'c', and it is a function of the density, 'ρ', and stiffness, 'k', of the medium, as shown in Equation 1.1:

$$c = \sqrt{\frac{k}{\rho}} \qquad (1.1)$$

Tissue with low density and high stiffness has a high speed of sound, whereas high density and low stiffness lead to low speed of sound. See Table 1.1 for speed of sound values in different tissue types and materials [2, 3].

In addition to speed of sound, the frequency, 'f', and the wavelength, 'λ', of the ultrasound wave are crucial parameters for medical ultrasound imaging. The frequency of a wave is the reciprocal of the time duration of a single oscillation cycle of the wave and carries a unit of Hz. The wavelength is the length of a single cycle of the wave and is linked to frequency and speed of sound, as in Equation 1.2:

$$\lambda = \frac{c}{f} \qquad (1.2)$$

In short, frequency has the timing information about the wave for a given space, and wavelength has the spatial (relating to physical space) information about the wave at a

Table 1.1 Ultrasound properties of common materials and tissue.

Material	Speed of sound c (m/s)	Acoustic impedance Z (MRayl)	Density, ρ (10^3 kg/m³)	Attenuation coefficient at 1 MHz (dB/cm)
Air	330	0.0004	0.0012	1.2
Blood	1570	1.61	1.026	0.2
Lung	697	0.31	0.45	1.6–4.8
Fat	1450	1.38	0.95	0.6
Liver	1550	1.65	1.06	0.9
Muscle	1590	1.70	1.07	1.5–3.5
Bone	4000	7.80	1.95	13
Soft tissue (mean)	1540	1.63	–	0.6
Water	1480	1.48	1	0.002

given time. Ultrasound image resolution is related to frequency/wavelength and is usually better at higher frequencies and shorter wavelengths. At a given ultrasound imaging frequency, the wavelength changes proportionally with the speed of sound. For medical ultrasound imaging, the speed of sound is usually assumed to be constant for the tissue and in order to change the image resolution, one needs to change the imaging frequency. For example, for an average speed of sound in soft tissues of 1540 m/s, the wavelength is 0.77 mm at 2 MHz and 0.154 mm at 10 MHz.

Acoustic Impedance

Acoustic impedance is the effective resistance of a medium to the applied acoustic pressure. For example, the particle velocity in soft tissue will be higher than the particle velocity in bone for the same applied pressure due to the difference in their acoustic impedance (see Table 1.1). The acoustic impedance, 'Z', of a material is determined by its density and stiffness values, as shown in Equation 1.3:

$$Z = \sqrt{\rho k} \tag{1.3}$$

Physical Processes That Affect Ultrasound Waves

Reflection

When an ultrasound wave travelling through a medium reaches an interface of another medium with a different acoustic impedance, some portion of the ultrasound wave is reflected, as shown in Figures 1.2 and 1.3. The amplitudes of the transmitted and reflected ultrasound waves depend on the difference between the acoustic impedances of both media, see Figure 1.3. This can be formulated as the reflection coefficient, shown in Equation 1.4:

$$R = \frac{Z_2 - Z_1}{Z_2 + Z_1} \tag{1.4}$$

The interfaces with higher reflection coefficients appear brighter on an ultrasound B-mode image, since a large portion of the ultrasound wave is reflected back. Reflection coefficients at some common interfaces are shown in Table 1.2.

It should be remembered that the underlying model for the equation of the reflection coefficient is based on specular reflection, which means a reflection from a perfectly flat surface or an interface.

In reality, the reflection of ultrasound waves can be considered either specular or diffuse (https://radiologykey. com/physics-of-ultrasound-2). When the ultrasound waves encounter a large smooth surface such as bone, the reflected echoes have relatively uniform direction. This is a type of specular reflection, as shown on the left of Figure 1.2. When the ultrasound waves reflect from a soft tissue interface, such as fat–liver, the reflected echoes can propagate towards different directions. This is a type of diffuse reflection, as shown on the right of Figure 1.2.

Refraction

Refraction is the bending of a wave when it enters a medium with a different speed. It is commonly observed with all types of waves. For example, when looked from above, a spoon appears to be bent in a glass full of water. The reason for this is that the light emerging from the water is refracted

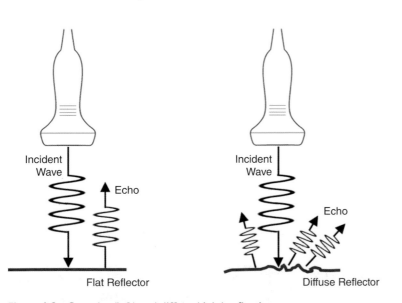

Figure 1.2 Specular (left) and diffuse (right) reflection.

away from the normal, causing the apparent position of the spoon to be displaced from its real position, due to the difference in the speed of light in water and in air.

Refraction of ultrasound waves occurs at boundaries between different types of tissue (different speeds of sound), as shown in Figure 1.3. In ultrasound imaging, this can cause displacement of the target from its true relative position. If the speed of sound is the same in both media, then the transmitted ultrasound wave carries on in the same direction as the incident wave.

Scattering

Human tissue has inhomogeneities. When these inhomogeneities are much smaller than the wavelength, then the ultrasound wave is scattered in many directions, as shown in Figure 1.3. Most of the ultrasound wave travels forward and a certain portion of the wave's energy is redirected in a direction other than the principal direction of propagation. Scattering reduces the amplitude of the initial propagating ultrasound wave, but the lost energy due to scattering is not converted to heat.

Scattering plays an important role in blood velocity estimation. Blood cells (e.g. erythrocytes are 6–8 μm) are usually much smaller than ultrasound imaging wavelengths (>100 μm). Therefore, blood does not reflect but scatter the ultrasound waves.

Absorption

Ultrasound waves are pressure waves. They change the local density by compression and rarefaction, where not all adjacent particles move together. When particles are moving towards each other they experience friction. In medical imaging, this friction is caused by the viscoelastic behaviour of human soft tissue, which is effectively the resistance against the motion.

When the local compression generated by the ultrasound waves are resisted by the friction of the soft tissue, heat is generated. In other words, there will be tiny differences in temperature between regions of compression and rarefaction. Tissue will conduct heat from the higher-temperature region to the lower. This overall process will result in a bulk rise in temperature of the tissue due to viscous losses. Consequently, the energy of the travelling ultrasound waves will be lost after propagation.

Attenuation

Attenuation means a reduction in the amplitude of ultrasound waves. In ultrasound imaging, attenuation of the transmitted waves is usually as a result of absorption, but other physical processes also attenuate the waves, such as reflection, refraction, scattering, and diffraction. The amount of attenuation is usually expressed in terms of the attenuation coefficient, as shown in Table 1.1.

Table 1.2 Reflection coefficients at some common interfaces.

Interface	R
Liver–air	0.9995
Liver–lung	0.684
Liver–bone	0.651
Liver–fat	0.089
Liver–muscle	0.0149
Liver–blood	0.0123

(a)

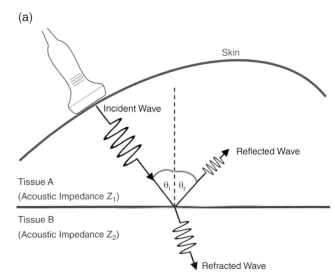

(b)

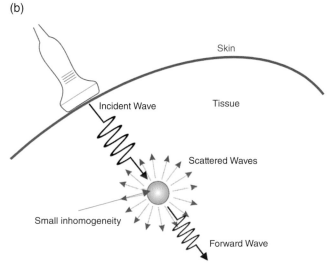

Figure 1.3   (a) Reflected, refracted, and (b) scattered waves.

The most important practical implication of attenuation is that it is hard to achieve good resolution in deep tissue. The image spatial resolution is better at higher ultrasound frequencies. However, the attenuation in tissue is also higher at higher frequencies. Over a given distance, higher-frequency sound waves have more attenuation than lower-frequency waves. This results in a natural trade-off between image resolution (frequency) and imaging depth (penetration). The functionalities to increase the signal amplification with depth in all ultrasound systems, known as time gain compensation (TGC), can, to a limited extent, recover weak signals in deep tissues.

Ultrasound Transducers

A transducer is a device that converts one type of energy into another. An ultrasound transducer generates ultrasound waves by converting electrical energy into mechanical energy. Conversely, an ultrasound transducer can convert mechanical energy into electrical energy. This duality is particularly useful for imaging applications, where the same ultrasound transducer can generate ultrasound waves and also sense the reflected echoes from the human body. Inside all ultrasound imaging probes there are transducer elements that convert electrical signals into ultrasound and, conversely, ultrasonic waves into electrical signals. There are several different methods to fabricate an ultrasound transducer. In this section, we will only explain the piezoelectric materials, which are used in most ultrasound probes.

Piezoelectric Effect

In precise terms, piezoelectric materials work with the principle of piezoelectric effect, which is the induction of an electric charge in response to an applied mechanical strain. The piezoelectric effect explains how ultrasound sensors can detect pressure changes. This effect may be reversed, and the piezoelectric material can be used to generate pressure waves by applying an electric field.

Ultrasound waves can be generated by applying an alternating current (AC) with a frequency closer to the working frequency of the transducer. The AC voltage produces expansions and contractions of the piezoelectric material, which eventually create the compression and rarefaction phases of the ultrasound waves, as shown in Figure 1.4. Usually the displacement on the surface of the piezoelectric material is proportional to the applied voltage. When pressure is applied to the piezoelectric material, it produces voltage proportional to the pressure.

Resonance Frequency

The frequency at which the transducer is most efficient is the resonance frequency. The transducer is also the most sensitive as a receiver at its resonance. If the applied voltage is at the resonance frequency of the transducer, it generates ultrasound waves with the highest amplitude, as shown in Figure 1.5.

The thickness and shape of the piezoelectric material determine the resonance frequency of the ultrasound transducer. The same piezoelectric material can be cut and shaped in different sizes to produce transducers working at different frequencies.

Transducer Bandwidth

Bandwidth is the range of frequencies at which the transducer can operate without significant loss. Piezoelectric materials are resonant systems that work well only at the resonance frequency, but this is not ideal for imaging applications. Imaging applications require a transducer that can work at a range of frequencies. For this reason, manufacturers apply damping to reduce the resonance behaviour.

Figure 1.6 shows the response of a resonant and a highly damped transducer. The undamped transducer has unwanted

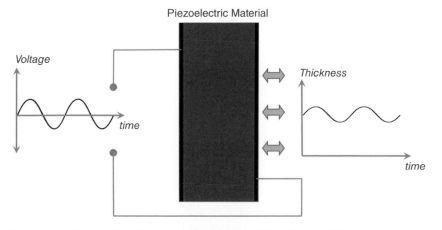

Figure 1.4 Changes in voltage across both sides of the piezoelectric material causes changes in the thickness.

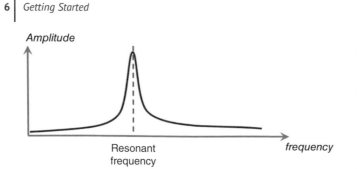

Figure 1.5 Resonance behaviour of piezoelectric ultrasound transducers.

ringing even after the electrical signal stops. This long-duration response of the transducer is not ideal for imaging. A good imaging pulse has a short duration in time, so it can be used to determine objects close to each other. A short pulse contains a range of frequencies and is better accommodated by a transducer with wide bandwidth, such as the damped transducer shown in Figure 1.6.

Single-Element Transducer

Single-element ultrasound transducers are fabricated by using one plate of piezoelectric material, as illustrated in Figure 1.7. A thin plate of piezoelectric material (shown in dark blue) is coated on both sides with a conductive layer,

forming electrodes. Both electrodes are bonded to electrical leads that are connected to an external system to transmit or receive ultrasound waves. The front electrode is usually connected to the metallic case of the transducer and the electrical ground for safety. The back electrode is the electrically active lead. In order to transmit an ultrasound wave, an oscillating voltage is applied to the electrodes. A matching layer is specifically designed for a target application, such as imaging the human body, and it increases the coupling efficiency of the transducer to the body. An acoustic lens may be placed in front of the matching layer to create a weak focal zone. This is particularly useful for small (small in comparison to the operating wavelength) transducers that diverge ultrasound waves outside the imaging region. The backing layer is specifically designed to absorb unwanted internal reverberations. It effectively dampens the resonance behaviour of the piezoelectric material and increases its bandwidth.

Imaging with a Single Element

A single-element transducer can act as a transmitter and also as a receiver. This makes it possible to measure the elapsed time between the transmission of an ultrasound pulse and the reception of its echo from a reflecting or scattering target. If the speed of sound in the medium is known, then the distance to the source of the echo can be

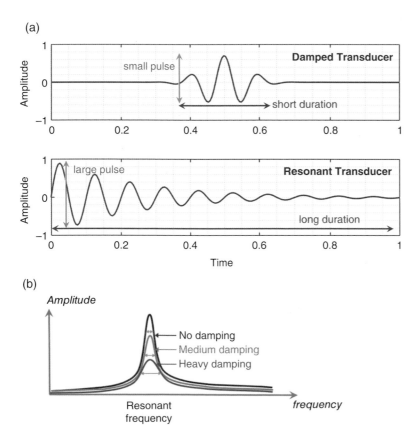

Figure 1.6 Response of a highly resonant transducer and damped transducer to a short electrical pulse. (a) Transducer response measured as a function of time. (b) The corresponding frequency response.

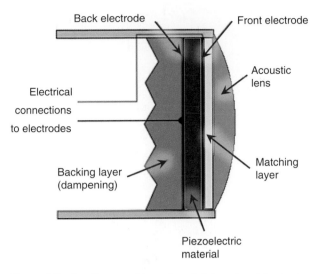

Figure 1.7 An ultrasound transducer's internal architecture.

calculated. After a single measurement, the depth and the amplitude of the echo, which are related to the ultrasonic properties of the target, can be calculated.

This measurement method is usually called a pulse–echo method or an A-scan. It is possible to generate an image by moving the transducer element and performing several A-scan measurements. However, this is not practical for imaging, since it requires a mechanical motion and knowledge of the exact transducer location in order to precisely combine the A-scan measurements. The mechanical scanning method is slower than the electronic scanning method, which will be explained in the next section.

Array Transducers and Transmit Beamforming

Most clinical ultrasound imaging probes consist of an array of transducer elements. Arrays provide flexibility as the transmitted ultrasound beam can be changed on the fly, which is not possible with solid apertures or single-element transducers. The array transducers usually have hundreds of elements with a single front electrode connecting all elements together to the electrical ground. This is important

for safety and also reduces fabrication complexity. Each element has individual electrodes at the rear, and these are connected to the imaging system with a separate cable, as shown in Figure 1.8. The ultrasound system can control each element individually during the transmit and receive cycles. By controlling the timing of transmission in each element, the ultrasound beam can be focused or steered electronically at different depths and directions in so-called transmit beamforming.

Line-by-Line Scan
The most common ultrasound imaging method is line-by-line image formation. In this method, the ultrasound energy is focused into a long and narrow region, as illustrated by the arrows in Figure 1.9 for different type of imaging probes. The received echoes from each transmission form a single line in the ultrasound image. After completing a transmit–receive sequence, the scan line is moved to the next position. The repositioning of the scan line is achieved electronically by controlling the timing of transducer elements. Electronically scanned arrays do not have any moving parts compared to mechanically scanned solid apertures, which are slow and require maintenance. It should be noted that the 'image line' is in reality a 3D volume, as shown in Figure 1.9d, narrower at the focal plane and wider elsewhere.

Ultrasound Image Formation

The transmitted ultrasound waves propagate through tissue and are reflected and scattered from tissue boundaries and small inhomogeneities wherever there is an acoustic impedance mismatch. A portion of these reflected and scattered ultrasound waves travels back to the transducer and is then converted to electrical signals by the transducer elements. Each element on the transducer provides a distinct electrical signal where the timing of each signal accommodates the distance information. Signals from each element are normally called channel signal. All channel

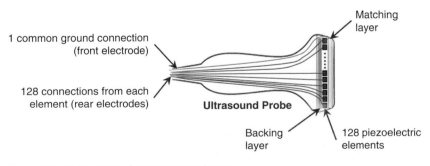

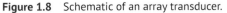

Figure 1.8 Schematic of an array transducer.

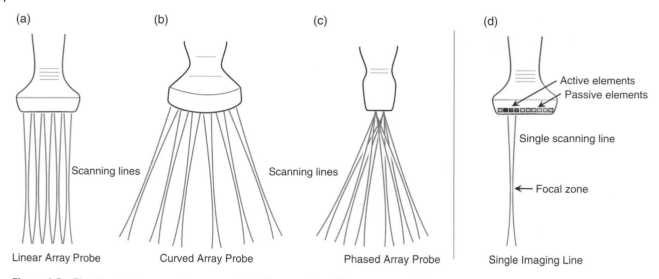

(a)   (b)   (c)   (d)

Scanning lines   Scanning lines

Active elements
Passive elements

Single scanning line

Focal zone

Linear Array Probe   Curved Array Probe   Phased Array Probe   Single Imaging Line

Figure 1.9 The line-by-line scanning approach is illustrated for different types of ultrasound probes used for liver scans. (a) Linear array. (b) Curvilinear array. (c) Phased array. (d) An imaging line.

signals are processed to reconstruct the images in different imaging modes with three main steps, pre-processing to amplify signals and remove noises, receive beamforming to reconstruct the image, and post-processing to enhance the image quality.

Pre-processing and Receive Beamforming

Pre-processing

Pre-processing is to enhance the received signals and remove noises for each channel signal before the receive beamforming. The first step is to amplify the received channel signals, as their amplitudes are generally too small to be processed directly by a beamformer. Besides the signal pre-amplifiers, to which users do not have access, there are two types of amplifiers that can be controlled by users: an overall amplifier and a TGC (Figure 1.10). The overall amplifier enhances the received signals as a whole, regardless of where these

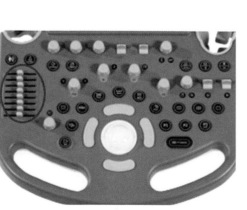

TGC controls

Figure 1.10 The typical time gain compensation (TGC) slide controls for different gains at different depths.

signals are originating from, while the TGC amplifies the signals based on the arrival time to have later-arriving signals from deeper regions being amplified more as they are more attenuated. Although these user-controlled amplifiers are to enhance the received signals, they also amplify the noise. To ensure a sufficient signal-to-noise ratio (SNR), a certain level of transmission power is required.

Band pass and other filters may also be used after the amplifications to remove some electrical noise in the signals. Signals received at each channel are analogue signals, which vary continuously. The beamforming and all post-processing in modern scanners are done in digital form. Therefore, analogue-to-digital conversion (ADC) is always required for digital processing.

Delay-and-Sum Receive Beamforming

In receive beamforming, the echoes received from all transducer elements are realigned in time through pre-determined time delays, so that only the echoes originating from the same spatial locations (pixels) are summed. In clinical ultrasound scanners, the images in all modes are typically formed with line-by-line transmitting and receiving, so signals from each transducer element are realigned to focus at specified depth(s) for each scanning line after the ADC. The realignment is done by compensating for the arriving delay time, which is determined by the path length between the specified depth and the individual elements, as shown in Figure 1.11. Then the realigned signals corresponding to a certain spatial location (pixel) are summed. This beamforming method is called delay-and-sum (DAS). In order for every pixel, or depth along the scan line, to be in focus in the reconstructed image, the delays to arrival time in DAS need to be adjusted dynamically to achieve

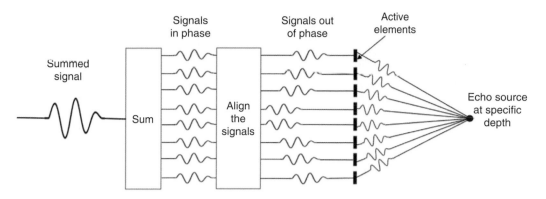

Figure 1.11 The delay-and-sum receive beamforming method for obtaining the in-phase summation of signals from individual active elements at a specific focusing depth. 'Dynamic focusing' means the delays need to be calculated for multiple depths.

continuous advancement of the focusing depth and have what it is called 'dynamic focusing in reception'.

Most ultrasound imaging modes, including B-mode ultrasound, Doppler ultrasound, and elastography, need to have the pre-processing and line-by-line receive beamforming procedure before the image display. The differences among those imaging modes start from post-processing after line-by-line beamforming, which will be explained in the following sections.

B-Mode Ultrasound

B-mode ultrasound in this chapter (B stands for brightness) refers to virtualising the tissue structures based on the brightness of received signals. According to the frequency components of the received signals selected for B-mode imaging, there is fundamental frequency imaging or harmonic imaging.

When an acoustic wave propagates in the human body, in addition to the attenuation of its amplitude, its initial shape and frequency compositions can also be gradually altered by the tissue as it propagates, a phenomenon called non-linear propagation. This is due to the fact that the local tissue density does not respond entirely proportionally to the local ultrasound compression or rarefaction pressure, especially at high acoustic pressures. Consequently, the propagating wave, as well as the received signals, not only has the same frequency components as the transmitted pulse (called fundamental frequency), but also harmonic frequencies, which are multiples of the transmitted frequencies. This distortion tends to occur when the transmitted pulse has high pressure or when there are ultrasound contrast media along the propagation path.

The different frequency components of the received signals have different characteristics, and the choice of which component to use forms the basis of the two imaging approaches, fundamental frequency imaging and harmonic imaging. Image reconstruction in both categories is to be explained in this section.

Fundamental Frequency B-Mode Imaging

This imaging approach assumes that the higher harmonic frequencies in the received signals can be discarded and only considers the fundamental frequency components. After the DAS beamforming, the summed signal is still in the radio frequency (RF) domain, oscillating at the transmitted frequency when non-linear propagation is ignored. This RF signal can be described as a modulated sinusoidal signal, which has the amplitude and phase information. In B-mode imaging, it is the amplitude information that determines the brightness of the image; the phase information is normally discarded. A procedure called amplitude demodulation is applied to extract this envelope information by removing the oscillating carrier frequency, as shown in Figure 1.12. Envelopes from each scanning line will be used to form a two-dimensional B-mode image.

Harmonic Imaging

In harmonic imaging, signals at the transmitted fundamental frequency are removed from the beamformed RF signal, and only the harmonic components are selected for extracting the envelope information and forming B-mode images. This is typically done by filtering out the fundamental components with a bandpass filter. One of the advantages of using harmonic components is that the beam width in the lateral direction is narrower than that of the fundamental components (Figure 1.13), which will give better lateral resolution, as explained in the next section. After removing the fundamental frequency components, amplitude demodulation is also needed to extract envelopes from harmonic components in each scanning line to form the 2D image.

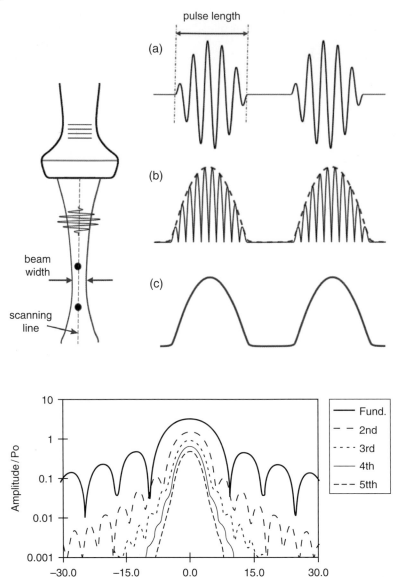

Figure 1.12 A pulsed ultrasound beam to image two point sources along one scanning line shown on the left. (a) The beamformed radio frequency signal. (b) Amplitude modulation applied to get the envelope of the two point sources. (c) The extracted envelope on this scanning line for the image display.

Figure 1.13 Computed harmonic beam profiles in the focal plane of a 2.25 MHz transducer, where lateral resolution is much improved with harmonic imaging. *Source:* Reproduced by permission from Duck, F.A., Baker, A.C., Starritt, H.C. (eds) (1998) *Ultrasound in Medicine*, Boca Raton, FL: CRC Press.

Image Resolutions

When evaluating the performance of an imaging system, the user should consider three different resolutions: temporal resolution, spatial resolution, and contrast resolution. The *temporal resolution* is to measure how many image frames can be reconstructed per second (fps). High temporal resolution is required to capture the fast-moving objects in the tissue, such as the moving heart and blood flow.

Spatial resolution is to evaluate the ability of an imaging system to distinguish the two closest points in a 3D object space. It includes the spatial resolution in the axial direction, lateral direction, and elevational direction in the ultrasound imaging coordinates (Figure 1.14). Spatial resolution in the axial direction is determined by the length of the transmitted pulse (Figure 1.12), which in turn is determined by the central frequency of the transmission and the bandwidth of the system. In the lateral direction, the resolution is related to the lateral beam width (Figure 1.12) and depends on the size of the transducer aperture and the imaging depth; it is typically between one and two wavelengths of the transmitted waves. In the elevational direction, the resolution is determined by the thickness of the scan plane, also called slice thickness, which varies with depth. Most transducers have a fixed focusing depth in the elevational direction, achieved by a cylindrical acoustic lens attached to the transducer face. Even with the lens focusing, the slice

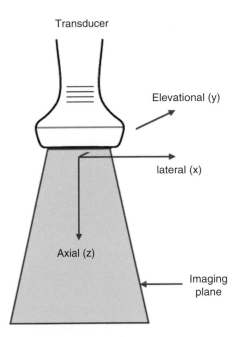

Transducer

Elevational (y)

lateral (x)

Axial (z)

Imaging plane

Figure 1.14 The conventional coordinate system in an ultrasound imaging system.

thickness is generally larger than the beam width in the lateral direction.

Contrast resolution defines the ability to differentiate an area of tissue from its surroundings. This ability is important in ultrasound diagnosis, since it can help identify different organs and monitor pathological change. Compared to magnetic resonance imaging (MRI), ultrasound imaging has relatively less contrast resolution due to the similar echogenicity of different soft tissues in the body.

Image Display

Before displaying the image on the screen, it is necessary to compress the signals into a certain dynamic range. This is because the reflected intensity from different tissues spreads over a large range. If all these intensities were displayed on the screen in a linear scale, the weak echoes scattered from most soft tissues would be dark in the image, and only the echoes from large surfaces/interfaces would stand out. To address this issue, the large-range intensity values of echoes are compressed to simultaneously display strong echoes from, for instance, organ interfaces and weak signals from within soft tissues. This compression process is normally a non-linear procedure such as logarithm compression, which amplifies the weak echoes more than it does the large echoes. In commercial ultrasound scanners, the non-linear compression curve can be adjusted to have a different dynamic range for the final image display.

After compression, the image can be displayed on the screen for diagnosis. From ultrasound transmission to final display the whole process can be in real time. Modern commercial systems may also use some advanced filters to reduce the speckle effect in the image or further smooth the image for an improved visual display.

Doppler Ultrasound

Medical Doppler ultrasound uses ultrasonic waves for measuring blood flow in the cardiovascular system as well as tissue motion. It has been widely used in clinical practice; its high temporal resolution and real-time imaging make it a unique modality for blood flow measurements. Over the past 50 years, most Doppler systems may be categorised as the continuous wave (CW) Doppler system and the pulsed wave (PW) Doppler system. The two types of system have their own advantages, but PW systems are more commonly used in modern scanners. In Doppler ultrasound, ultrasonic waves are transmitted through a transducer and are scattered by the moving red blood cells and then received by the same aperture (in a PW system) or a separate one (in a CW system) for extracting the blood flow velocities with signal processing algorithms. Both CW and PW systems are based on the Doppler effect for the estimation of blood flow or tissue motion velocities.

Doppler Effect

The Doppler effect refers to the shift in the observed frequency of a wave as a result of motion from the wave source or from the observer. In ultrasound flow imaging the ultrasound transducer, which is fixed in one position, transmits a sound wave at a frequency of f_t and this sound wave will hit blood cells; meanwhile the blood cells are moving at a velocity of v. The frequency f_r of the sound wave scattered by blood cells and received by the transducer will have the relation shown in Equation 1.5:

$$f_d = f_t \cdot \frac{2v}{c} \qquad (1.5)$$

If the blood flow is static, the received wave and transmitted wave have the same frequency, so the Doppler frequency shift will be zero (Figure 1.15). The received wave will have a higher frequency than the transmitted wave if the blood cells are moving towards the transducer, producing a positive Doppler frequency shift, and vice versa. When there is an angle θ between the direction of the moving blood cells and the ultrasonic sound wave beam direction, a triangular relation needs to be considered, giving the final Doppler frequency in Equation 1.6:

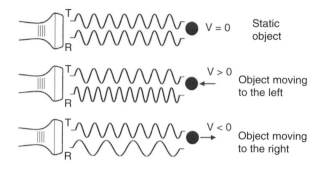

Figure 1.15 Doppler effect occurring due to blood cell motion.

$$f_d = f_t \cdot \frac{2vcos(\theta)}{c} \qquad (1.6)$$

From this relation, it is clear that the angle between the transmitted sound beam and the flow must be smaller than 90° to generate a shift in frequency. To avoid a 90° beam incident, the transmitted beam sometimes is intentionally steered to have a small angle to the vessel wall. From Equation 1.6, it can also be seen that a typical blood velocity of 1 m/s will only produce a Doppler frequency of about 6.4 kHz when the transmitted frequency is 5 MHz, which is a very small fraction of the transmitted frequency (about 0.1%).

Flow Measurement and Imaging Using Doppler

There are different types of clinical Doppler techniques, depending on the way ultrasound waves are transmitted and echo data processed. CW Doppler transmits a constant wave with one transducer (or a group of transducer elements) and receives with another, while PW Doppler uses the same transducer element(s) for both transmission and reception.

Once the echo signals are received they need to be processed to extract the blood flow information. While some processing is different between the Doppler techniques, the processing steps in common include demodulation and tissue clutter filtering. The demodulation is to remove the transmitted carrier frequency in the RF signal so that only the frequency changes caused by motions are kept. This procedure is similar to that in B-mode imaging, but in Doppler imaging the phase information also needs to be extracted. In practice, motions of the tissue within the path of the ultrasound beam, which could be introduced by pulsatile flow in blood vessels and the pumping heart or breathing, also generate Doppler signals together with the moving blood. Doppler signals caused by tissue motions need to be removed to have an unbiased estimation of blood flow velocities. Typically, signals from moving tissues have about 40 dB (100 times) higher amplitude than

signals from moving blood cells. In contrast, the Doppler frequency components arising from tissue motions are lower than those from moving blood cells, as blood cells can move at a velocity as high as a few metres per second (up to ~5 m/s), while even the myocardium and the heart valves normally move at a speed of less than 0.1 m/s. The differences in frequency between Doppler signals from moving blood cells and moving tissues make it possible to separate them. Clutter in Doppler ultrasound refers to tissue signals that interfere with the detection of moving blood cells, and can be filtered out by a high-pass filter in the frequency domain. This is also called a 'wall filter', although it is not limited to removing signals coming from the moving vessel walls. The hypothesis is that clutter has lower-frequency components, so a high-pass filter in the frequency domain can remove the clutter by choosing the right frequency threshold. This frequency filter will remove any signals below that threshold, meaning signals from slow-moving blood cells are also cut off altogether. In modern ultrasound scanners, the cut-off threshold can be adjusted by the user depending on different clinical applications.

Continuous Wave Doppler System

In a CW system, ultrasound waves are continuously transmitted by one set of elements in the transducer and received continuously by a separate set of elements, as shown in Figure 1.16. The biggest disadvantage of the CW system is that it does not provide specific depth information about where the blood flow is being measured. The measurements are made within the whole sensitive region, which is the overlap region of the transmitted and received beams (Figure 1.16), and depends on the positions of transmitting and receiving apertures and the transmitting beam steering angle. The CW system is still commonly used in clinical practice, as it has the advantage of being able to measure blood flow with very high velocity.

After demodulation and clutter filtering, what remains are the Doppler signals arising from the moving blood cells from within the sensitive region, as shown in Figure 1.16. The next step is to estimate the frequency components, which are related to the blood flow velocities. In the CW

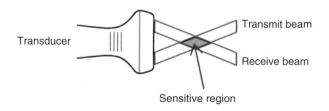
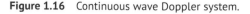

Figure 1.16 Continuous wave Doppler system.

system, the estimator used is called fast Fourier transform (FFT), which takes a segment of 5–20 ms of the Doppler signal samples to generate one frequency spectrum. Frequency components in this spectrum are converted into velocities according to Equation 1.6. A series of FFTs need to be done to process all the received signals for a real-time display.

The flow velocity display in a CW system is called a sonogram, as shown in Figure 1.17. In a sonogram, the horizontal axis represents the time and the estimated velocity is shown along the vertical axis. Each column of the sonogram is one spectrum estimated by the FFT estimator. The brightness of each pixel in the sonogram relates to the number of blood cells travelling at a particular velocity within the sensitive region. The horizontal baseline corresponds to zero velocity, which is the defining line for positive and negative flow with regard to the transducer. Normally, it is designed to have positive velocity (blood moving towards the transducer) locate above this baseline and negative velocity (blood moving away from the transducer) below the baseline. This convention can be changed by the operator in the scanner's settings. The Doppler shift frequency in medical imaging is generally within the audible range so that it can also be played by a speaker for clinicians to listen to.

Pulsed Wave Doppler System

In a PW system, pulsed waves are transmitted and the same transducer can be used both for transmission and reception. A PW system is shown in Figure 1.18.

The advantage of PW Doppler is that both the depth and size of the region of interest for acquiring Doppler signals (also called sample volume or range gate) are known, and can be adjusted manually by the operator on the screen of the scanner in real time. The transmitting time of each pulse can be used as a reference to retrieve the depth information of the received signal by assuming that the speed of sound in tissue is constant and known. There are three different

Doppler imaging modes that are based on the PW system: spectral Doppler, colour Doppler, and power Doppler.

Spectral Doppler

Spectral Doppler in the PW system is very similar to CW Doppler in terms of signal processing in demodulation, clutter filtering, frequency estimation, and display, making them indistinguishable to some degree. The only difference is that the signal is not received continuously but in a pulsed way. It is also this difference that allows the operator to adjust the sensitive region (depth and length of the range gate) in PW spectral Doppler, and a velocity sonogram can be displayed in real time. The ability to have these real-time adjustments and the availability of quantitative velocity information makes spectral Doppler one of the most common Doppler techniques in clinical practice. The disadvantage of a PW system compared to a CW system is that it has an aliasing problem when the blood flow to be measured is moving at high speed. This issue will be explained later.

In PW spectral Doppler, samples within the echoes corresponding to consecutive pulses originating from the chosen depth are combined in sequence to form a sampled Doppler signal. Then the same processing as in CW Doppler is applied to generate spectra for sonogram display (Figure 1.17). The chosen depth in the sampling procedure corresponds to a fixed spatial position, and it is adjustable by the user.

The sampling procedure in pulsed signals could cause aliasing when the blood flow is moving at high speed. This is similar to that in sampling theory, where a higher sampling rate is required to keep the higher-frequency components in a signal (the Nyquist theorem). In the PW system, each received pulse provides the Doppler signal with one sample. Blood flow moving at high speed will generate high-frequency components in the Doppler signal, as explained in Equation 1.5, meaning that a higher sampling frequency is required to avoid aliasing. The sampling rate in the PW system is the pulse repetition frequency (PRF) of the system, which is limited by the speed of sound for a specific imaging depth. According to the Nyquist rule, the PRF must be at least twice as high as the maximum Doppler shift frequency component.

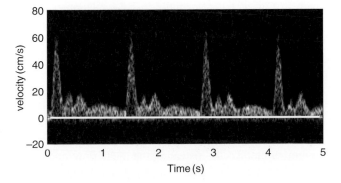

Figure 1.17 A sonogram of continuous wave Doppler and pulsed wave spectral Doppler.

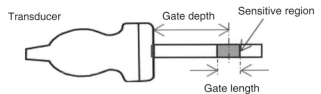

Figure 1.18 Pulsed wave spectral Doppler system.

According to Equation 1.5, the Doppler shift frequency is 6.4 kHz when the blood cells move at 1 m/s and the transmitted frequency is 5 MHz, so the PRF must be more than 12.8 kHz. It is difficult to achieve such a high PRF for a PW system, as it is always interleaved with B-mode and/or colour Doppler to obtain a duplex or triplex mode in clinical practice. One way to mitigate this issue is to use a lower transmitted frequency to have a proportionally lower Doppler shift frequency under the same blood velocity. This is the reason the transmitted frequency in PW spectral Doppler is normally lower than 5 MHz, to avoid aliasing for high-speed blood flow applications. Another way is to adjust the baseline in the sonogram to give a larger range in the direction (positive or negative) where the flow velocity is larger.

Colour Doppler

Spectral Doppler can only measure the blood flow velocities from within a range gate. It is not able to cover a larger region of interest, although it allows the user to adjust the location of the range gate. Colour Doppler is for a 2D blood velocity visualisation, and it always works together with B-mode imaging to have the colour-coded velocity map superimposed on the B-mode image. In most modern scanners, it is also possible to combine anatomical B-mode image, spectral Doppler sonogram, and colour-coded velocity map into one image on the scanner's screen, as shown in Figure 1.19. This is possible because all these three modes are based on pulsed wave transmitting and receiving, so interleaving strategies can be designed to allow them to work in a dedicated sequence.

In CW Doppler and spectral Doppler, there is only one received ultrasound beam to estimate the flow velocity along one scanning line. In colour Doppler, a series of beams sweeping along the transducer's element array are transmitted and received, forming an 2D region of interest

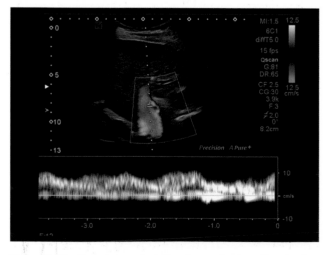

Figure 1.19 B-mode, spectral Doppler, and colour Doppler in a triplex mode assessing flow in the portal vein.

in a similar way as is done in standard B-mode imaging. Each of these beams is transmitted and received in the same way as in spectral Doppler, but it contains multiple adjacent range gates along its scanning line rather than only one range gate. Within each range rate, it is the mean velocity component (instead of a spectrum in CW or PW Doppler) along the beam direction that is being estimated in colour Doppler. The same demodulation and clutter filtering are done here as in CW Doppler and spectral Doppler. In principle, the mean velocity in each range gate can also be derived by FFT of the demodulated Doppler signal to the frequency domain, followed by extracting the mean frequency shift in the spectrum. However, this is not how it is done in most commercial scanners, since this method would take too much time to have a 2D mean velocity map in real time.

Instead, an autocorrelation estimator is adopted in colour Doppler, which can directly obtain the mean flow velocity through estimating the mean 'phase shift' at each location with an ensemble of consecutive received echoes. The number of pulses required along each scanning line is important for the estimation. Typically over 10 pulses per scan line are necessary for an acceptable mean velocity estimation, especially for low-level velocities. This means the frame rate in colour Doppler will be reduced by ≥ 10 times compared with B-mode imaging. The compromise between the frame rate and the quality of velocity estimation in colour Doppler presents challenges in dealing with fast flow while maintaining the real-time imaging frame rate. Two measures can be taken to increase the frame rate in colour Doppler without compromising velocity estimation. The first one is to restrict the imaging field of view by defining a colour box, and only estimating the colour-coded velocities within the colour box. The size and position of this colour box can be adjusted by the user. In this way, the number of scanning lines is reduced to only fill up the colour box, and each scanning line does not need to cover the whole depth on the B-mode image. The second method could be to have a lower line density, meaning less time needed for each imaging frame. A typical colour box is given in Figure 1.19. Normally in colour Doppler, red is used to represent the blood flow moving towards the transducer and blue for the flow moving in the opposite direction, but this can be changed by the user in the settings.

Power Doppler

Most of the basics discussed in colour Doppler remain the same in power Doppler, except that power Doppler displays the power of the blood flow signals, a measure of the amount of blood cells, instead of the mean flow velocity of the blood cells as in colour Doppler. The calculated signal power is proportional to the square of the amplitude of the demodulated and clutter-filtered Doppler signal, and this

Figure 1.20 A typical colour-coded box estimated from power Doppler superimposed on a B-mode image. *Source:* Reproduced by permission from Hoskins, P.R., Martin, M.K., Thrush, T.A. (2019) *Diagnostic Ultrasound: Physics and Equipment*, London: Taylor & Francis.

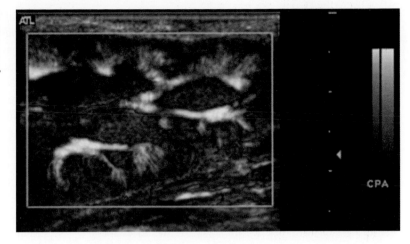

power information can also be estimated by the autocorrelation estimator used in colour Doppler.

An example of power Doppler is shown in Figure 1.20, where the colour relates to the local density of moving blood cells. Since there is no directional information about the moving blood cells in the signal power, the conventional power Doppler method does not contain information on the blood flow direction. The instrument settings for displaying colour Doppler and power Doppler are usually the same.

Compared to colour Doppler, which can image the flow dynamics, power Doppler does not generate velocity information and could be optimised, for instance through temporal averaging, to have better sensitivity for visualising vascular morphology. Temporal averaging can reduce the noise level in the image, making it possible to distinguish small vessels. Flow direction information can also be introduced to power Doppler, for example by incorporating flow direction estimation from colour Doppler.

Challenges with Doppler Flow Imaging

While tissue signals can be suppressed and blood flow can be specifically imaged using Doppler techniques, there are significant limitations. Doppler techniques depend on the echoes from blood cells that are very weak, more than an order of magnitude weaker than surrounding tissues. Therefore, Doppler signals are usually noisy, and it is difficult to detect the signal from small vessels such as small arterioles, venules, and capillaries.

Microbubble Contrast Agents

Microbubble contrast agents are micro-sized gas bubbles. They are sufficiently small that after being introduced, typically through intravenous injection, they are able to cross the capillary bed of the pulmonary circulation. At the same time, these bubbles are big enough that they do not cross the vascular endothelium, making them true intravascular

agents compared to the MRI or CT agents, which often can leak out of the vasculature. In order to prevent the bubbles from rapidly dissolving and/or agglomerating, they are stabilised by a coating of a biocompatible surfactant or polymer (see Figure 1.21), most commonly phospholipids or proteins. This coating both lowers the interfacial tension at the bubble surface and also provides a barrier to gas diffusion.

Despite being similar in size to red blood cells, bubbles are much more efficient scatterers of ultrasound owing to the fact that they are filled with gas. The gas presents a significant interface with acoustic impedance mismatch where strong scattering occurs. Furthermore, due to the gas being highly compressible, bubbles undergo volumetric oscillations in response to the oscillatory ultrasound pressure changes, and can absorb and reradiate the incident sound efficiently rather than merely acting as passive reflectors. This makes bubbles highly sensitive agents, and it has been well demonstrated that with the appropriate imaging parameters, a single micro-sized bubble can be detected by an ultrasound scanner. Following injection, the bubbles circulate throughout the vascular space and greatly increase the amplitude of the scattered signals from within the blood, making the blood flow from very small vessels and even capillaries detectable.

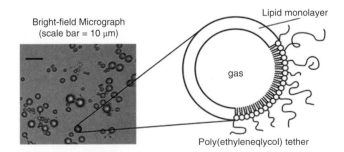

Figure 1.21 Microbubble contrast agents. Left: bright-field micrograph of a microbubble population; right: the compositions of a typical microbubble contrast agent.

While Doppler signals can be significantly enhanced by microbubbles, imaging small vessels presents an extra challenge, as the flow velocity in such small vessels is low. Doppler techniques rely on the difference in velocity between flow and tissue to remove the tissue clutter from Doppler signals. Within small vessels where flow can be as low as millimetres per second, it is difficult to distinguish flow from tissue clutter based only on Doppler velocity estimation, particularly when tissue is also in motion.

Non-linear Behaviour of Microbubbles

Microbubbles' behaviour under ultrasound heavily depends on the amplitude of the ultrasound. The transmit amplitude of the ultrasound is usually indicated by the mechanical index (MI) displayed on the scanner screen. MI is a measure of the potential for mechanical bioeffects (cavitation) in tissue owing to ultrasound exposure, and is defined as the peak negative ultrasound pressure in kPa divided by the square root of the ultrasound frequency in MHz. At a very low MI, the microbubbles undergo volumetric oscillation with radius change approximately proportional to the ultrasound pressure; that is, the oscillation is linear. As the MI increases some microbubbles starts to oscillate, with greater radius changes that are no longer proportional to the ultrasound pressure changes. This is a non-linear process and higher harmonic signals with frequencies at multiples of the fundamental ultrasound frequency can be generated by the microbubble oscillation, even at an MI as low as 0.05. When the MI goes above a certain level (typically between 0.1 and 0.3 depending on the bubble types and ultrasound frequency), some microbubbles start to be destroyed by ultrasound, resulting in reduced contrast enhancement.

Bubble Imaging: High Mechanical Index Destructive Imaging versus Low Mechanical Index Bubble-Specific Imaging

At a high MI microbubbles are easily destroyed and hence the contrast enhancement only happens in the very first few imaging frames with a 'flash' in image intensity. This is due to the fact that the microbubbles can generate strong echo signals while being destroyed. However, in order to maintain the contrast enhancement, lower MIs have to be used. Currently in clinical practice, depending on the different parts of the body and the agent type, the MI typically ranges from 0.04 to 0.3.

While microbubbles can significantly enhance the signal from within the blood, the amplitude of the echoes from within the blood is still at a similar level to those of surrounding tissues. Doppler can be used to separate blood flow from the tissue depending on the motion (blood flow). However, there is a lower limit in flow velocity for Doppler detection: when the flow velocity is close to tissue motion (due to the heart or breathing), blood flow can no longer be separated from surrounding tissue using Doppler, even when microbubble contrast agents are present.

Bubble-specific imaging techniques have been developed to separate the bubble echoes from tissue echoes based on the harmonic signals in the echoes. At a low MI, tissue generally does not produce higher harmonic signals and only bubbles do. Such harmonic signals specifically from microbubbles can be separated from tissue by using multiple pulse transmissions such as pulse inversion or amplitude modulation, as shown in Figure 1.22. In pulse inversion, positive pulse and its inverse are transmitted, and the corresponding received pulses can be summed to form a signal for the image reconstruction. The summed signal will only contain the harmonic components that from tissue are caused by microbubbles even when they are stationary, as fundamental components from tissue are cancelled out due to the linearity. In amplitude modulation, two pulses are transmitted at different levels of amplitude (normally the amplitude of one pulse is doubled, as shown in Figure 1.13); received echo 1 is first multiplied by a factor of two and subtracted from echo 2 to remove the fundamental components from tissue.

Quantification Based on Contrast-Enhanced Ultrasound

In contrast-enhanced ultrasound (CEUS), a time series of contrast-specific images can be obtained, and the tissue

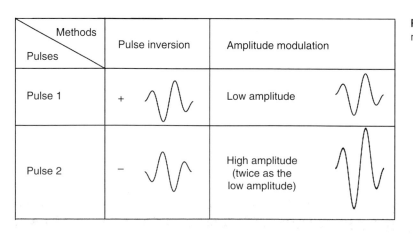

Figure 1.22 The pulse inversion and amplitude modulation methods for harmonic imaging.

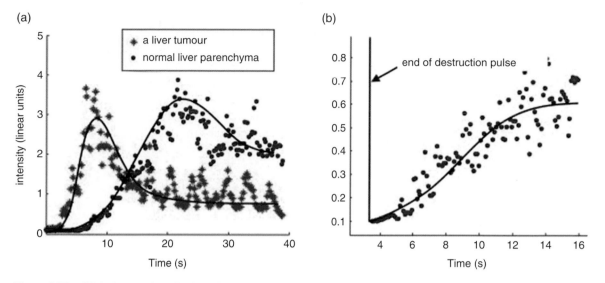

(a)

(b)

end of destruction pulse

a liver tumour

normal liver parenchyma

intensity (linear units)

Time (s)

Time (s)

Figure 1.23 Clinical examples of a time–intensity curve for (a) a bolus injection in a liver; and (b) constant infusion with destruction–replenishment in the myocardium. Oscillations in the signals were mainly caused by tissue motion during imaging, while in (b) cardiac systole may also have contributed to the oscillation. Note that the *y*-axes between (a) and (b) are not comparable as they were acquired with different scanner settings on different patients. *Source:* Tang, M.-X., Mulvana, H., Gauthier, T. et al. (2011), *Interface Focus*, 1(4): 1520–1539. Reproduced with permission of The Royal Society.

uptake of the bubbles can thus be measured as a function of time. Quantification of CEUS can be based on image intensity or the timing of the tissue uptake of the bubbles. A curve of image intensity versus time (the so-called time–intensity curve, TIC) can be produced for any pixel or region of interest within the image plane. Such a curve contains information on tissue perfusion. Two types of TIC can be obtained, depending on whether the bubbles are administered as a bolus injection or via a constant infusion. A bolus is relatively simple to administer and more common in clinical practice, while a constant infusion is often combined with a 'destruction–replenishment' mode in which higher-MI ultrasound pulses are used to destroy the bubbles in the imaging plane, followed by low-MI ultrasound pulses to monitor replenishment in the tissue. This technique is unique to ultrasound, as no other clinical imaging modalities can deactivate their contrast-enhancing agents to create a new input function. Examples of the two types of TIC are shown in Figure 1.23.

Elastography

Tissue stiffness carries diagnostic information: for example, cancerous tissue is usually harder than normal tissue. Manual palpation, such as in the breast, has been proven to be effective, but only for shallow targets, and it is subjective. Elastography uses imaging to non-invasively detect internal tissue displacement as a result of applied forces, based on which a map of tissue elasticity property can be obtained. For example, in Figure 1.24, if we have an imaging tool to show

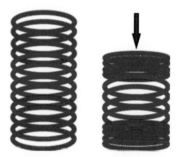

Figure 1.24 Principle of elastography: the blue spring, which simulates soft tissue, compresses more under force than the red spring, which simulates harder tissue. An elastography system can measure the compression of different tissue under force and hence detect their stiffness.

that the red part of the spring is harder to compress, then we will know that part is stiffer than the rest of the spring.

There are a few key quantities in tissue elastography. The first is tissue displacement, which can be measured using imaging and target tracking. The second is stress, which is the applied force per unit area and has units of pressure. The third is strain, ε, which is the fractional change in length, that is, the ratio of total deformation to the initial dimension of the material body, $\varepsilon = \Delta L/L$. Here L is the initial dimension and delta L is the deformation due to the applied force.

An elastography was initially defined as a strain image, but it is not quantitative, and the strain value does not only depend on tissue stiffness. Young's modulus (E), $E = \sigma/\varepsilon$, which describes longitudinal deformation in terms of strain ε in response to longitudinal stress σ, and the tissue shear modulus, which relates transverse strain to transverse stress, are found to be useful tissue stiffness parameters. Such parameters can be obtained by matching the displacements measured from ultrasound images before and after force is applied with those calculated based on a theoretical tissue deformation model with tissue stiffness parameters.

Shear Wave Elastography

A more recent advance to quantitatively measure tissue stiffness is shear wave elastography. In a shear wave, tissue oscillates perpendicularly to the direction of wave propagation. This is in contrast to a longitudinal wave, where tissue oscillates in the same direction as wave propagation. Such a shear wave can be generated through an external mechanical force, or via a push within the tissue remotely generated by ultrasound. When ultrasound is scattered, reflected, or absorbed, energy and momentum are transferred to the medium, inducing a force, termed an acoustic radiation force (ARF). Such an ARF can be used to remotely push tissue at a certain location and generate shear waves originating from this location non-invasively.

Shear wave elastography is based on the relationship in Equation 1.7 between tissue shear modulus μ, tissue density ρ, and shear wave velocity c:

$$c_{SH} = \sqrt{\frac{\mu_{SH}}{\rho}} \qquad (1.7)$$

Assuming a known and constant density of the tissue, the tissue shear modulus μ can be calculated if we know the shear wave velocity c. This velocity can be obtained by ultrasound imaging of the tissue displacement due to the shear waves. Tissue displacement can be obtained by comparing the beamformed image data between consecutive frames through cross-correlation, for instance. When the shear wave passes a certain spatial location in the image, its tissue displacement will increase and decrease over time, as shown in Figure 1.25. If we observe the tissue displacements over time at two chosen spatial positions with known distance, we can calculate the shear wave velocity

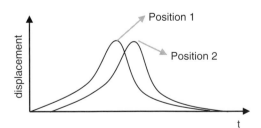

Figure 1.25 Principle of shear wave elasticity estimation: the two curves show tissue displacements at two spatial positions over time, measured by the imaging system. As the spatial distance and time of peak displacement between the two positions are known, shear wave velocity can be calculated, based on which the average shear modulus between the two spatial points can be estimated.

by dividing the distance by the time difference between the two peaks in Figure 1.25.

Given that typical shear wave velocity in soft tissue is in at least metres per second, and an ultrasound imaging field of view is typically a few centimetres, a very high image frame rate, typically at thousands of frames per second, is required to capture the shear wave propagation in the tissue in order to calculate the spatially resolved local velocity distributions.

Ultrasound Imaging Artefacts

Ultrasound images usually contain not only information on tissue structure and function, but also some features and interferences, including speckle, noise, and artefacts. These three features exist in almost all ultrasound imaging modes due to the underlying physics and assumptions made in the imaging. It is important for users to understand these features so that the images can be better interpreted in the diagnosis.

Noise

In a broad sense, there are two types of noise in ultrasound imaging, electronic noise and acoustic noise. The first type is the noise generated by the electronics and can be measured by the SNR. Averaging between consecutive frames of the images could increase the SNR, but it will also bring down the frame rate (temporal resolution). The SNR could also be increased by transmitting at a higher acoustical power, up to the safety limit. The second type of noise is called acoustic noise, which is commonly referred to as the speckle pattern, explained below.

Speckles

Speckles refer to the granular texture in images generated due to the scattering of waves by multiple and closely situated sub-wavelength scatters. As explained previously, an ultrasound system has certain spatial resolutions in a 3D space, which is typically of an order of more than a wavelength. This means that any objects/scatters much smaller than a wavelength cannot be resolved as separate objects. This volume is often called the sample volume. As a result, the brightness of the corresponding pixel in the image is formed by the coherent addition of echoes from all scatters within the sample volume. This coherent addition produces a granular texture called speckle in B-mode images (Figure 1.26). It is tempting to imagine that the speckle pattern represents the true structure within the sample volume. However, this is not the case, and the speckle patterns appear random and are often perceived as noisy, although this pattern is determined once the positions of the scatters and the transducer are determined. Therefore, the speckle patterns do contain information on the underling tissue

(a) (b)

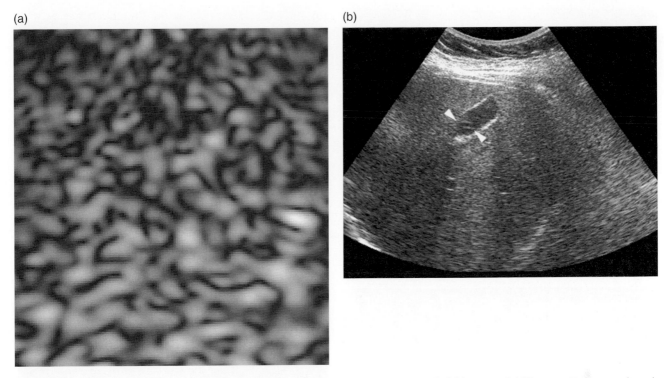

Figure 1.26 (a) The ultrasound B-mode speckle pattern of scatterers within a tissue-mimicking material. These scatterers are densely distributed and their size is smaller than the sound wavelength. (b) An ultrasound image showing some reverbration artefacts (arrows) due to highly reflective tissue interfaces above.

structure. While work has been done to reduce or remove the speckles to generate seemingly less noisy images, some other studies have also been trying to use the speckle pattern to detect the abnormalities by tissue characterisation algorithms, since the speckle pattern will change in a statistical sense if there is abnormal structure in the sample volume.

Artefacts

In ultrasound image formation there are several assumptions regarding ultrasound propagation in and its interaction with tissue. Artefacts could be produced if those assumptions are violated. These assumptions include (i) the speed of sound is constant (1540 m/s in soft tissue); (ii) the ultrasound pulse travels in a straight line; (iii) all energy is confined in the ultrasound beam, whose shape is straight and narrow in 3D space; (iv) the attenuation in tissue is constant; and (v) the pulse travels only to targets that are on the beam axis and back to the transducer, and hence echo signals at each point in time are only dependent on the reflection/scattering characteristics of the corresponding on-beam point in space. Each of these assumptions, when broken, can bring visible image artefacts. Detailed explanations and illustrations of various artefacts arising from these assumptions can be found in [3]. A good understanding of artefacts is important in interpreting the reconstructed images for diagnosis.

B-Mode Artefacts

In the formation of B-mode images, artefacts, which mainly include reverberation, double reflection, side lobes, acoustic shadowing, and post-cystic enhancement, are explained in what follows.

Reverberation

Multiple reflections of the ultrasound wave between the transducer piezoelectrical material surface and a strongly reflecting structure at depth create 'ghost' reflections. Such multiple reflections appear later in time and since the ultrasound scanner does not account for such multiple reflections, it 'thinks' there are similar-looking objects below the reflecting structure deeper in the tissue, at integer multiples of depth. Such reverberation image artefact is also seen close to the transducer surface, especially when the imaging transducer is in the air/not in contact with skin, due to the highly reflective transducer casing–air/skin interface. Figure 1.26b shows an example of reverberation artefact within the gallbladder, depicted by the arrowheads owing to the highly reflective tissue interfaces closer to the transducer.

Double Reflections

A mirror image of an object can be formed, when the ultrasound wave is strongly reflected by a tissue interface (e.g. a vessel wall, as shown in Figure 1.27) before reaching a target

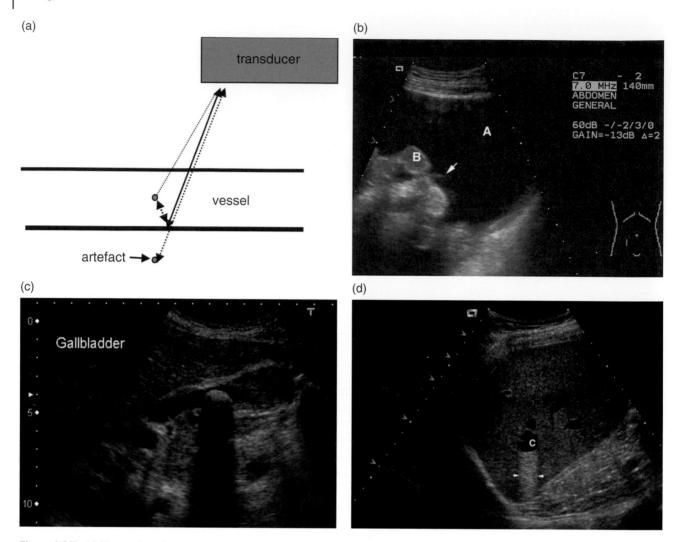

Figure 1.27 (a) Illustration of double reflection artefact. (b) A, ascites; B, bowel; the arrowhead depicts a sidelobe artefact. (c) An image of a gall bladder with a highly attenuating object casting a 'dark'/acoustic shadow posteriorly. (d) An image of a liver with a liquid filled cavity indicated by letter c, which casts a 'bright' shadow or 'through transmission' posteriorly owing to the reduced attenuation of the sound waves by the 'cavity'.

and scattered back to the transducer. In this case echoes are received by the transducer from the target, which is off beam. As the ultrasound scanner assume the echoes are always from the targets on beam, the off-beam object in this case appears as a fake on-beam object deeper in the image.

Side Lobes

While ultrasound scanners assume that the ultrasound imaging pulse travels in a single straight line and the shape of the beam is straight and narrow, in reality the cross-section of the ultrasound beam in the lateral direction has not only a peak (called the main lobe), but also long tails with ripples in them (called side lobes, see Figure 1.13). This means there is some off-beam energy potentially generating detectable echoes from off-beam targets. The transducer/machine cannot differentiate between echoes

from the main beam versus those returning from these off-beam sidelobes, which results in the generation of multiple images of the same object at different (wrong) spatial location(s) (see Figure 1.27b).

Acoustic Shadowing

One assumption by the ultrasound scanner is that the attenuation coefficient of the tissue is constant, so that the compensation of the attenuation is only a function of depth/time, the so-called TGC. However, tissue attenuation is not constant and any region of very high attenuation effectively blocks the beam path, so that very little signal gets through, causing loss of detail or even any signals in image below this region. Figure 1.27c shows an example of such acoustic shadowing in the gallbladder caused by a stone.

Post-cystic Enhancement

The principle of this post-cystic enhancement artefact is the same as acoustic shadowing, except that instead of a region of very high attenuation, the presence of any region of abnormally low attenuation (e.g. a fluid-filled cyst) causes over-compensation of gain below this low attenuation region, making deeper structures too bright. Figure 1.27d shows an example of such post-cystic enhancement (cyst labelled as c).

Artefacts in Doppler Ultrasound

Generally, the artefacts introduced in B-mode imaging also have similar effects on Doppler ultrasound. On top of that, there are some other artefacts that are associated with the estimation of blood flow velocities. For PW Doppler systems, an aliasing issue always exists when the flow is moving too fast. Aliasing will result in high velocities wrapping around the top of the display being shown as flow in the opposite direction (Figure 1.28). In colour Doppler, the aliasing will cause the high-velocity positive flow to be displayed as a negative flow with the wrong colour (Figure 1.29). It should be noted that this aliasing problem does not exist in CW systems.

Another well-known artefact in Doppler imaging is its angle dependence, which applies to most Doppler modes. The underlying reason is that Doppler-based methods can only detect the velocities projected in the acoustic beam direction. As a result, the angle between the beam direction and the real flow direction must be known to derive the real flow velocity. However, this angle information normally is not available due to the complexities of flow in the cardiovascular system. In practice, it is often assumed that the blood is moving parallel to the vessel's long axis, so the angle

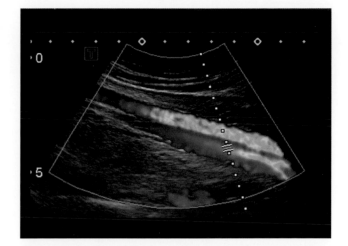

Figure 1.29 The pulse repetition frequency is not high enough and the aliasing issue causes the colour in the high-velocity area to be displayed as the wrong colour.

between the acoustic beam and the vessel's long axis is used to derive the true flow velocity. This beam–vessel angle is obtained by displaying the beam path on the screen together with an indicating bar manually adjusted to be parallel to the vessel (Figure 1.19) in spectral Doppler. In colour Doppler, since the dynamic velocity colour map is of more interest than the absolute velocity values, the angle independence is not as important as it is in spectral Doppler, as long as the colour box is steered to have a non-normal angle to the vessels inside. Power Doppler only detects the power of the motion to distinguish flow from static tissue. The angle dependence issue has little effect in this case, unless the angle between the flow and the beam direction is close to 90°.

In PW spectral Doppler, an inverted mirror image of the Doppler spectrum may be observed if the gain for PW spectral Doppler is set too high (Figure 1.30). A high gain could cause the system to be overloaded and not be able to separate the forward and reverse flows. The mirror image in the sonogram is not from the true reverse flow and it can be removed by turning down the Doppler gain. In colour Doppler, even though the clutter filter is applied to remove the signals from moving tissue, it cannot remove all of them. These unwanted Doppler shifts will produce patterns of colours not associated with blood flow within regions of tissue. The clutter filter could also remove some low-frequency Doppler signals arising from slow-moving blood flow near the vessel wall. Also, some unexpected movements from the transducer or the human body could produce the so-called flash artefact, which appears as false areas of colour on the colour image.

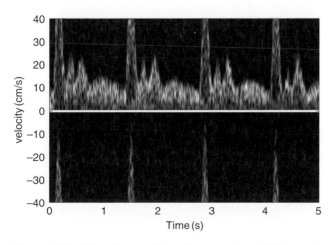

Figure 1.28 The pulse repetition frequency is not high enough and the aliasing issue causes the high positive velocities wrapping around the display to be shown as negative velocities in the opposite direction.

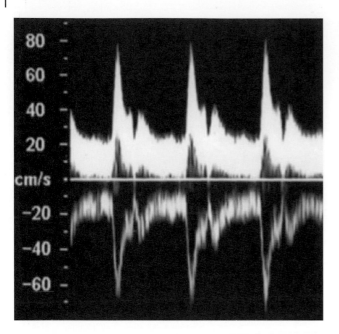

Figure 1.30 The inverted mirror sonogram is observed in pulse wave spectral Doppler due to a high gain. *Source:* Reproduced by permission from Hoskins, P.R., Martin, M.K., Thrush, T.A. (2019) *Diagnostic Ultrasound: Physics and Equipment*, London: Taylor & Francis.

References

1 Leighton, T.G. (2007). What is ultrasound? *Prog. Biophys. Mol. Biol.* 93: 3–83.

2 Dunn, F. (1986). Attenuation and speed of ultrasound in lung: Dependence upon frequency and inflation. *J. Acoust. Soc. Am.* 80: 1248–1250.

3 Hoskins, P.R., Martin, K., and Thrush, A. (2019). *Diagnostic Ultrasound: Physics and Equipment*. London: Taylor & Francis.

2

Knobology and Terminology

Adrian K.P. Lim

Department of Imaging, Imperial College Healthcare NHS Trust, London, UK
Department of Metabolism, Digestion and Reproduction, Imperial College London, UK

Ultrasound scanners come in a multitude of size and types. The more advanced higher- and premium-end scanners can initially look daunting, but all scanners have the same basic image controls. While these controls may be given slightly different names, they have similar image icons and are typically in similar positions on the main control panel to optimise user ergonomics. This chapter provides a guide on the functionality of ultrasound scanner controls and how to utilise them in routine clinical scanning. The aim is for the recently initiated to understand the basic scanner controls in order to optimise the ultrasound image and obtain useful diagnostic information.

Getting Started

On/Off Switch

There is usually an 'On/Off' control button on the keyboard console, but on some scanners this is on the panel near the port for the transducers, and occasionally on the back of the scanner where all the output cables feed into.

Patient Details

Entering the patient details is the next key step after configuration of the scanner is complete, and this is usually denoted by a 'face' icon or 'ID' in letters. When connected to the hospital network, the user should select 'worklist' and highlight the correct patient from the worklist.

Transducer

The transducer icon is standard and an image of the transducer is usually on a touch screen monitor on the main console. The abdominal probe for imaging is typically a curvilinear probe with a frequency range between 1 and

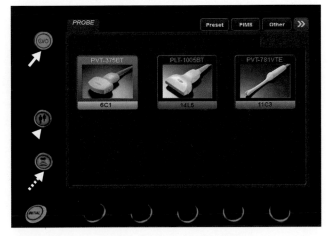

Figure 2.1 This outlines the essential buttons on a typical ultrasound console (arrow = on/off button, arrowhead = patient data symbol, dashed arrow = symbol for transducer). Note the images of the transducer to choose from that are on the touch screen panel.

8 mHz and are usually labelled based on their frequency range number, for instance C5–2 or C6–1, where the letter denotes the curved probe and the numbers are the frequency range of the probe (see Figure 2.1).

Preset

All manufacturers will have optimised preset/start-up configurations so that most settings are pre-selected and initialised for the user. This is particularly useful for new users of ultrasound, and for the liver the abdominal preset is typical, although there may be sub-presets for more penetration in the larger patient. These preset configurations include initialisation of the transducer, power output (usually set to maximum), depth, focal position, dynamic range, degree of smoothing, persistence and many other controls.

Image Optimisation

Depth/Zoom/Width

The 'depth' and 'zoom' controls are clearly marked and feature as control buttons or levers, which can be incrementally adjusted to increase or decrease depth and size. The zoom feature is generally located close to the depth knob and typically has a symbol similar to a magnifying glass. When the zoom feature is selected, a region of interest (ROI) box typically appears on the image, the position and size of which can be modified using the trackball (see Figure 2.2).

Focal Zone and Position

The focal zone number and position can be controlled by a knob or lever, usually labelled 'focus' and located near to the 'depth' and 'zoom' buttons. The position of the focus is indicated by an arrow on the side of the image or a line indicating a range if 'range focus' is employed. The user can usually select multiple foci, but the trade-off is a significantly reduced frame rate, sometimes for only a small increment in image resolution (see Figure 2.3).

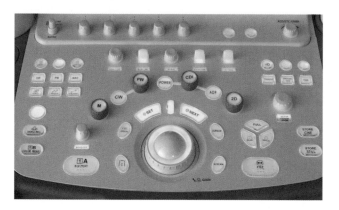

Figure 2.2 A typical console for a high-performing ultrasound scanner. Most of the knobs and levers have been appropriately labelled. Note the central tracker ball and body mark icon at the bottom left. The console has been laid out for ergonomic ease. 2D, gain; ABC, annotation; CDI, colour Doppler imaging; PW, pulsed wave Doppler.

2D Gain and Time Compensation

The 2D gain is usually marked on a knob, which can be turned to adjust the overall brightness of the image. The time gain compensation (TGC) is used to provide a uniformly bright image for the user and consists of 5–9 individual slider controls, which are located on one side of the control panel of the scanner. On some scanners these are electronically displayed on the touch screen console.

State-of-the-art scanners now employ an automated TGC and many also work in the background, optimising the quality and brightness of the image, often without the user realising that this is occurring during real-time scanning (Figures 2.4 and 2.5). Manufacturers have acronyms for their automated TGC, such as 'QScan' (Canon Medical Systems), 'iScan' (Philips Medical Systems) and 'TEQ' (Siemens Healthineers).

Useful Tools

Measurement

The measurement button is usually a symbol of either a ruler or callipers joined by dots. There is also a scale on the side of the image, which is in 0.5 or 1 cm increments depending on the size/depth of the image (Figure 2.3).

Trackball/Freeze/Cineloop

The trackball or touchpad functions as the 'mouse' of the ultrasound scanner and is the common operating form of the screen cursor. Most scanners also have a 'select' or unlabelled push button adjacent to the trackball, which is similar to the left- and right-hand 'click' functions found with a computer 'mouse' (Figure 2.2).

The freeze function is used to pause the moving live image and there is also an automatic cineloop function between two 'freeze' button clicks. This enables the user to scrutinise individual frames acquired previously more precisely. This is particularly advantageous for locating structures that were only briefly visible in the moving image and can elude targeted freezing attempts.

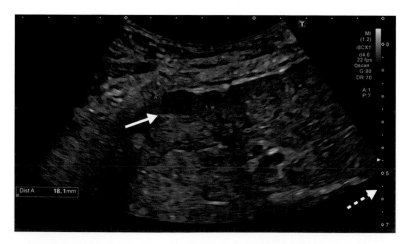

Figure 2.3 The measurement callipers outlining a hepatocellular carcinoma (white arrow). Note the scale in cm on the right-hand side of the image (dashed arrow). The small white arrowhead by the scale indicates the position of the focal zone.

The length of the cineloop depends on the system used and can usually be modified by the user, longer loops being associated with ultrasound studies where contrast agent is injected. The cineloop can be stored retrospectively (i.e. between two freeze frames) or prospectively, starting once the 'video' function has been activated. The length of these clips varies depending on the manufacturer, but can usually be altered to suit user preference.

Image/Clip Store

This is an important function to indicate the body part that is scanned and also to delineate any relevant abnormality. This is treated as a legal medical document and such images are typically stored for at least seven years depending on the laws of the respective country. The button usually features a camera or the word 'store' or 'print' and, in the case of a videoclip/cine loop, a picture illustrating a 'reel of film' or the word 'cine' (Figure 2.2).

Annotation/Body Marking

It is important that the body part that is being scanned is indicated on the image. The ability to annotate is usually performed by pressing the 'annotate/text' button or, on occasion, by an 'ABC' icon. Alternatively, some manufacturers have specific function keys assigned to this or text will appear as soon as the keyboard is activated.

Sometimes it may be easier to indicate the position of the probe on the body part diagram. Each manufacturer will have a body part figure and the user can just select the appropriate body part and move the position of the probe using the trackball (Figure 2.2).

Advanced Applications

Colour/Power/Spectral Doppler Controls

Many of the controls discussed for optimising spectral Doppler are also used to optimise colour Doppler imaging (CDI). The scale of the colour Doppler can be adjusted to ensure that the full range of velocities is displayed in the image. The gain and

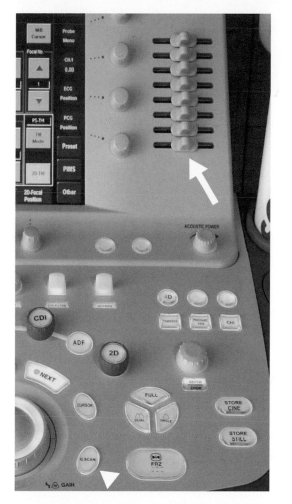

Figure 2.4 Time gain compensation (TGC; arrow) and automated TGC (arrowhead) buttons.

(a) (b)

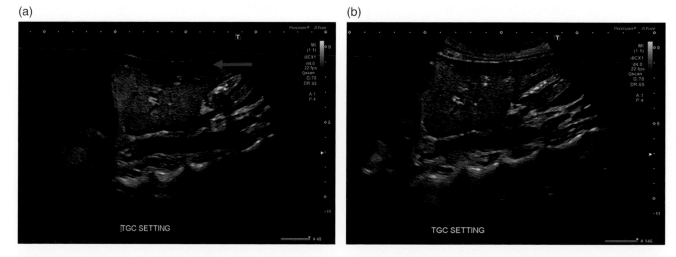

Figure 2.5 (a) No time gain compensation (TGC) adjustment – note that the near field of the liver is darker compared with the deeper segment (arrow). (b) After TGC adjustment.

power output can be adjusted so that the vessel is full of colour, with minimal colour outside the vessel walls. Owing to the angle dependence of Doppler imaging, the colour or power Doppler ROI box can also be steered using the 'STEER' button to ensure that insonation is not at 90° to the vessel. In many high-end scanners, the manufacturers have also set a single optimisation key for user ease, and this is typically the same as the TGC/brightness optimisation button (Figure 2.2).

Contrast-Enhanced Ultrasound

The contrast-enhanced ultrasound (CEUS) control is typically labelled contrast or contrast harmonic imaging (CHI). Pressing this button will typically launch the contrast ultrasound twin mode setting. The timer button to start the clock will also be in close proximity (Figure 2.6).

Shearwave Elastography

The shearwave elastography (SWE) control is commonly under Elastography or 'E'. The user has the option of selecting the type of elastography mode they wish to enable: strain, point shearwave elastography (pSWE), or 2D-Shearwave elastography (2D-SWE) (Figure 2.6).

Useful Terminology

Echotexture/Echogenicity

This is usually the ultrasonic description of the greyscale appearance of the organ or lesion and is dependent on the returning echoes.

Hyperechoic/Echogenic/Hyperreflectivity

This indicates more returning echoes from the organ/ lesion of interest. It makes the organ/lesion appear brighter and 'whiter' than the adjacent structures.

Hypoechoic/Echopoor/Hyporeflectivity

This indicates fewer returning echoes from the organ/ lesion of interest. It makes the organ/lesion appear darker and 'blacker' than the adjacent structures.

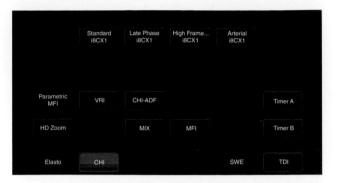

Figure 2.6 Note functional buttons when choosing advanced presets and two timer buttons (Timer A and Timer B) are in close proximity for ease of use. Other advanced functionalities include parametric microflow imaging (MFI) for contrast-enhanced ultrasound (CEUS) and vector imaging (VRI). ADF, annular dark field; CHI, contrast harmonic imaging, i.e. CEUS; Elasto, strain elastography; SWE, shearwave elastography; TDI, time delay integration.

Anechoic

This indicates no returning echoes within the structure or lesion. It is typical for simple fluid where the echoes pass directly through the medium.

Acoustic Shadowing

This describes when a lesion or tissue attenuates the ultrasound beam (typically dense, fibrous, or calcified lesion), which will form an artefactually echopoor region posterior to it.

Acoustic through Transmission

This describes when a lesion does not attenuate any of the transmitted or returning echoes. The tissue deep to the lesion (typically fluid-filled structures) will have more returning echoes and artefactually appear echogenic compared with the adjacent tissue.

Further Reading

Allan, P.L., Baxter, G.M., and Weston, M.J. (ed.) (2011). *Clinical Ultrasound*, 3e. London: Churchill Livingstone.

Dresser, T., Jedzejewicz, T., and Bradley, C. (2000). Native tissue harmonic imaging: basic principles and clinical applications. *Ultrasound Q.* 16 (1): 40–48.

Hoskins, P.R., Martin, K., and Thrush, A. (2019). *Diagnostic Ultra-sound Physics and Equipment*, 3e. Abingdon: Taylor & Francis.

McDicken, W.N. (1991). *Diagnostic Ultrasonics: Principles and Use of Instruments*, 3e. London: Churchill Livingstone/Wiley.

ter Haar, G. (2012). *The Safe Use of Ultrasound in Medical Diagnosis*, 3e. London: British Institute of Radiology.

Zander, D., Hüske, S., Hoffmann, B. et al. (2020). Ultrasound image optimization ('knobology') using B-mode and Doppler techniques. *Ultrasound Int. Open.* 6 (1): E14–E24.

3

Normal Liver Anatomy

How to Perform a Liver Ultrasound Scan

Adrian K.P. Lim[1,2], Ivica Grgurevic[3], and Matteo Rosselli[4,5]

[1] Department of Imaging, Imperial College Healthcare NHS Trust, London, UK
[2] Department of Metabolism, Digestion and Reproduction, Imperial College London, UK
[3] Department of Gastroenterology, Hepatology and Clinical Nutrition, University Hospital Dubrava, University of Zagreb School of Medicine and Faculty of Pharmacy and Biochemistry, Zagreb, Croatia
[4] Department of Internal Medicine, San Giuseppe Hospital, USL Toscana Centro, Empoli, Italy
[5] Division of Medicine, Institute for Liver and Digestive Health, University College London, Royal Free Hospital, London, UK

Ultrasound is considered one of the first-line diagnostic tests for liver imaging. Based on its findings, decisions that have a direct impact on the patient pathway are made, leading to further investigations, follow-up, or discharge. Along these lines, it should be kept in mind that greyscale ultrasound images lay out an anatomical and structural view of the liver, and therefore it is important to have a significant knowledge of abdominal anatomy and to ensure that the whole liver is assessed thoroughly. This chapter provides an overview of normal liver anatomy and its sonographic transposition, as well as a practical guide on how to start scanning the liver, with probe position and obtaining the standard recorded ultrasound images that should form the backbone of any liver ultrasound scan. A guide on how to report on a liver ultrasound study is also provided.

Anatomy of the Liver and Ultrasound Appearance

Location, Shape, and Borders

The liver is the largest parenchymal organ in the abdominal cavity. It is located below the diaphragm, extending from the right hypochondrium to the epigastrium, usually reaching the left subcostal edge (Figure 3.1). It has a smooth, dome-shaped diaphragmatic surface and a visceral, more irregular one, moulded by the adjacent organs and indented by the left, right, and interlobar fissures (Figure 3.2). Normally during respiration, the liver moves following the diaphragm. This movement is important and can be increased with deep inspiration to optimise liver visualisation during ultrasound imaging in a subcostal view. The magnitude of these excursions depends on the individual's lung capacity as well as body habitus and the mechanical properties of the thoracic wall (obesity and some structural diseases of the musculature or bone of the thoracic wall reduce this oscillation). Owing to the liver's high anatomical variability, it is generally accepted to compare its size to the right kidney to gauge whether it is enlarged, normal, or atrophic, rather than taking an exact measurement of its diameter [1]. A subcostal maximal length of 16 cm taken in the mid-clavicular is considered the upper limit of normal.

In normal conditions, the liver has smooth margins and regular contour, the echotexture is homogeneous, and the echogenicity is almost equal to or slightly brighter than the cortex of the right kidney (Figure 3.3). The liver is enveloped within the fibrous Glisson's capsule, which contains sensitive nerve endings supplied by the phrenic nerve. The capsule can be barely seen on ultrasound as a hyperechoic line that permeates the liver in direct contact with the peritoneum and is therefore more easily distinguished when there is ascites (Figure 3.4).

The suspensory system of the liver is constituted by ligaments that are seen on ultrasound as hyperechoic linear structures of different widths that fix the liver to the diaphragm, abdominal wall, and adjacent organs. Other ligaments envelope vascular and biliary structures and provide useful landmarks for the description of the complex liver

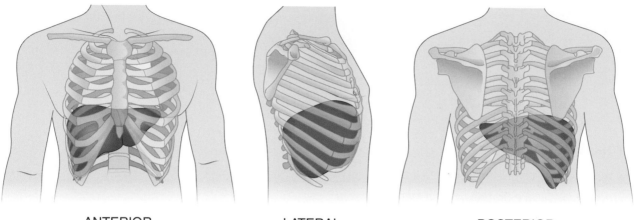

ANTERIOR   LATERAL   POSTERIOR

Figure 3.1 The liver is located below the diaphragm, extending from the right hypochondrium to the epigastrium, usually reaching the left subcostal edge. The liver is shown here from three different angles: anterior, right lateral and posterior. As explained in the chapter, in order to explore the liver appropriately, different angles of insonation are necessary. More specifically, a transverse and longitudinal scan view, in both the subcostal and intercostal approaches, is routine. A longitudinal scan parallel to the intercostal spaces allows assessment of the lateral segments of the liver and rarely, if needed, a posterior acoustic window can also be used.

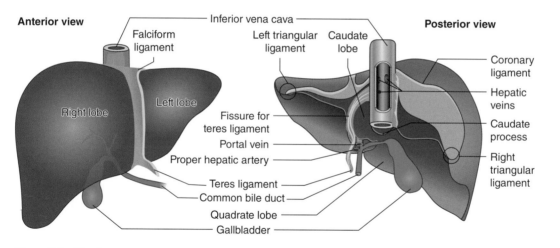

Figure 3.2 The liver has a smooth, dome-shaped diaphragmatic surface and a mildly irregular visceral one, which is moulded by the adjacent organs and indented by the interlobar fissures.

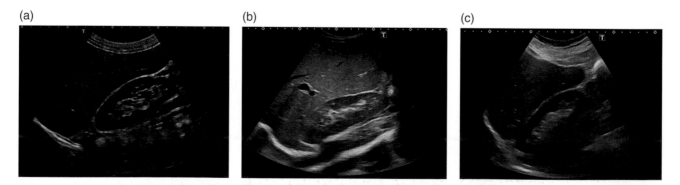

Figure 3.3 Examples of liver size compared to the right kidney. (a) Normal size of the right lobe compared to the right kidney. (b) Enlarged right liver lobe with subtle increase in echogenicity compared to the cortex of the right kidney. (c) The right liver lobe is smaller and has rounded margins and an irregular outline, in keeping with fibrotic retraction.

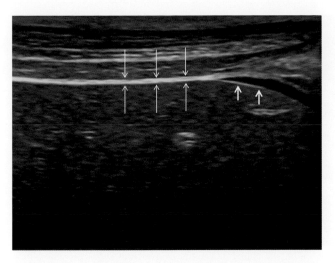

Figure 3.4 The Glisson's capsule can barely be seen surrounding the liver, since it is in direct contact with the peritoneum (thin arrows point to the interface of the peritoneum and Glisson's capsule). Note is made of a small amount of intraperitoneal fluid that detaches the liver from the peritoneum, highlighting a subtle hyperechoic line surrounding the liver corresponding to the Glisson's capsule (thick arrows).

structure. More specifically, the falciform ligament connects the dorsal surface of the liver to the diaphragm and to the anterior abdominal wall dividing the liver into the anatomic right and left lobes. Its free margin continues with the remnant of the obliterated umbilical vein, which is known as the ligamentum teres (or round ligament) and runs along the ventral surface of the liver, coming into direct contact with the left branch of the portal vein (PV) (Figure 3.5). The obliterated remnants of the ductus venosus constitute the venous ligament, which is seen on

ultrasound as a thin hyperechoic line that surrounds the parenchyma adjacent to the retrohepatic inferior vena cava (IVC) defining the borders of the caudate lobe (Figure 3.6). The lesser omentum attaches the liver to the lesser curvature of the stomach through the hepatogastric ligament and to the duodenum through the hepatoduodenal ligament. The latter envelopes the portal triad running from the porta hepatis to the very first portion of the duodenum. It contains the liver lymphatics and is often the site of lymphadenopathies that can be seen in infective, inflammatory, or neoplastic liver diseases.

Gallbladder and Biliary Tree

The gallbladder (GB) is a pear-shaped structure located in the GB fossa along the inferior surface of the right liver lobe, lateral to the second portion of the duodenum and anterior to the right kidney (Figure 3.7). Its position is variable according to the patient's body habitus [2]. Four anatomical variants are described and should be borne in mind, since anatomical landmarks and GB positioning might vary considerably:

- Hypersthenic body habitus: the diaphragm, liver, GB, and stomach tend to lie high in the abdomen and the ultrasound examination is often limited due to the presence of overlying bowel gas and food residue.
- Sthenic: the liver and GB lie as expected in the right upper quadrant and the GB has an oblique position.
- Hyposthenic: the liver and GB lie lower, often in the lumbar region, and the GB is more vertically oriented.
- Asthenic (extremely hyposthenic): the liver and GB might lie as low as in the right iliac fossa and the GB is vertically oriented [2].

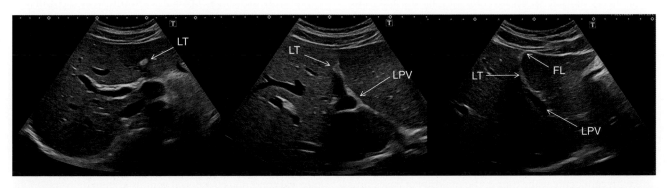

Figure 3.5 Ligamentum teres (LT) or round ligament takes direct contact with the left branch of the portal vein (LPV). LT runs along the ventral surface of the liver continuing with the falciform ligament (FL) along the dorsal surface of the liver. By changing the plane of insonation from transverse to longitudinal scan view (left to right image) the LT will be seen elongating in full extent to join the FL (right side image).

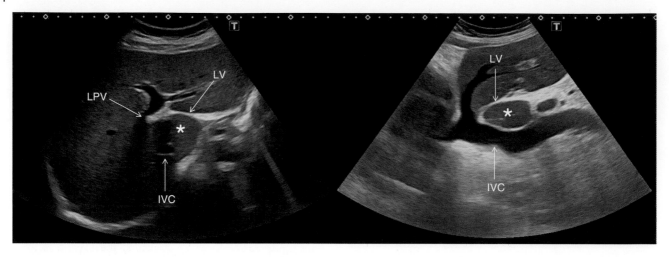

Figure 3.6 The boundaries of the caudate lobe (asterisk) are defined by the retrohepatic inferior vena cava (IVC), the ligamentum venosum (LV), and the left branch of the portal vein (LPV) that is better seen when imaging in transverse section (left side image).

(a)

(b)

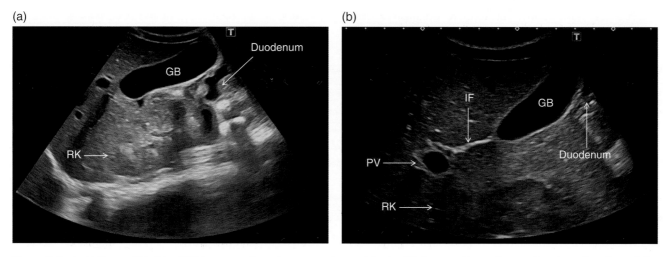

Figure 3.7 (a, b) The gallbladder (GB) is a pear-shaped structure located in the GB fossa, a depression on the visceral surface of the liver between the right and left lobe. The GB is usually lateral to the second part of the duodenum and anterior to the right kidney (RK). (b) Note is made of the main interlobar fissure (IF) between the portal vein (PV) and the GB.

The biliary tree can be divided into intrahepatic and extra-hepatic segments. The intrahepatic ducts run across the liver from the periphery to the liver hilum, converging in larger ducts, and are in tight anatomical connection with the hepatic arterial supply and the portal venous system. In proximity to the liver hilum, the cystic duct that drains bile from the GB joins the main hepatic duct to form the common bile duct (CBD). The CBD terminates with the pancreatic duct at the ampulla of Vater within the second portion of the duodenum.

In normal physiological conditions, the CBD is the only biliary duct that can be clearly seen as a thin tubular structure with echogenic walls that in the majority of cases runs anteriorly and parallel to the PV at the level of the hepatic hilum (Figure 3.8). However, the anatomical relationship of the biliary ducts and the portal vessels may vary along their course, and usually the peripheral biliary ducts (which are only clearly visible when dilated or significantly thickened) run posteriorly to the PV (Figures 3.9 and 3.10).

The CBD measures between a minimum of 2–3 mm and an upper limit of 6–7 mm. Larger calibres are observed, especially post cholecystectomy and with age, where it is generally accepted that the calibre may increase by 1 mm each decade after 70 years [3].

Liver Vascular Anatomy

The PV is formed by the confluence of the superior mesenteric vein and the splenic vein, draining the blood of the whole digestive system and spleen (Figure 3.11). Under physiological conditions the portal venous system delivers 75% of the total hepatic inflow, whereas the hepatic artery (HA) is responsible for the remaining 25%. It is important to keep in mind the physiology and pathophysiology of the hepatic blood inflow, since during the progression of liver disease, especially when cirrhosis and portal hypertension develop, the portal venous inflow is reduced while the arterial hepatic

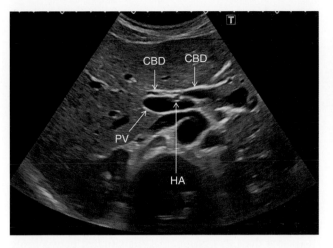

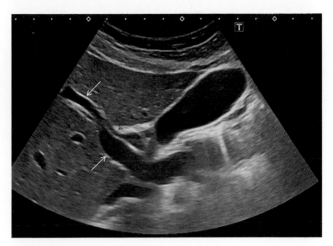

Figure 3.8 The common bile duct (CBD) can be seen as a thin tubular structure with echogenic walls that, in the majority of cases, runs anteriorly and parallel to the portal vein (PV) at the level of the hepatic hilum. The hepatic artery (HA) is often seen at this level in transverse section, hence it is visualised as a small rounded or ovoid structure (depending on the angle of insonation) with echogenic walls between the CBD and the PV.

Figure 3.9 In the majority of cases the portal vein (white arrow) lies posterior to the common bile duct (red arrow) at the hepatic hilum. Note that shortly after entering the liver, its position becomes anterior to the bile ducts.

(a) (b) (c)

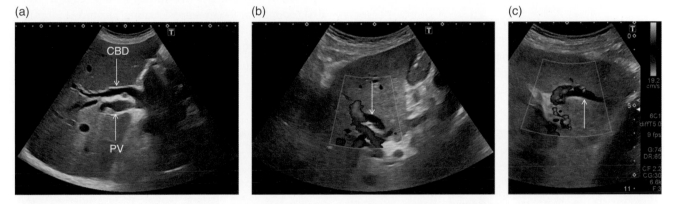

Figure 3.10 In this sequence of images, the dilated bile ducts help to clearly delineate their anatomical relationship with the portal venous system. At the level of the hepatic hilum the portal vein (PV) is posterior to the common bile duct (CBD) (a). As the portal venous tree progresses within the liver, its position gradually changes (b), crossing over to run anteriorly to the bile ducts in the more peripheral regions of liver parenchyma. Bile ducts are identified in (b) and (c) by white arrows, while the color signal highlights the portal venous blood flow.

Figure 3.11 Pictorial view of the portal venous system draining blood from the digestive system and the spleen.

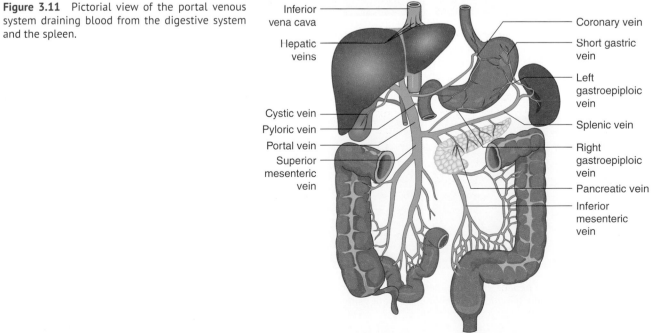

inflow is increased (See Chapter 8). The PV can be recognised on ultrasound as a tubular structure with a variable normal calibre of approximately 8–12.5 mm, with thick echogenic walls that enters the liver together with the HA at the level of the hepatic hilum. It is followed by the HA and the biliary system in its whole intrahepatic course and for a short portion in its extrahepatic tract at the level of the porta hepatis, where it is contained within the hepatoduodenal ligament. Upon entering the liver, the PV and HA divide into the left and right branches, with further divisions providing the blood supply to each of the eight main liver segments (Figure 3.12). At the periphery of the liver lobules the arterial and venous blood mix and enter the sinusoids, terminating finally in the central veins that converge to form the right (RHV), middle (MHV), and left hepatic veins (LHV) that finally drain into the IVC (Figure 3.13). It is of note that the caudate lobe is drained independently by a main or multiple small pericaval veins. Its independent venous drainage system is the reason why the caudate lobe typically hypertrophies in advanced chronic liver disease. In Budd–Chiari syndrome, this compensatory mechanism is even more pronounced, since while the main three hepatic veins are obstructed, the pericaval ones often remain patent, leading to an abnormally hypertrophied caudate lobe (See Chapter 11).

Vascular Segments of the Liver

Based on the divisions of the portal and hepatic veins, the liver may be divided into eight segments, as first suggested by the French surgeon Claude Couinaud in 1957 (Figure 3.14) [4]. This classification relies on the fact that each of these segments has its own individual blood supply and might be resected without jeopardising the viability of other segments. In this classification, the liver segments II and III are situated to the left of the LHV and falciform ligament, and the left branch of the PV (LPV) divides them into segment II (above the PV) and segment III (below the LPV). Segment IV is situated between the LHV and the MHV and the LPV divides them into segment IVA (above the LPV) and segment IVB (below the LPV). Segments V and VIII are located between the MHV and RHV, whereas segments VI and VII represent most lateral segments situated to the right of the RHV. The right branch of the RPV divides segment V (caudal) from VIII (cranial) and segment VI (caudal) from VII (cranial) (Figure 3.15). On the dorsal, central part of the liver, between the IVC and the venous ligament, lies the caudate lobe that corresponds to segment I (Figures 3.6 and 3.12c).

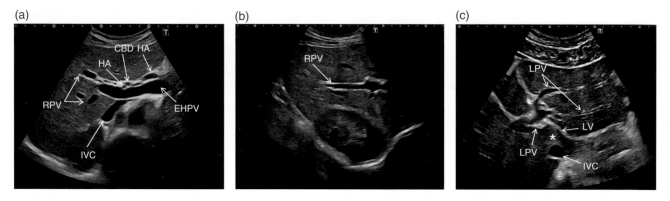

Figure 3.12 The portal venous system can be recognised on ultrasound as a tubular structure with echogenic walls that enters the liver together with the hepatic artery (HA) at the level of the hepatic hilum (a), and reaches the more distal liver segments. (b) Posterior branch of the right portal vein (RPV); (c) left portal vein (LPV) branches. (c) The caudate lobe can be clearly visualised in this scanning plane (asterisk) between the inferior vena cava (IVC), the ligamentum venosum (LV), and LPV. CBD, common bile duct; EHPV, extrahepatic portal vein.

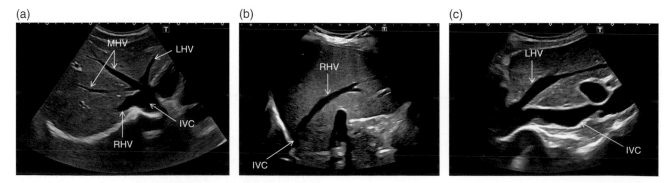

Figure 3.13 (a–c) The hepatic veins originate from the periphery of the liver, converging into the inferior vena cava (IVC). LHV, left hepatic vein; MHV, middle hepatic vein; RHV, right hepatic vein.

Figure 3.14 Liver segmentation following Couinaud classification. IVC, inferior vena cava.

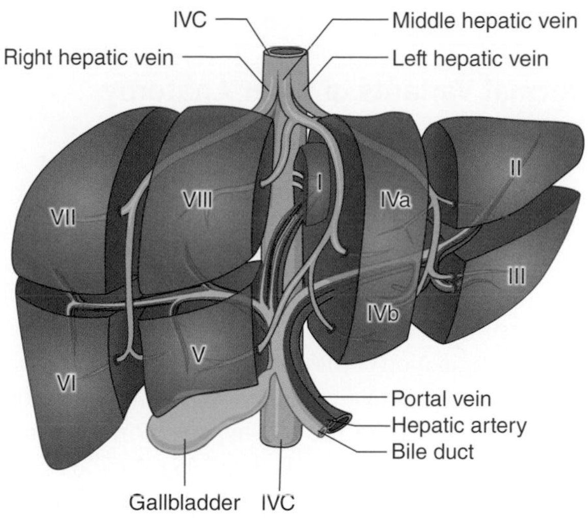

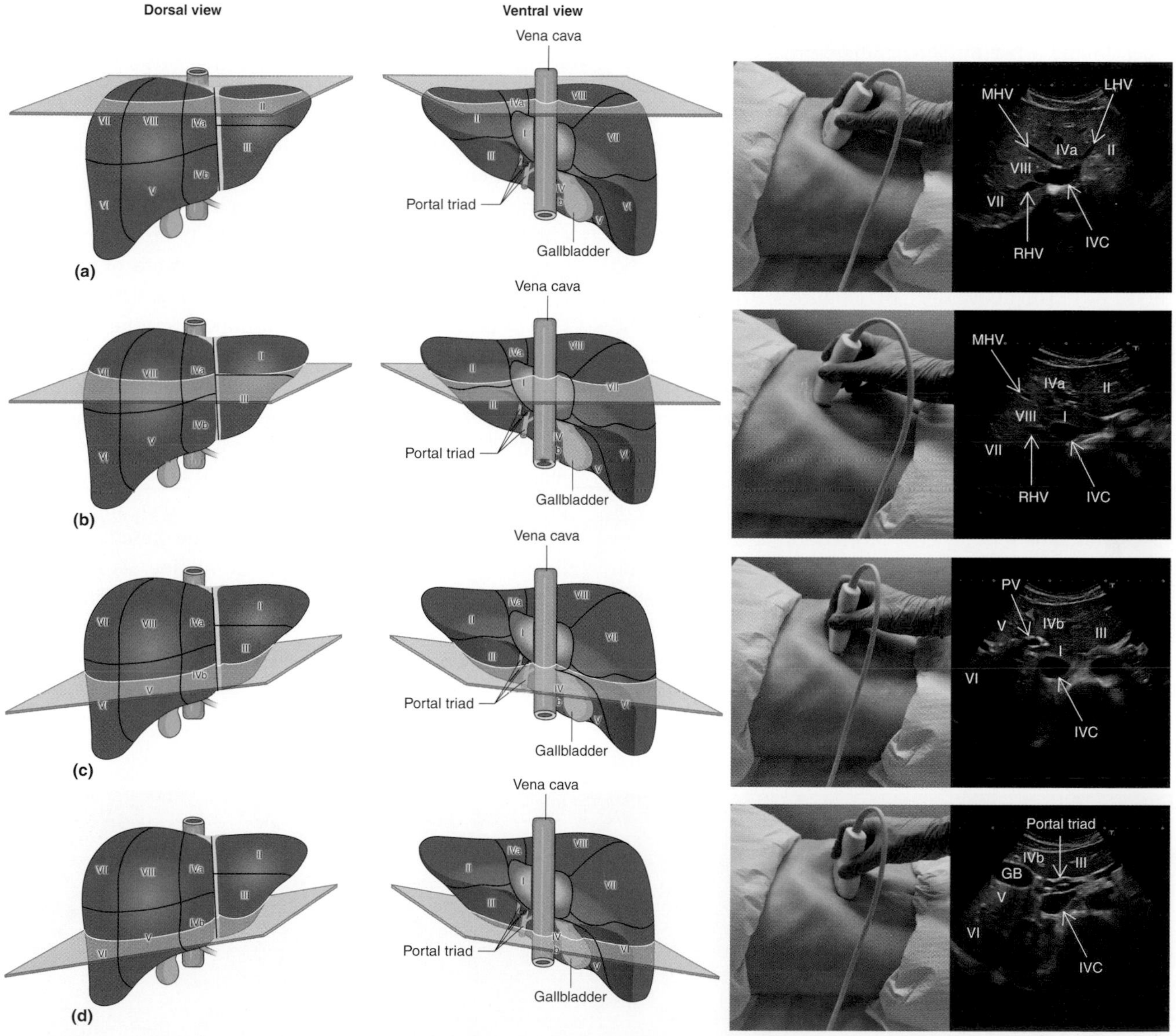

Figure 3.15 (a–d) This sequence of images shows how the ultrasound beam transverses the liver along sequential axial planes when moving the probe craniocaudally (i.e. from top to bottom) and how the hepatic and portal veins serve as reference landmarks, in line with Couinaud classification. Note is made of a pictorial view of the dorsal and ventral surfaces of the liver, with an adjacent right hand image of the corresponding liver segments seen ultrasonically. The sectional planes correspond to the orientation of the ultrasound beam. RHV, right hepatic vein; MHV, medium hepatic vein; LHV, left hepatic vein; IVC, inferior vena cava; PV, portal vein; GB, gallbladder.

Normal Variants of Liver Anatomy

Liver anatomical variants might be related to the shape, size, and vasculature, as well as the GB and biliary tree. Parenchymal variants include diaphragmatic slips, sliver of liver, Riedel's lobe, and papillary process of the caudate lobe [5]. Diaphragmatic slips represent incomplete accessory fissures at the site of the diaphragmatic liver surface due to invagination of the diaphragm (Figure 3.16). A sliver of the liver refers to an anatomical variant where the left liver lobe extends to the left hypochondrium, wrapping around part of the spleen (Figure 3.17). Another common variant is a Riedel's lobe, represented by a downward tongue-like projection of the lower anterior edge of the right liver lobe (segment VI), sometimes so pronounced as to extend along the right paracolic space up to the iliac fossa (Figure 3.18) [6]. The papillary process is an anterior and medial extension of the caudate lobe, which might resemble a lymph node or mass next to the pancreatic head or IVC (Figure 3.19).

Other anatomical variants include the position of the PV, HA, and CBD at the level of the hepatic hilum. In the majority of cases the PV lies posteriorly, and the HA lies between the PV and the above CBD, while less frequently the HA will run above the CBD (Figure 3.20) or below the PV. The main trunk of the PV usually bifurcates at the porta hepatis into a main left and right branch and a further anterior and posterior branch of the right trunk. Alternatively the PV might have a trifurcation that might be extrahepatic or intrahepatic. The hepatic veins can also show some anatomical variants. With regard to the RHV, this is usually single and dominant, while in a minority of cases there might be an early bifurcation or trifurcation or multiple small RHVs entering the IVC. The most common variant is an accessory right inferior hepatic vein. Both the MHV and LHV can be double and sometimes form a common trunk that drains independently into the

IVC. When the hepatic veins are duplicated, typically the larger is used for segment classification. The caudate lobe might have a single vein or several small hepatic veins that drain independently and directly into the IVC. The HA can have several anatomical variants, especially with regard to its origin. The most common is directly from the aorta or the superior mesenteric artery. All these vascular variants do not have pathological implications, but should be kept in mind since they have important technical implications in a case of liver transplant, resection, or embolic treatment of liver tumours [7]. Rare vascular anatomical variants include congenital portal venous shunting (see Chapter 11).

Practical Approach for How to Scan the Liver

In Chapter 2, the optimisation of the scanner to achieve the best image quality was outlined. However, this not only relies on the scanner capabilities, but also on the operator- and patient-related factors. It is very important that the operator has anatomical, physiological, and good clinical knowledge, as well as the ability to interpret the sonographic images. They should also be aware of potential artefacts and pitfalls in order to corroborate their findings. One of the cornerstones of ultrasound scanning technique compared to other modalities is its dynamic nature.

In order to ensure that an organ has been fully assessed, the operator must continuously adapt the angle/plane of insonation. Every organ should be assessed in at least two planes, since some of the findings that are present on one plane can sometimes disappear on another, highlighting their artefactual nature. Alternatively, the presence on multiple planes may confirm a specific finding. Artefacts can also mask an underlying pathology and thus it is important to change the angle of insonation or the patient's position. In general, moving the patient can significantly improve

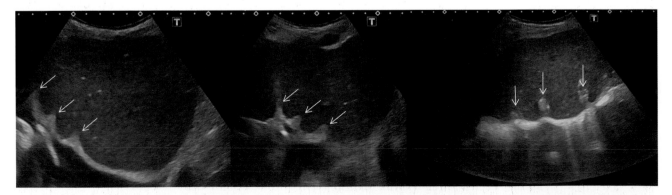

Figure 3.16 Diaphragmatic slips (arrows) represent incomplete accessory fissures at the site of the diaphragmatic liver surface due to invagination of the diaphragm.

(a)

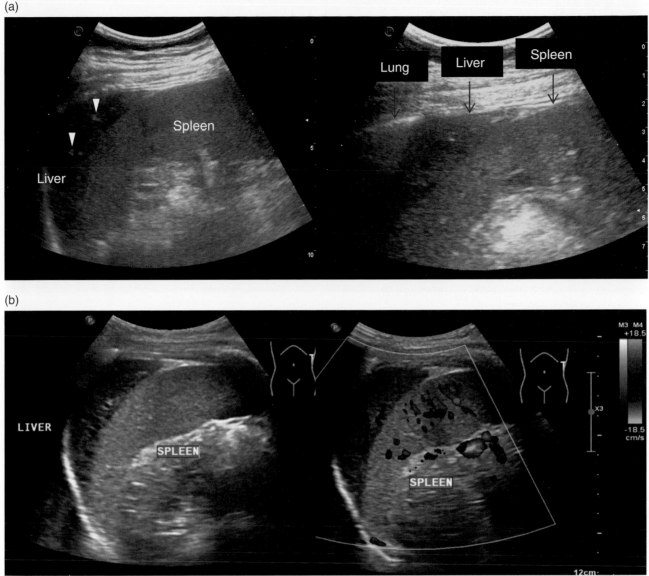

(b)

Figure 3.17 An anatomical variant known as beaver tail liver or a sliver of liver, more commonly found in females. An elongated left liver lobe extends to left upper quadrant, making contact with and sometimes surrounding the spleen. In case of hepatic steatosis, echogenicity might almost be identical to the spleen, giving the false appearance of a double layer. (a) However, the presence of different vasculature, in particular the hyperechoic outline of portal tracts (arrowheads) is usually sufficient and useful for differentiating the two organs. (b) Colour Doppler highlights the differences of the hepatosplenic vasculature.

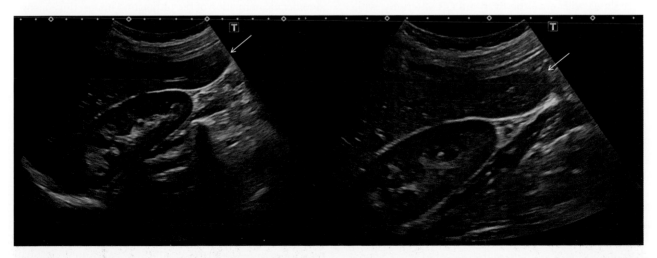

Figure 3.18 A Riedel's lobe is represented by a downward projection of the lower anterior edge of the right liver lobe, corresponding to a tongue-like elongation of segment VI (arrow). Sometimes this is so pronounced that it extends along the right paracolic space up to the iliac fossa. Of note is that, in the presence of hepatomegaly, segment VI might well go beyond the lower pole of the right kidney and might be confused with a Riedel's lobe. Nevertheless, in that case the whole liver is enlarged, while in the presence of a true Riedel's lobe, the left lobe is usually normal.

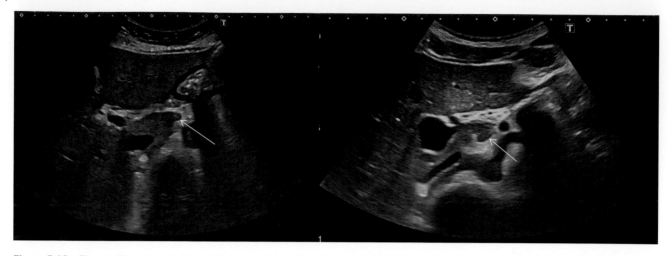

Figure 3.19 The papillary process (arrow) is an anterior and medial extension of the caudate lobe, which might resemble a lymph node or mass next to the pancreatic head or inferior vena cava.

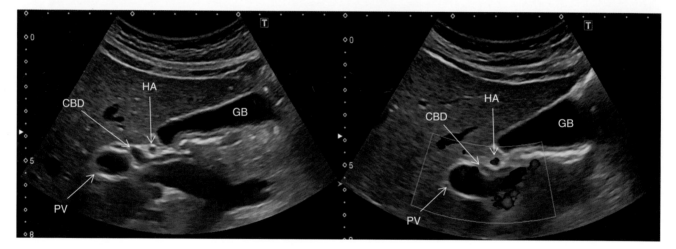

Figure 3.20 Anatomical variant of the hepatic artery (HA) running anteriorly to the common bile duct (CBD) instead of between the CBD and the portal vein (PV) at the level of the hepatic hilum.

ultrasound imaging. For example, rotating the patient to the left decubitus will move the liver and GB anteriorly, while overlying bowel loops flop downwards, optimising liver visualisation. Deep inspiration extends the liver beyond the costal margin, allowing further assessment of the deep segments, a manoeuvre that can be very helpful, especially in patients with hypersthenic body habitus.

It is very important to highlight that despite the availability of excellent equipment and a highly skilled operator, the diagnostic confidence in excluding pathological findings can be severely limited by patient-related factors. It is crucial to acknowledge these limitations and highlight them in the ultrasound report, since a suboptimal image may lead to an inconclusive scan and thus the need for further investigations to aid patient management.

Patient-related factors include constitutional limitations such as obesity, narrow intercostal spaces, and severe kyphosis. Obese patients might be challenging because of thick subcutaneous tissue with reverberation artefacts limiting the

visualisation of parenchymal organs. Severe steatosis leads to significant attenuation of the ultrasound image, thus making it difficult to visualise the most posterior and deep liver segments. Within limits, adjusting the gain, harmonics, increasing penetration, and the availability of new software and probes may enable some improvement in image resolution. However, not all ultrasound machines are equipped with new-generation software or dedicated ultrasound transducers specifically designed for the larger patient.

Very narrow intercostal spaces and severe kyphosis found in some physical conditions, and particularly in elderly patients, limit the intercostal acoustic window for assessing the right and left lobes.

Poor patient compliance can also often be encountered, leading to difficult scanning and suboptimal imaging. The reasons for this include patients' mental status, abdominal pain, or respiratory distress. All these conditions are challenging. For example, a patient might need an ultrasound scan for abdominal pain, which may be exacerbated by increased pressure exerted by the ultrasound transducer during the examination. A dyspnoeic patient is always challenging, since the optimal scanning position would be in a supine or lateral decubitus position. These patients will have difficulty in maintaining these positions and a degree of innovation is needed sometimes, for instance by scanning posteriorly. For some patients it may be difficult to hold a deep breath, even for a few seconds, thus excluding this useful manoeuvre in optimising liver parenchymal visualisation. Patient compliance secondary to psychological issues may also be encountered and the operator may find a non-cooperative patient refusing to undergo the required examination. Specifically, patients with advanced cirrhosis are sometimes encephalopathic, which could lead to a very challenging interaction during the exam. Finally, gas in the gastrointestinal tract is one of the most common and difficult limitations to abdominal ultrasound imaging. The recommendation is that patients undergo a period of at least six hours of fasting to maximise GB distension and also reduce food residue and gas in the upper gastrointestinal tract to optimise scanning conditions [2].

Liver Parenchyma Assessment

Liver ultrasound assessment requires careful scanning of all segments while evaluating the echotexture, echogenicity, margins, and contour. There are no strict rules on how to scan the liver, but rather a suggestion of a systematic approach in order to provide a concise description of liver anatomy and ensure that the whole liver and associated vascular and biliary structures are assessed completely.

Start by scanning in the longitudinal scan (LS) plane within the epigastrium, showing segments I and II of the liver, the aorta, and the IVC. Ensure that you sweep from right to left of these liver segments to assess for any focal lesions, contour abnormalities, or biliary tree dilatation. When sweeping left (towards the right side of the patient), the IVC will be more clearly visible, with the caudate lobe well defined between the IVC and the ligamentum venosum (Figure 3.21a); when sweeping right (towards the left side of the patient) the aorta will appear running posteriorly to the left lobe (Figure 3.21b) (see Videos 3.1a and b). Of note are the possibility of accessory lobes (normal anatomical variants), particularly of segment II,

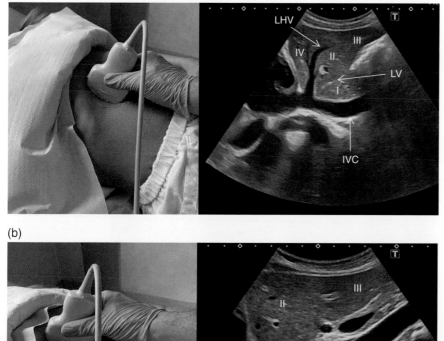

Figure 3.21 (a) Longitudinal scan view at the epigastric level, showing segments II, III, and I between the ligamentum venosum (LV) and the inferior vena cava (IVC). Segment IV is also visualised just medially to the left hepatic vein (LHV). (b) By slightly moving the probe towards the left side of the patient, segments II and III are visualised but with the aorta running just below.

which can extend to the left upper quadrant and around the spleen (Figure 3.17).

Next, bearing in mind that the LHV represents the boundary between segments II/III and IV, turn the probe into the transverse scan (TS) plane and then sweep up and down, ensuring that these liver segments are also visualised in the orthogonal plane. By doing so segment IVA will be visualised in the most cranial plane next to segment II, and segment IVB will be visualised just below, next to segment III (Figure 3.22). Segment IV should also be imaged in LS view (Figures 3.21 and 3.23) (Videos 3.2 and 3.3). Be aware of the appearance of the ligamentum teres in the TS plane, since it may mimic a hyperechoic focal lesion, and keep in mind that all structures need to be visualised in at least two planes (Figure 3.5) (Video 3.4).

The right liver lobe includes segments V–VIII, which should be assessed in both the LS and TS planes via a subcostal and intercostal approach, as shown in Figures 3.24–3.26 (Video 3.5). Start again by keeping the probe in the epigastric region in a TS view. By angling upwards, you will visualise the most cranial liver segments (from left to right of the patient will be segment II, IV, VIII) and you will image part of the heart, eventually excluding or highlighting the presence of a pericardial effusion. Then, remaining in the subcostal scanning position, turn the probe oblique (rotating anticlockwise) and slowly angle downwards, making small adjustments as required. By doing so you will visualise the confluence of the three hepatic veins and the IVC from two slightly different angles, with the oblique scan favouring the visualisation of the right hepatic vein

(a)

(b)

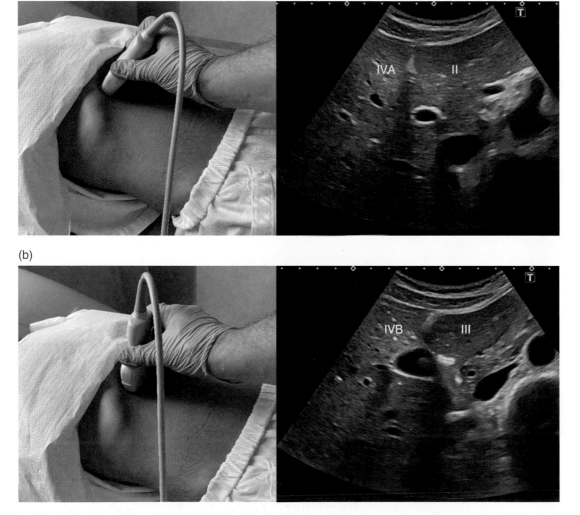

Figure 3.22 (a) Epigastric transverse scan view showing cranial segments IVA and II. (b) By tilting the probe downwards, segment IVB and III are imaged just below.

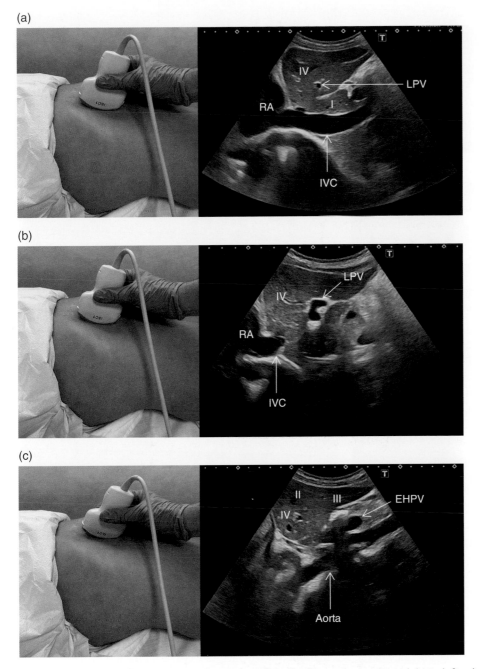

Figure 3.23 (a–c) Different images of segment IV obtained by sweeping from right to left using an epigastric longitudinal scan view. RA, right atrium; LPV, left portal vein; IVC, inferior vena cava; EHPV, extrahepatic portal vein.

(Figure 3.24) (Video 3.5). Maintaining the same probe position and slowly moving downwards, you will visualise first the GB and left branch of the PV and then, eventually turning the patient left side down and making small adjustments, you will visualise the PV crossing and 'dividing' the liver in a cranial and caudal region (Figure 3.25)

(Videos 3.6 and 3.7). Bear in mind that according to body habitus, when sweeping downwards the PV might appear before the GB or viceversa. Representative images of the right lobe should also be obtained intercostally, moving the probe from one intercostal space to another angling upwards and downwards in order to have a complete view

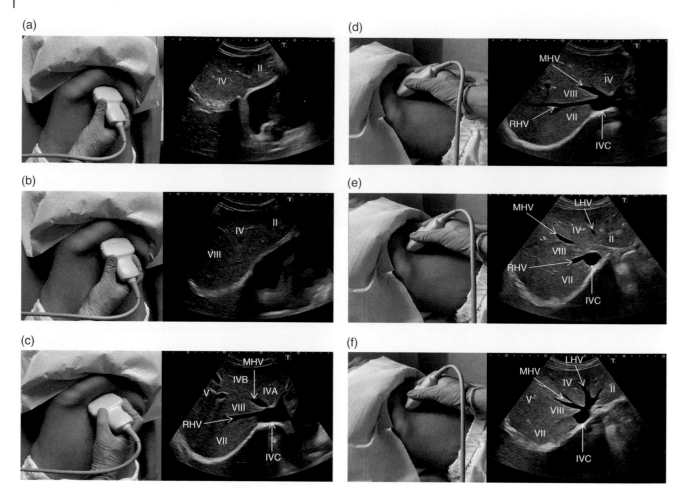

Figure 3.24 Transverse subcostal (TS) epigastric view. The higher TS view will ensure the visualisation of the most cranial subcapsular segments and part of the heart (a, b). Tilting the probe downwards will open up to the inferior vena cava (IVC) and hepatic vein confluence (c–f). By making small adjustments and moving the probe subcostally and anticlockwise towards the right side of the patient, a better view of the middle (MHV) and right hepatic veins (RHV) will be ensured (c, d). Conversely, if the probe is still kept subcostal but is rotated slowly clockwise instead, the left (LHV) and MHV confluence will be visualised (e, f).

from each angle (Video 3.5). A representative image of the liver with the right kidney is important to allow comparison of its echogenicity to the cortex of the right kidney to diagnose or exclude steatosis. This image can be obtained in the LS plane, starting along the mid-clavicular line and sweeping outwards (laterally) until the kidney is visualised, or intercostally in case of bowel gas interference (Figure 3.26) (Video 3.8).

Gallbladder and Common Bile Duct

The GB is assessed in the subcostal position, in two orthogonal planes, and also intercostally. As a first approach, place the transducer on the anterior abdominal wall along the mid-clavicular line, adjusting its position until the GB is located. Ask the patient to take a deep breath to lower the diaphragm and push the liver downwards below the costal margin; this will facilitate GB visualisation. It is essential to image the GB in its entire long axis and to angle the transducer so that it is also imaged transversally. The longitudinal intercostal approach will complete the GB visualisation, also offering an alternative to a sometimes challenging subcostal view in case of bowel gas interposition (Figure 3.27) (Video 3.9). In other circumstances, especially in the presence of narrow intercostal spaces, an intercostal approach might not be ideal. The CBD is best visualised with the patient supine or slightly turned with the left side down. Start with the probe obliquely

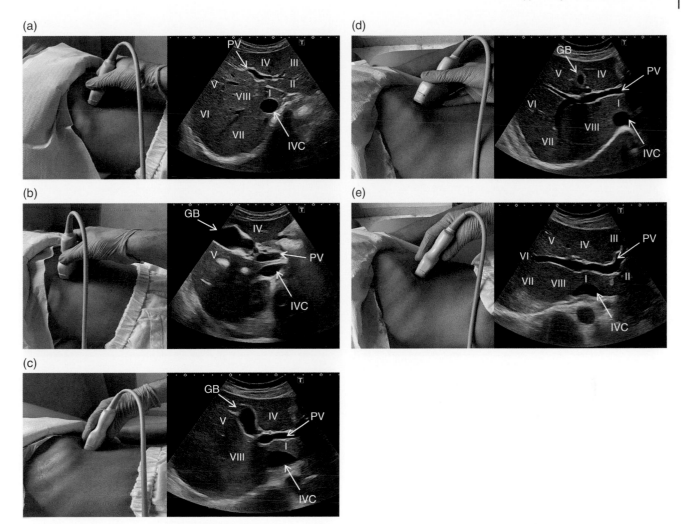

Figure 3.25 By further angling the probe downwards the portal vein (PV) appears (a), followed by the gallbladder (GB) (b, c). By turning the patient's left side down and making small adjustments, using a subcostal transverse/oblique plane, the PV is better visualised dividing the liver into cranial and caudal segments (d, e). The bifurcation of the right PV in its anterior and posterior branches is clearly visible (d). IVC, inferior vena cava.

positioned in the epigastrium, in line with the anatomical plane of the CBD. Sweep subcostally and outwards until you see the image of the portal triad (Figure 3.28). This may require some fine adjustments of the probe position (Video 3.10). The CBD is usually measured longitudinally where the HA intersects the CBD and PV; nevertheless, if the CBD shows some size variations it should be measured at the level of its maximal calibre (Figure 3.29). As for the GB, there may be occasions, owing to bowel gas, in which the CBD is better visualised in the anterior intercostal plane (Figure 3.30).

Although GB ultrasound assessment can be easily carried out, there are a few important tips and pitfalls that

should be kept in mind. Before starting the scan, check if the patient has undergone a cholecystectomy that might be associated with CBD dilatation, or endoscopic retrograde cholangiopancreatography requiring Oddi's sphincterotomy that usually leads to aerobilia. Both these findings after these procedures should be considered paraphysiological, unless the clinical picture and laboratory results suggest that an underlying pathological obstructive/infective process is also present.

If the GB cannot be visualised, consider an ectopic position and check lower down within the pelvis. Always be sure that the patient has truly fasted for at least six hours, since a contracted GB can mimic cholecystitis and in

(a)

(d)

(b)

(e)

(c)

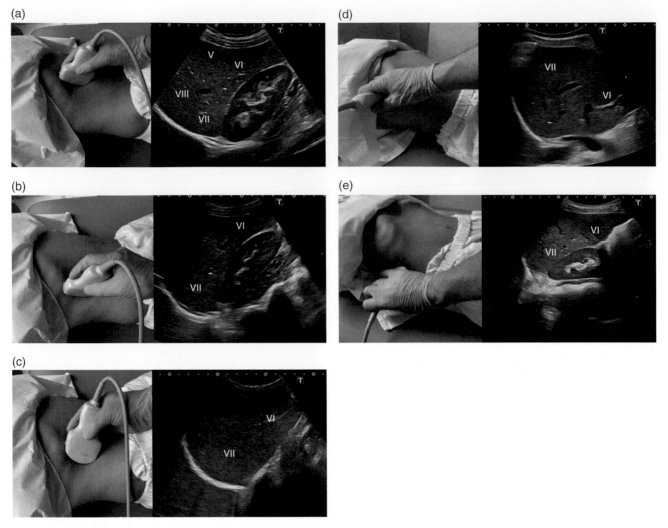

Figure 3.26   The most lateral segments of the liver are visualised by scanning longitudinally along the midclavicular line (a) and then moving more laterally (b,c). This acoustic window is important since it allows a comparison of the echogenicity of the liver parenchyma to the cortex of the right kidney to assess for steatosis, and also because it favours better visualisation of segment VII. The latter in the intercostal view may not be entirely visible owing to lung interface which acts as a 'curtain' (d). For completion a longitudinal intercostal view can also be used to assess the posterolateral segments and their relationship to the right kidney (e).

general does not allow correct evaluation of its wall thickness and content, thus carrying a risk of missed pathology. Some congenital variants can make its visualisation or assessment difficult (see Chapter 6). It is important to keep in mind that the main interlobar fissure is a useful landmark to identify the GB fossa. Follow the fissure from the right branch of the PV to its other extremity that ends with the GB fossa (Figure 3.7) [6]. This will help to locate and identify the GB, especially when it is small or contracted.

Be aware of the presence of near-field artefact, which may obscure the anterior wall of the GB; the proximity of the duodenum may bulge against the posterior wall, mimicking pathology or limiting its correct assessment. Changing the patient's position may also help to move the duodenum's position and content and improve GB visualisation (Figure 3.31). Partial volume artefact can mimic the presence of sludge that accumulates in the infundibulum or a 'side-lobe artefact' with posterior acoustic shadowing can

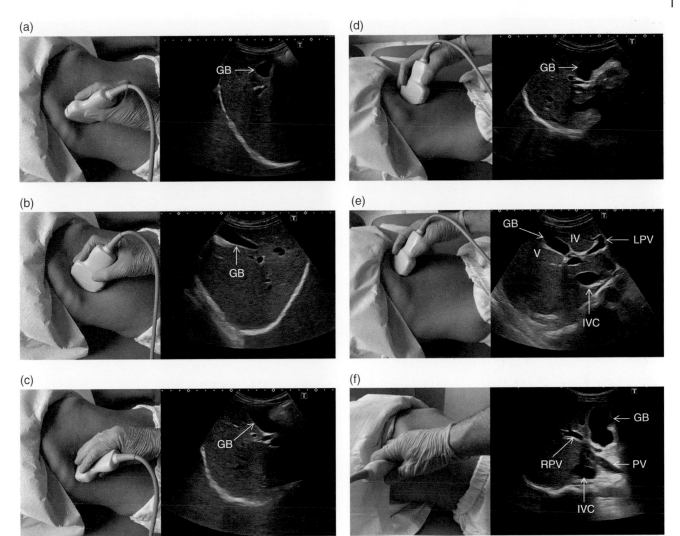

Figure 3.27 The gallbladder (GB) ultrasound assessment starts with a subcostal longitudinal scan in the mid-clavicular line (a) and then sweeping through, in deep inspiration, with an oblique and transverse subcostal view (b–d). A further subcostal transverse scan view allows evaluation of a large portion of the right and left lobes with a good view of the GB, left branch of the portal vein (LPV) with segment IV on the left side of the GB (medially) and segment V on the right side of the GB (laterally) (e). A longitudinal intercostal plane completes the GB visualisation (f). IVC, inferior vena cava; PV, portal vein; RPV, right portal vein.

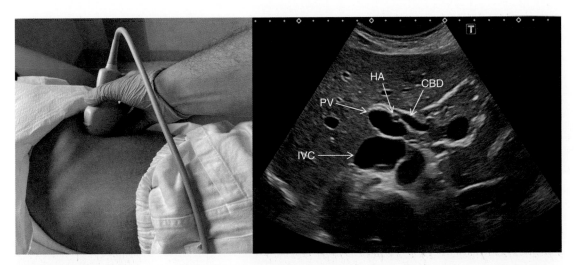

Figure 3.28 The probe is obliquely positioned in the epigastrium and it is moved subcostally and outwards until the image of the portal triad appears. IVC, inferior vena cava; PV portal vein; CBD, common bile duct.

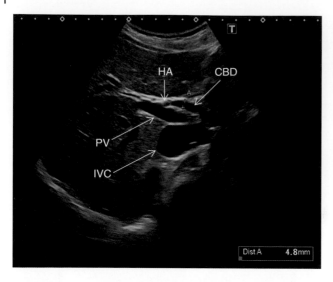

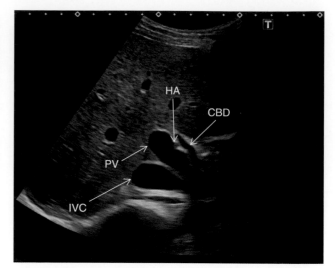

Figure 3.29 A subcostal epigastric view of the hepatic hilum and porta hepatis. The common bile duct (CBD) should be measured at the level of its maximum diameter. In this case it is measured near to the crossing of the hepatic artery (HA). PV, portal vein. IVC, inferior vena cava.

Figure 3.30 Intercostal longitudinal scan showing the hepatic hilum and the portal triad with a clearly visible common bile duct (CBD). HA, hepatic artery; PV, portal vein. IVC, inferior vena cava.

(a)

(b)

(c)

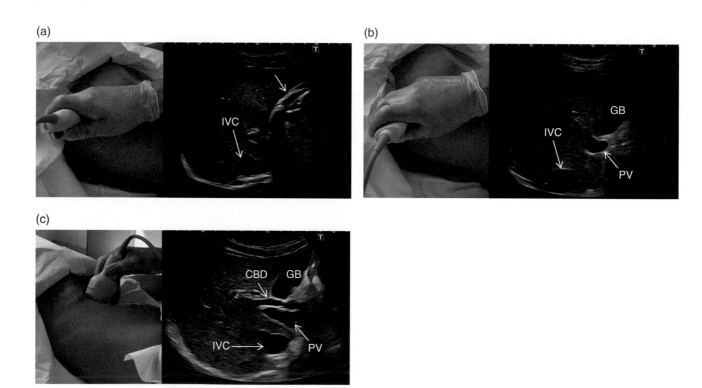

Figure 3.31 An intercostal longitudinal scan view (a) usually provides a good gallbladder (GB) view. However, in this case the interference of air in the duodenum gave a false image of a contracted GB (white arrow) and a 'stone' at the level of the infundibulum/neck (red arrow). Tilting the probe upwords allowed a better view of the GB (b). However, the best view in this case was obtained with an oblique subcostal approach (c). The hepatic hilum is now visible and the GB is nicely seen as well as the common bile duct (CBD) and the portal vein (PV). IVC, inferior vena cava.

give a false image of a stone lying in the neck of the GB. As previously mentioned, changing angle and plane of insonation will clarify the actual presence or absence of underlying pathology and confirm if the sonographic findings are artefactual.

Portal Vein, Hepatic Artery, and Hepatic Veins

The PV is best assessed in the intercostal position, typically when scanning through the right liver segments. When scanning intercostally be sure to visualise the hepatic hilum and the main PV (the main trunk will appear as the more posterior structure) (Figure 3.32a). Alternatively the main PV can be visualised maintaining a subcostal oblique approach (Figure 3.32b). In order to visualise the origin of the main extrahepatic PV, start by searching the splenic vein with a transverse subcostal epigastric view. The splenic vein will be seen lying below the pancreas and above the superior mesenteric artery in its transverse section (Figure 3.33a). Once the splenic vein is visualised, slowly turn the probe clockwise approximately 90° in order to visualise the superior mesenteric vein (Figure 3.33b). Next turn the probe anticlockwise by 45°, maintaining an oblique subcostal position. By doing so the confluence of the splenic vein and superior mesenteric vein will be seen forming the extrahepatic PV entering the liver (Figure 3.33c) (Video 3.11). It is important to remember that there may be subjective variability in the visualisation of hepatic structures, especially of the vessels, according to the angle of insonation. Therefore, it is advised to follow the mentioned landmarks moving slowly, since small movements of the probe can lead to considerable changes in ultrasound imaging.

The PV calibre is measured at the hepatic hilum at the crossing with the HA, where a diameter up to 12.5–13 mm is considered normal (Figure 3.34).

The HA has echogenic walls, it runs anteriorly to the PV and posteriorly to the CBD, and its normal calibre at the hepatic hilum measures up to 3 mm in diameter (Figure 3.34). The hepatic veins have thinner and less echogenic walls [8] and have a straighter and linear course compared to the portal venous system. Although the measurement of the hepatic veins is usually not performed on a routine basis, the cut-off value of their calibre is approximately 8 mm, measured at about 2–3 cm from their confluence into the IVC [9]. It should be kept in mind that in lean subjects both IVC and hepatic veins may be more ectatic. When performing a liver ultrasound scan it is important to keep in mind that the echogenicity of both hepatic veins and PV walls changes according to the angle between the ultrasound beam and the vascular wall. The more acute is the angle of insonation, the closer it is to being parallel to the longitudinal axis of the vessel. Therefore, despite there being clear differences between the thick perivascular collagen of the portal venous system and the thin walls of the hepatic veins (Figure 3.35), if the angle of insonation is low between the ultrasound beam and the PV walls, these could appear very thin or even not be visible. On the other hand, if the angle of insonation with the hepatic veins is close to 90°, the walls will appear thick and echogenic. It is always important to keep in mind this physical principle, remembering the anatomical landmarks and tracing the vessels to their origin: the PV to the hepatic hilum and the hepatic veins to their confluence into the IVC.

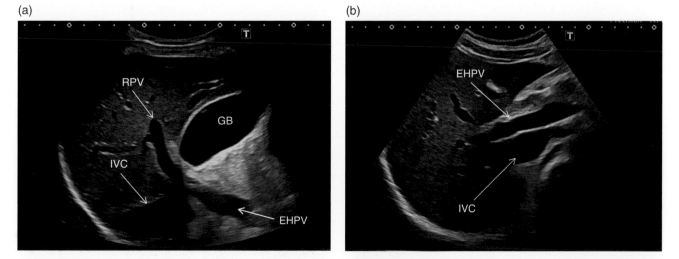

Figure 3.32 The portal vein can be assessed by using (a) an intercostal longitudinal scan or (b) a subcostal transverse oblique scan approach. IVC, inferior vena cava; GB, gallbladder; RPV, right portal vein; EHPV, extrahepatic portal vein.

(a)

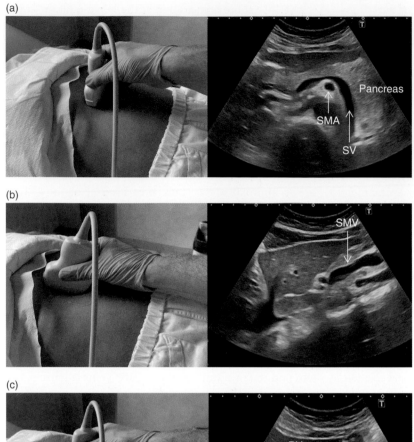

(b)

(c)

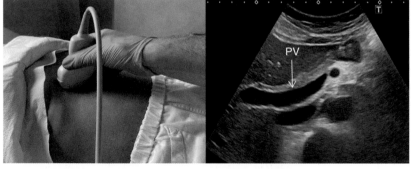

Figure 3.33 (a) To assess the portal venous system, start by using an epigastric transverse scan plane, carefully angling the probe downwards until the splenic vein (SV) is imaged lying below the pancreas and above the superior mesenteric artery (SMA). (b) By rotating the probe approximately 90° clockwise (a degree of variation may be found in different individuals) a longitudinal view of the superior mesenteric vein (SMV) will appear. (c) The confluence of both SV and SMV into the main extrahepatic portal venous trunk is obtained by using an intermediate position of approximately 45°. In order to follow the portal vein (PV) entering the liver, using an oblique subcostal scan view, carefully move the probe downwards just below the right subcostal margin. In case of bowel interposition, try to move the patient into the left lateral decubitus position and ask them to take a deep breath. This manoeuvre usually facilitates the movement of bowel loops inferiorly and also pushes the liver below the costal margin.

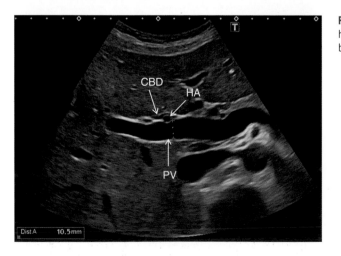

Figure 3.34 The portal vein (PV) calibre is measured at the hepatic hilum at the crossing with the hepatic artery (HA). CBD, common bile duct.

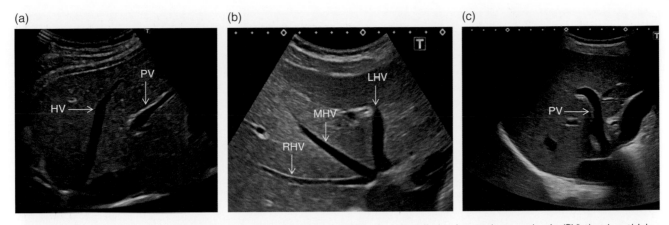

Figure 3.35 The hepatic veins (HV) have a thin wall that is barely visible, in contradistinction to the portal vein (PV) that has thicker, visible echogenic walls. However, the angle of incidence between the ultrasound beam and the insonated structure can modify the appearance of the image. (a) The normal thin-walled HV can be compared to the thick-walled PV. (b) The right hepatic vein (RHV) lies perpendicular to the ultrasound beam, appearing to have a thicker echogenic wall compared to the medium (MHV) and left hepatic veins (LHV) that are respectively oblique and parallel to the ultrasound beam. (c) The PV's long axis is almost parallel to the ultrasound beam, significantly 'reducing' the width of its wall (arrow).

The following is a liver assessment check-list with probe position for segment visualisation:

- Segments I–III and segment IVA/IVB: Longitudinal and transverse subcostal epigastric view.
- Confluence Segments IVA and IVB and confluence of hepatic veins: mainly transverse subcostal epigastric view but also longitudinal subcostal view to focus on the left hepatic vein draining into the IVC.
- Segments V and VI right subcostal transverse view and right intercostal longitudinal view.
- Segment VII and VIII: epigastric/right subcostal view and right intercostal longitudinal view.
- GB and CBD measurement at porta hepatis: right intercostal longitudinal view or transverse epigastric and transverse/oblique right subcostal view.

Doppler Studies of the Liver

A more in-depth assessment of the PV may be needed, and this is usually traced from the confluence of the superior mesenteric vein and splenic vein forming the main PV, as previously described. This should then be traced to its intrahepatic division into the main right and left lobes of the liver (Video 3.6). These vessels should be assessed with greyscale, colour, and spectral Doppler flow (see Chapter 1). Portal venous flow is usually monophasic or mildly phasic and hepatopetal in direction (Figure 3.36). Portal flow velocity may be influenced by obstruction and increased intrahepatic resistance, particularly in the presence of PV thrombosis and cirrhosis or severe heart failure/increased central venous pressure. In the latter case, the portal venous flow is typically pulsatile (see Chapters 8 and 12).

The confluence of the hepatic veins in the subcostal oblique view provides a good starting point to visualise their patency. From there the LHV, MHV, and RHV can be visualised along their entirety to the IVC with B-mode and colour Doppler. These should also be assessed with spectral Doppler, best in the longitudinal plane, primarily to assess the flow phasicity (Figure 3.37) [9]. An assessment of the HA is usually not performed for routine clinical purposes. However, there has been much work assessing the Doppler flow of the HA in research studies for chronic liver disease [10–12]. The HA is typically visualised at the porta hepatis and in the longitudinal plane. A spectral Doppler trace allows measurement of the velocities and resistive index (Figure 3.38). Note that there are anatomical variants of the origin of the hepatic artery, which can be difficult to ascertain on occasion especially with ultrasound.

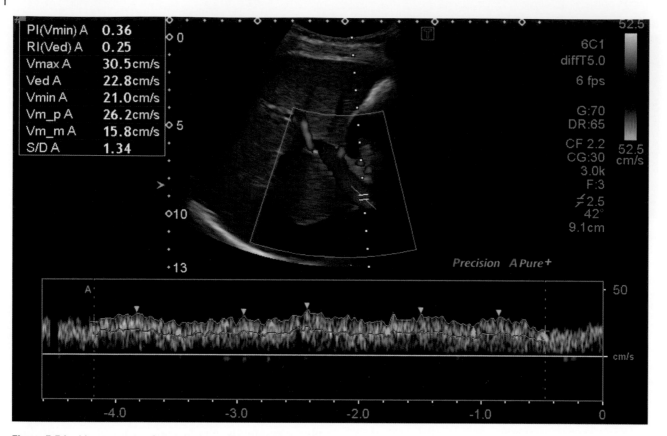

PI(Vmin) A	0.36
RI(Ved) A	0.25
Vmax A	30.5 cm/s
Ved A	22.8 cm/s
Vmin A	21.0 cm/s
Vm_p A	26.2 cm/s
Vm_m A	15.8 cm/s
S/D A	1.34

Figure 3.36 Measurement of portal venous flow at the level of the main portal vein. Colour Doppler shows hepatopetal slightly phasic flow with normal velocities. Usually the portal venous flow is monophasic or might show some subtle phasicity as in this case.

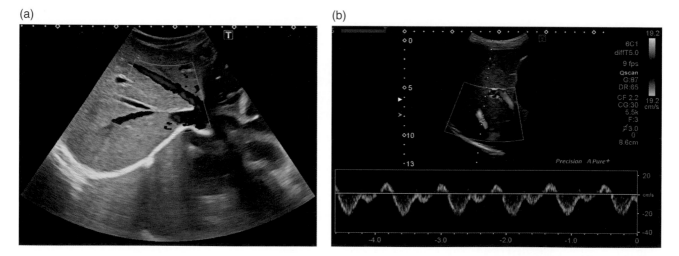

(a)   (b)

Figure 3.37 (a) Colour Doppler of the hepatic veins. (b) Spectral analysis of the right hepatic vein imaged using an intercostal longitudinal scan view shows normal triphasic flow.

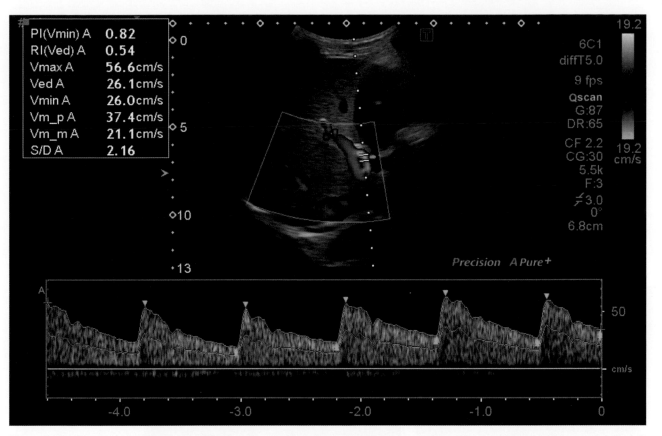

PI(Vmin) A	0.82
RI(Ved) A	0.54
Vmax A	56.6cm/s
Ved A	26.1cm/s
Vmin A	26.0cm/s
Vm_p A	37.4cm/s
Vm_m A	21.1cm/s
S/D A	2.16

Figure 3.38 The hepatic artery is visualised using a longitudinal intercostal plane where it runs anterior to the portal vein. A few seconds of suspended respiration will ensure stability and quality of the arterial trace with no sampling displacement.

The Spleen

The spleen is a very important organ in liver disease, since it is linked anatomically and physiologically to the liver through the portal venous system. Its increase in size is described as one of the hallmarks of significant portal hypertension in cirrhosis (see Chapter 8), although extrahepatic causes of splenomegaly should always be borne in mind. Therefore, when performing a liver ultrasound scan, the size of the spleen must always be described, highlighting both longitudinal and anteroposterior diameters (respective cut-offs ≤13 cm and ≤4 cm). However, splenic parenchymal evaluation is also very important in addition to the splenic size, where textural differences can be seen with different pathological conditions ranging from infectious diseases, haematological and immune/inflammatory-related pathologies as well as congenital and acquired vascular malformations. Moreover, splenic parenchyma can also be the site of benign and primary or secondary malignancies manifesting as discrete focal lesions.

Of note, accessory spleens (splenunculi) are relatively common (Figure 3.39). These are typically rounded or ovoid small lesions with similar splenic echotexture and vascularity. They are a result of the incomplete fusion of splenic tissue into a single organ during its embryonal development and thus can occur anywhere along the splenic bed. Occasionally, these can be difficult to distinguish from peritoneal or renal lesions and thus may require contrast ultrasound or further imaging for confirmation.

The spleen is assessed intercostally through the left lateral intercostal spaces with the patient lying supine. Keep in mind that in some cases the spleen is more posterior and difficult to visualise entirely (Figure 3.39). In case of splenomegaly, the spleen can be assessed with a longitudinal subcostal scan; alternatively, in case of a normal-sized spleen the intercostal approach remains the best option. Imaging may be improved sometimes by turning the patient right side down, although sometimes bowel loops and the lung might interfere, leading to suboptimal imaging.

(a)

(b)

(c)

(d)

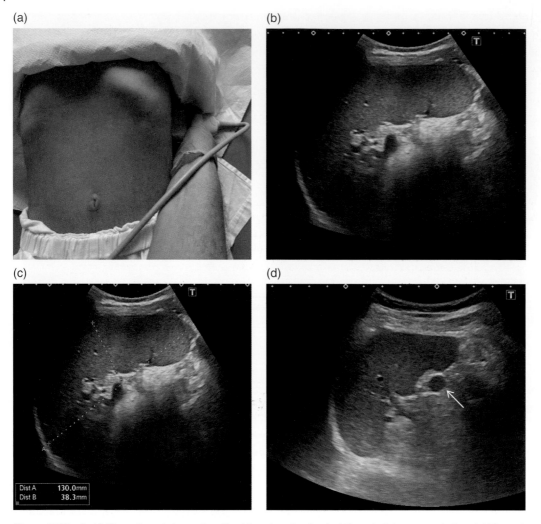

Figure 3.39 (a, b) The spleen is best visualised in a longitudinal oblique left intercostal view. (c) The spleen size is measured in this plane, allowing to evaluate its longitudinal bipolar and anteroposterior diameter. (d) An example of a small accessory spleen is also shown (white arrow). Accessory spleen or splenunculus is a round or ovoidal area of the same splenic echostructure usually adjacent to the splenic hilum, although it can lie anywhere within the splenic bed. It will typically have vascularity similar to the main splenic tissue.

Liver Ultrasound Report

The ultrasound report is an official document, a proof of findings that has medical and legal implications. Hence, for clarity, it is best to follow a standardised 'checklist'. This has the advantage of being a point of reference for the operator, but also makes for ease of reading and interpretation by the referring clinical team. Ideally, the report should be clear, concise, simple to read, and, importantly, it should answer the clinical question.

The name and date of birth of the patient as well as the clinical history-specific request for the scan should be documented within the report. A misleading result of a 'normal scan' should be avoided. Therefore, if for any reason imaging is suboptimal or the scan inconclusive, this should be clearly documented in the report,

owing to the potential for a missed pathology. In some instances, the types of transducer used may also be specified.

The ultrasound report should start describing the size, echotexture, echogenicity, and contour of the liver. Note should be made of any anatomical variants. A normal liver typically has a homogeneous echotexture, with angular margins and a smooth contour. The liver contour is best assessed using the highest-frequency linear transducer possible. The liver echogenicity is equal to or subtly brighter than the cortex of the right kidney.

The echotexture of the liver is a very important feature to describe, because it is related to the potential presence of underlying chronic liver disease. However, it is a sensitive but not specific observation, since it is also seen in other conditions, hence careful integration with other parameters and patient information is warranted before jumping to conclusions.

Finally, the observation of hepatic parenchyma should include the description of focal liver lesions or highlight their absence. If a focal lesion is found, several parameters should be described: the location, in terms of right or left lobe and the relative liver segment; the shape and size (maximum diameter); the echogenicity as well as the homogeneous or heterogeneous appearance; the presence of calcifications; the presence of a peripheral halo. If present, the displacement of vessels or biliary tracts adjacent to the lesion should also be described. The use of colour/power Doppler may be useful in some cases, as well as the description of some artefacts that may help with a differential diagnosis.

The GB assessment requires the description of its size, appearance of its lumen (if it has a distended or contracted appearance), as well as the wall width and content. Signs of inflammation or sinister pathology and indications for further imaging should be outlined. The biliary tree should be described with respect to the intra- and extrahepatic ducts and the calibre of the CBD should always be reported. If dilatation of the biliary tree is noted, information on the site of the obstruction or calibre change should be documented. The pancreas should also be commented on, especially if there is dilatation of the CBD and pancreatic duct.

When describing the portal venous system, the calibre, patency, and flow direction of the intra-and extrahepatic PV should be reported, together with the splenic and superior mesenteric veins if these can be clearly visualised. If features of PV thrombosis are found, the extent, echogenicity, and partial or complete occlusion of the vessel should be reported.

The HA usually is not described on a routine scan unless specific abnormalities are found, such as dilatation and areas suspected of shunting. In conditions such as hepatic trauma or liver transplantation, focal dilatations need to be excluded, since they may be complicated by pseudoaneurysms, while flow velocities and resistive indices may highlight the presence of stenosis or other post-transplant complications (see Chapter 13).

The IVC and hepatic veins should always be described because of their haemodynamic cardiac relationship and potential underlying pathology, which may directly cause an outflow obstruction syndrome. The IVC should always be traced up to the atrio-caval junction (see Chapters 8 and 12).

The spleen is an important organ in liver pathology and in general its echotexture, size, and presence of focal lesions including splenunculi, should always be described. In cirrhosis, the presence of perisplenic porto-systemic vascular shunts suggesting clinically significant portal hypertension should always be reported.

Even if the ultrasound request is focused on liver imaging, in general, an upper abdominal ultrasound scan should also include both kidneys. The right kidney is commonly evaluated since it serves as a comparison of liver parenchyma echogenicity to highlight the possible presence of steatosis, as mentioned previously.

Lastly, the presence or absence of ascites needs to be highlighted, describing if there is a small, moderate, or marked amount of fluid. If present, the sonographic characteristics of the ascitic fluid should also be described, especially if it has a multiloculated appearance, as that may be a result of infection, bleeding, or underlying malignancy. Moreover, it has therapeutic implications where drainage may prove challenging.

It is also worth commenting on observations above the right hemidiaphragm, most commonly a pleural effusion or lobar consolidation.

Overall, a good ultrasound study is tailored to the clinical history and question to be answered. It is beneficial that the operator should have sufficient knowledge and skill to be able to assess the other respective upper abdominal organs and not just the liver. If not, then the operator should be aware of their own limitations and put pathways in place for referral to an appropriate person with the required skills.

Videos

Videos for this chapter can be accessed via the companion website: www.wiley.com/go/LiverUltrasound.

References

1 Dietrich, C.F., Serra, C., and Jedrzejczyk, M. (2020). *Ultrasound of the Liver*. London: European Federation for Ultrasound in Medicine.

2 Jenssen, C., Bridson, J.-M., Barreiros, A.P. et al. (2020). *Ultrasound of the Gallbladder and Biliary System*. London: European Federation for Ultrasound in Medicine.

3 Neumyer, M.M. (2017). Ultrasound evaluation of the hepato–portal system. *J. Vasc. Ultrasound* 41 (2): 76–86.

4 Couinaud, C. (1957). *Le foie: Etudes anatomiques et chirurgicales*. Paris: Masson.

5 Caseiro-Alves, F., Seco, M., and Bernardes, A. (2013). Liver anatomy, congenital anomalies, and normal variants.

In: *Abdominal Imaging* (ed. B. Hamm and P.R. Ros), 983–1000. Berlin: Springer.

6 Glennison, M., Salloum, C., Lim, C. et al. (2014). Accessory liver lobes: anatomical description and clinical implications. *J. Visc. Surg.* 151: 451–455.

7 Catalano, O.A., Singh, A.H., Uppot, R.N. et al. (2008). Vascular and biliary variants in the liver: implications for liver surgery. *Radiographics* 28 (2): 359–378.

8 Wachsberg, R.H., Angyl, E.A., Klein, K.M. et al. (1997). Echogenicity of hepatic versus portal vein walls revisited with histologic correlation. *J. Ultrasound Med.* 16 (12): 807–810.

9 McNaughton, D.A. and Abu-Yousef, M.M. (2011). Doppler US of the liver made simple. *RadioGraphics* 31: 161–188.

10 Lim, A.K., Patel, N., Eckersley, R.J. et al. (2005). Can Doppler sonography grade the severity of hepatitis C-related liver disease? *Am. J. Roentgenol.* 184 (6): 1848–1853.

11 Park, H.S., Desser, T.S., Jeffrey, R.B., and Kamaya, A. (2017). Doppler ultrasound in liver cirrhosis: correlation of hepatic artery and portal vein measurements with model for end-stage liver disease score. *J. Ultrasound Med.* 36 (4): 725–773.

12 Piscaglia, F., Gaiani, S., Calderoni, D. et al. (2001). Influence of liver fibrosis on hepatic artery Doppler resistance index in chronic hepatitis of viral origin. *Scand. J. Gastroenterol.* 36 (6): 647–652.

4

An Introduction to Contrast-Enhanced Ultrasound

Adrian K.P. Lim[1,2], Chris J. Harvey[1], and Matteo Rosselli[3,4]

[1] Department of Imaging, Imperial College Healthcare NHS Trust, London, UK
[2] Department of Metabolism, Digestion and Reproduction, Imperial College London, UK
[3] Department of Internal Medicine, San Giuseppe Hospital, USL Toscana Centro, Empoli, Italy
[4] Division of Medicine, Institute for Liver and Digestive Health, University College London, Royal Free Hospital, London, UK

Ultrasound Contrast Agents

Microbubbles form the basis of ultrasound contrast agents (UCAs), where one of the first agents used was agitated saline. Following on from this was an agent that consisted of tiny microbubbles of air stabilised with a surfactant layer, which had the trade name Levovist (Schering, Berlin, Germany). It had a stability of only 30 minutes once constituted. However, it has now been superseded by more stable agents. These typically contain a perfluorocarbon gas and a phospholipid outer shell for improved stability, and can be used for diagnostic purposes for up to six hours once they have been mixed. Many of the agents are constituted by mixing a prepared syringe of a solvent into a vacuum-sealed vial containing a powder and the perfluorocarbon gas. The mixing and shaking of the two produces microbubbles that range in size, typically between 1 and 10 μm.

The most commonly used agent in Europe is SonoVue, but there are several others licensed for clinical use. Currently there are four agents that are available internationally:

- Definity®/Luminity® (Lantheus Medical Imaging, North Billerica, MA, USA)
- SonoVue®/Lumason® (Bracco Suisse, Geneva, Switzerland)
- Optison™ (GE Healthcare, Oslo, Norway)
- Sonazoid® (GE Healthcare)

The approval of these agents varies throughout the world along with the approved indications, and is dependent on the regulatory agency of the country of use.

Pharmacokinetics

UCAs remain in the intravascular space and do not diffuse out into the extracellular fluid. The advantage of their being confined to the vascular compartment is that this provides improved delineation of the microvasculature, better than the iodinated or gadolinium-based agents used in computed tomography (CT) and magnetic resonance (MR) imaging, respectively [1].

Interestingly, although there is no renal excretion unlike CT/MR agents, a couple of these agents where either phagocytosis by Kuppfer cells has been reported or they remain stationary for a period of time within the sinusoidal spaces of the liver [2]. These days there are target-specific microbubbles such as those conjugated with an anti-vascular endothelial growth factor receptor-2 monoclonal antibody. These could potentially help image the vascularisation of a tumour. Much of the work has been on animal models, but some are currently being trialled for prostate tumours [3, 4].

Interaction with Ultrasound Waves

When UCAs are insonated they contract, expand, and contract, producing oscillations that are asymmetrical in diameter. These generate harmonic signals and it is fortuitous that microbubbles resonate at the lower frequency range used in diagnostic imaging. The propagation of the ultrasound wave also demonstrates similar non-linear behaviour in biological tissue, but to a lesser extent than with UCAs. It is this property that ultrasound manufacturers have utilised to tease out the signal difference between tissue and microbubbles.

Scanning Modes

Many scanners have a contrast mode, which utilises a pulse inversion or pulse modulation technique or sometimes a combination, to amplify the signals by UCAs while cancelling those from tissue. These are low power modes, typically one-tenth of that used for the greyscale image. At higher powers, the microbubbles will burst and could lead to a loss of signal, with apparent non-enhancement or washout. Each manufacturer has its own acronym for contrast mode, usually with 'harmonic imaging' in the name. Some have simplified this to just 'contrast' and many have also ensured that all the buttons necessary to perform the contrast study are ergonomically positioned close together. They also ensure that adequate cineloops of at least 60 seconds or more are enabled for storage. The preferred on-screen display is a split-screen set-up, where one half depicts the microbubble and the other side is the greyscale localiser (Figure 4.1). The option of having just the microbubble signature display is also possible, as is an overlay of this mode on the greyscale image. The microbubble display is usually a bright, distinct colour to enable easy visualisation, typically with a gold/chrome hue. On some scanners a dual cursor also allows the more accurate localisation of a small lesion, ensuring that the enhancement pattern can be accurately assessed (Figure 4.2).

Injecting Ultrasound Contrast Agents (Microbubbles)

These are typically injected through either a cannula or a butterfly placed within a vein. This would ideally be at least 22 gauge. A three-way tap is helpful to ensure ease when flushing with normal saline. The shorter the connecting tubing, the lower the volume of saline that is needed. If possible, avoid any filters at the end of the cannula. These filters and smaller-bore needles will cause some destruction of the microbubbles and thus if they are unavoidable, a larger volume of injectate may be needed to produce diagnostic images. This can be easily gauged after the first injection. Owing to the improved sensitivity of state-of-the-art scanners in detecting the microbubble 'signature', only between 0.5 and 1.5 mL of contrast agent is needed to produce diagnostic images; this volume is dependent on the patient's size. In contrast, some UCA manufacturers used to advocate two to three times that quantity. It should be noted that too high a dose can occasionally produce a 'block' on the visualised depth within the liver; that is, the depth where the microbubbles can be detected is limited by the quantity of contrast in the nearfield effectively 'blocking' the ultrasound beam.

Most agents are easy to prepare. Figure 4.3 illustrates the usual packaging and set-up, where a powder and the sulfur hexafluoride guide are within a vacuum-sealed bottle. A syringe with a solvent (provided in the pack) is injected via a spike and the mixture is shaken vigorously for at least 10 seconds. This action forms the microbubbles within the vial and this fluid can then be withdrawn and injected. Once constituted, the mixture can be used for typically up to six to eight hours.

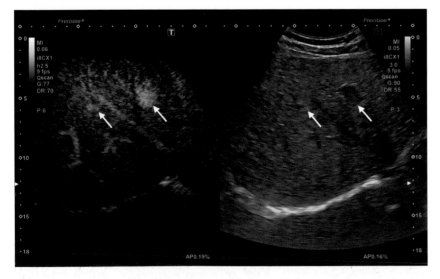

Figure 4.1 The preferred split-screen mode where the microbubble-specific mode is depicted in a golden hue. Note the easily distinguishable arterially hyperenhancing lesions (arrows) on the background of a cirrhotic liver, thus likely representing multifocal hepatocellular carcinoma. The hepatic venous confluence with the inferior vena cava is also depicted.

Figure 4.2 (a, b) The measurement callipers can be a useful aid when trying to determine the enhancement characteristic of the focal lesion (arrow) in question with respect to the adjacent liver, especially when lesions are of iso-enhancement. In this case of focal nodular hyperplasia, the callipers outline the lesion in the portal venous and late phases, where there is no washout of contrast, and the boundaries are better seen on the B-mode image (b).

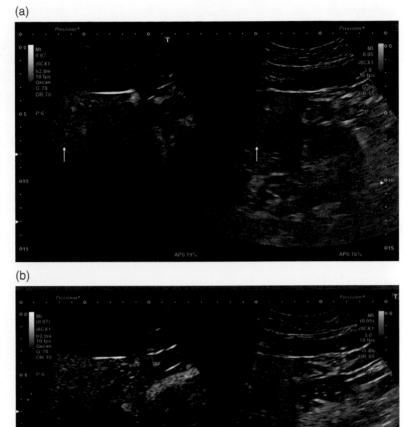

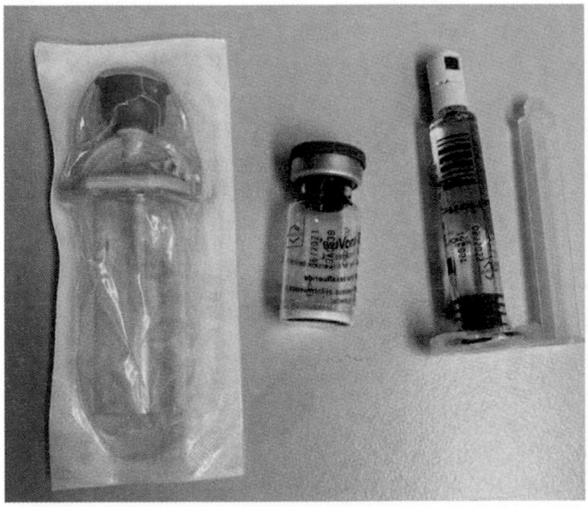

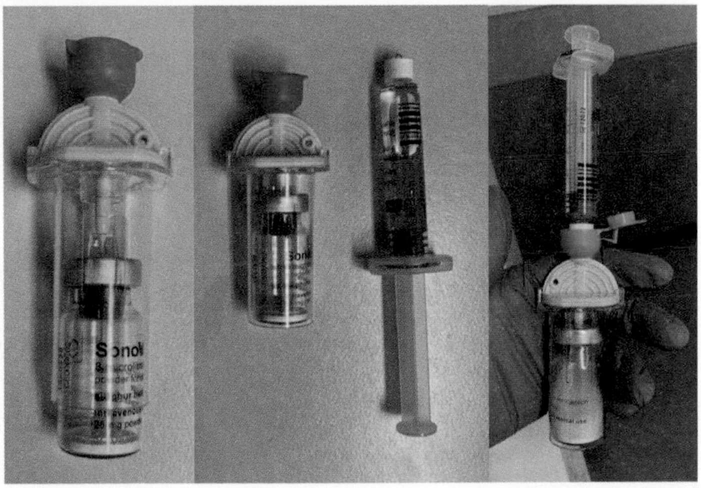

Figure 4.3 (a, b) The typical packaged items provided to constitute microbubbles. In this case it is SonoVue. Note that the solvent is injected into a powder-containing and gas vial via a 'spike introducer', which will fit the Luer-lock end of the syringe. Once the solvent is injected into the vial, shake vigorously for at least 10 seconds and the contrast is ready for use. A single vial usually makes up to 4.8 mL and only 1.0–1.5 mL of contrast agent is typically needed to obtain a diagnostic set of images. For this agent, there have been no reports of any symptoms with overdose but usually no more than 4.8 mL (1 vial) is needed for assessment of the liver. Note in paediatrics, this is titrated to weight, usually 0.03 mL/kg up to a maximum of 2.4 mL for imaging the liver.

Safety

UCAs are extremely safe when compared with iodinated or gadolinium-based contrast agents. They are not nephrotoxic and can be safely administered to patients with renal insufficiency, with no risk of contrast-related nephropathy or nephrogenic systemic fibrosis. There is no need for a renal profile prior to injection, and there is no evidence of any effect on thyroid function. UCAs also have a very low reported rate of anaphylactoid-type reactions (1/7000 patients, 0.014%) [5–7], which is significantly lower than the rate with current iodinated CT agents (35–95/100000 patients, 0.035–0.095%) [8] and comparable to the rate of severe anaphylactoid reactions associated with gadolinium-based contrast agents at 0.001–0.01% [9]. Serious anaphylactoid-type reactions to UCAs are observed in approximately 1/10000 exposures [5–7].

The most frequent adverse events reported are headache, nausea, chest pain, and chest discomfort. These adverse events are typically mild and resolve spontaneously within a short time, without any lasting effects. Most cases of allergy-like events and hypotension occur within a few minutes following injection of the agent.

Contrast-enhanced ultrasound (CEUS) is also used in the paediatric population, mostly as off-label use. However, the US Food and Drug Administration (FDA) recently approved the use of Lumason for paediatric liver imaging. This is an important development in paediatric imaging, where a significant reduction of ionising radiation exposure is likely to be achieved in many areas by using CEUS.

State of the Art

All the latest scanners utilise a low mechanical index mode to visualise microbubbles and this is typically in the split-screen format. It is also now available on the medium-range scanners and some manufacturers also have it available on their portable scanners. The sensitivity of this mode and image resolution will vary. Premium-end scanners with the latest probe technology ensure a homogeneous image and range focusing. Many also have a 'bubble burst' function to allow reperfusion in the same plane; however, the kinetics are not entirely comparable to the first pass. There are 3D functions for CEUS, but the images are of lower resolution than the standard 2D images and while some images may be aesthetically pleasing, they do not typically add much in terms of diagnostic value. Maximum-intensity projections of lesions where multiple images are slowly built up over one another during a set time limit can also be useful at outlining the typical enhancement characteristics of a lesion. This function can colour code the arriving bubbles by time, thus providing a clearer image of which portions of the lesions enhance first, which can be crucial for characterising lesions.

One area of research is the ability to plot time-intensity curves of these lesions, which has shown some promise in assessing response to disease and also for characterising chronic liver disease [10–12]. There are now typically in-built programs within the ultrasound scanner to allow this, where previously such calculations needed to be performed off-line.

There have also been significant improvements in microbubble technology in terms of stability and dosage, which is related to the average size of the microbubbles. One of the latest agents, Sonazoid, has a liver-specific phase, and there are also targeted microbubbles in development that are likely to play a significant role in hepatic ultrasound diagnostic and therapeutic capabilities.

The most recent guidelines on the latest clinically available UCAs and how best to utilise them within the liver have been nicely summarised in a document jointly written by CEUS experts within the European and World Federations of Societies in Ultrasound in Medicine and Biology (EFSUMB and WFUMB, respectively) [9].

References

1 Krix, M., Plathow, C., Kiessling, F. et al. (2004). Quantification of perfusion of liver tissue and metastases using a multivessel model for replenishment kinetics of ultrasound contrast agents. *Ultrasound Med. Biol.* 30 (10): 1355–1363.

2 Cosgrove, D. (2006). Ultrasound contrast agents: an overview. *Eur. J. Radiol.* 60 (3): 324–330.

3 Lyshchik, A., Fleischer, A.C., Huamani, J. et al. (2007). Molecular imaging of vascular endothelial growth factor receptor 2 expression using targeted contrast-enhanced high-frequency ultrasonography. *J. Ultrasound Med.* 26 (11): 1575–1586.

4 Wu, H., Rognin, N.G., Krupka, T.M. et al. (2013). Acoustic characterization and pharmacokinetic analyses of new nanobubble ultrasound contrast agents. *Ultrasound Med. Biol.* 39 (11): 2137–2146.

5 Cochran, S.T., Bomyea, K., and Sayre, J.W. (2001). Trends in adverse events after IV administration of contrast media. *Am. J. Roentgenol.* 176: 1385–1388.

6 Piscaglia, F. and Bolondi, L. (2006). The safety of SonoVue in abdominal applications: retrospective analysis of 23188 investigations. *Ultrasound Med. Biol.* 32: 1369–1375.

7 Tang, C., Fang, K., Guo, Y. et al. (2017). Safety of sulfur hexafluoride microbubbles in sonography of abdominal and superficial organs: retrospective analysis of 30,222 cases. *J. Ultrasound. Med.* 36: 531–538.

8 Hunt, C.H., Hartman, R.P., and Hesley, G.K. (2009). Frequency and severity of adverse effects of iodinated and gadolinium contrast materials: retrospective review of 456,930 doses. *Am. J. Roentgenol.* 193: 1124–1127.

9 Dietrich, C.F., Nolsøe, C.P., Barr, R.G. et al. (2020 Oct). Guidelines and good clinical practice recommendations for contrast-enhanced ultrasound (CEUS) in the liver-update 2020 WFUMB in cooperation with EFSUMB, AFSUMB, AIUM, and FLAUS. *Ultrasound Med. Biol.* 46 (10): 2579–2604.

10 Lim, A.K., Taylor-Robinson, S.D., Patel, N. et al. (2005 Jan). Hepatic vein transit times using a microbubble agent can predict disease severity non-invasively in patients with hepatitis C. *Gut* 54 (1): 128–133.

11 Park, M.S., Hong, S., Lim, Y.L. et al. (2018). Measuring intrahepatic vascular changes using contrast-enhanced ultrasonography to predict the prognosis of alcoholic hepatitis combined with cirrhosis: a prospective pilot study. *Gut Liver* 12 (5): 555–561.

12 Sugimoto, K., Moriyasu, F., Saito, K. et al. (2013). Hepatocellular carcinoma treated with sorafenib: early detection of treatment response and major adverse events by contrast-enhanced US. *Liver Int.* 33 (4): 605–615.

5

Focal Liver Lesions – Characterisation and Detection

Chris J. Harvey[1], Adrian K.P. Lim[1,2], and Matteo Rosselli[3,4]

[1] *Department of Imaging, Imperial College Healthcare NHS Trust, London, UK*
[2] *Department of Metabolism, Digestion and Reproduction, Imperial College London, UK*
[3] *Department of Internal Medicine, San Giuseppe Hospital, USL Toscana Centro, Empoli, Italy*
[4] *Division of Medicine, Institute for Liver and Digestive Health, University College London, Royal Free Hospital, London, UK*

There is a wide spectrum of benign and malignant focal liver lesions. Their detection and characterisation are of paramount clinical importance to direct appropriate management. Their sonographic appearances may be variable, even within a given pathology, with a large overlap between benign and malignant lesions [1, 2]. B-mode (brightness-mode) ultrasound can confidently diagnose a sub-centimetre simple cyst, which may not be possible on computed tomography (CT) or magnetic resonance (MR) because of the ultrasound's superior spatial resolution. Unfortunately, this is not true for the majority of focal solid liver lesions, where ultrasound is restricted to a description of size, echogenicity and Doppler findings, which commonly does not accurately characterise a lesion. Prior to ultrasound contrast agents, the finding of a focal solid liver lesion would have prompted referral for a CT or MR. Since the development and licensing of ultrasound contrast agents, the characterisation of focal liver lesions has become their most important application, with sensitivities and specificities rivalling those of contrast-enhanced computed tomography (CECT) and contrast-enhanced magnetic resonance (CEMR) [3–7]. This has led to the formulation of guidelines by ultrasound societies [8] and the UK National Institute for Health and Care Excellence (NICE) [9].

Ultrasound of the liver must be performed with full knowledge of the clinical history and any prior imaging. It is especially important for lesion characterisation, because the potential lesion types differ between cirrhotic and non-cirrhotic livers. Similarly, if there is a known primary carcinoma the onus is on detection of liver metastases. An incidental focal liver lesion detected in the absence of cirrhosis or a known malignancy is most likely to be benign.

Liver Contrast-Enhanced Ultrasound Protocol and Image Optimisation

All major ultrasound vendors have dedicated contrast-enhanced ultrasound (CEUS) software on their systems. Curvilinear transducers are most commonly used, but high-frequency linear transducers are better for superficial lesions. Focal lesions up to 10 cm in depth are optimally imaged with CEUS. At greater depths there is insufficient power due to beam attenuation. This can be overcome by decreasing the transmit frequency to improve penetration or by increasing the acoustic power, although the latter will increase microbubble destruction. Once the target lesion is identified, the optimum acoustic window should be sought such that the lesion can be imaged during quiet respiration with the patient in a comfortable position [8]. A longitudinal plane is best rather than transverse so that the lesion can be imaged throughout respiration (to avoid out-of-plane motion) during the whole CEUS study. CEUS is subject to the same limitations as conventional ultrasound, so if the lesion is difficult to view on baseline B-mode it is likely that the CEUS will be suboptimal. CEUS may also be suboptimal in high body mass index (BMI) patents and in marked hepatic steatosis. Similarly, sub-diaphragmatic and deep-seated lesions may be difficult to visualise on CEUS, but this may be overcome by scanning in the left lateral position. Small lesions (<5 mm) may be difficult to resolve on CEUS. Another limitation is that the whole liver cannot be adequately assessed in the arterial phase and repeat injections may be necessary to image multiple lesions.

The contrast agent is preferably administered by a cannula or butterfly (18–22g). Typical doses are 1.5–2.4 mL of

SonoVue/Lumason and 0.1–0.2 mL of Definity/Luminity. The timer should be started with the contrast injection.

The liver demonstrates three phases of enhancement after an intravenous (IV) bolus injection: the arterial, portal-venous, and late phases (Table 5.1). The late phase occurs as the vascular phases subside, when the microbubbles are sequestered in the sinusoids and reticuloendothelial system of the liver. In contrast to the real time of CEUS, CECT and CEMR images are 'snapshots' in time, which can be suboptimal due to differences in cardiac output that can deleteriously affect enhancement.

CEUS is visualised in real time using a co-registered dual-screen display alongside B-mode fundamental grey-scale images. This latter B-mode is of reduced resolution compared to conventional B-mode because of the lower acoustic power (mechanical index) used in microbubble-specific modes. The dual-screen format allows anatomical guidance and ensures that the target lesion is kept within the field of view during imaging. The focal zone should be set just deep to the lesion.

CEUS protocols are usually based on a combination of continuous imaging in the arterial phase and intermittent imaging in the late phases to obtain a diagnostic scan while minimising bubble destruction. Imaging is usually performed

continuously from contrast injection until at least peak arterial-phase enhancement. Imaging can be continued after this time to determine timing of early washout. Thereafter imaging should be performed intermittently (5–10 seconds every 30–60 seconds) to detect and assess late washout. Video recording of the study is optimally performed from contrast arrival through peak arterial phase until 60 seconds. Thereafter static images can be recorded intermittently (every 30–60 seconds) to document the presence, timing and degree of washout. Late-phase scanning may need to be performed for longer in suspected hepatocellular carcinoma (HCC), as discussed below. Sweeps through the liver in the late phase are useful to identify defects that may signify malignant lesions not seen earlier in the scan. If detected, the arterial and portal phases of these lesions can be characterised by a second injection. Repeat injections can safely be performed in accordance with manufacturer guidelines.

This chapter discusses the enhancement characteristics of benign and malignant focal liver lesions encountered in clinical practice (their typical features are summarised in Tables 5.2 and 5.3). Enhancement should be assessed in all phases in order to fully characterise a lesion. The presence, intensity (hyper, iso-, hypo-, or non-enhancing), and pattern of arterial-phase enhancement (diffuse, rim, peripheral globular, or stellate) should be documented as well as the presence, timing, and pattern of washout. As a general rule, however, lesions that do not washout in the late phase showing sustained enhancement (i.e. they remain hyperenhancing or isoenhancing to liver parenchyma) tend to be benign (with the exception of simple cysts, haematomas, ablation cavities, and necrotic abscess-related areas, which do not enhance in any phase), whereas lesions that do not retain contrast in the late phase (i.e. they demonstrate washout) are usually malignant [8–11].

Table 5.1 Time windows for the three phases of liver enhancement on contrast-enhanced ultrasound.

Phase	Time window
Arterial	10–30 seconds
Portal venous	>30–120 seconds
Late vascular phase	>120 seconds–5 minutes

Table 5.2 A summary of the typical enhancement characteristics of benign liver lesions on contrast-enhanced ultrasound.

	Arterial phase	Portal venous phase	Late vascular phase
Haemangioma	Peripheral 'nodular' enhancement	Partial/complete centripetal fill-in	Complete enhancement or central non-enhancing areas
Focal nodular hyperplasia	Early centrifugal enhancement	Hyper/isoenhancing 50% central scar	Hyper/isoenhancing 50% central scar
Hepatic adenoma	Hyperenhancing (heterogeneous)	Isoenhancing	Isoenhancing
Focal fatty sparing/change	Isoenhancing	Isoenhancing	Isoenhancing
Regenerative and dysplastic nodule	Isoenhancing	Isoenhancing	Isoenhancing
Hepatic cyst	Non-enhancing	Non-enhancing	Non-enhancing
Hepatic abscess	Enhancing periphery/septa	Hyper/isoenhancing rim Enhancing septa No central enhancement	Hypoenhancing rim No central enhancement

Table 5.3 A summary of the typical enhancement characteristics of malignant liver lesions on contrast-enhanced ultrasound.

	Arterial phase	Portal venous phase	Late vascular phase
Hypovascular metastases (e.g. colon, pancreatic cancer)	Peripheral rim enhancement	Hypo- or non-enhancement	Hypo- or non-enhancement
Hypervascular metastases (e.g. neuroendocrine)	Hyperenhancement	Hypo- or non-enhancement	Hypo- or non-enhancement
Hepatocellular carcinoma	Hyperenhancement	Hypo- or non-enhancement*	Hypo- or non-enhancement*
Cholangiocarcinoma	Variable hyperenhancement	Hypo- or non-enhancement	Hypo- or non-enhancement
Lymphoma	Variable hyperenhancement	Hypo- or non-enhancement	Hypo- or non-enhancement

*can be iso-enhancing if a well-differentiated tumour or demonstrate very late washout i.e., >5 mins.

The enhancement characteristics of the majority of liver lesions at CEUS are similar to those seen on CECT and CEMR imaging, but microbubbles are confined to the vascular space, whereas CT and MR contrast media diffuse into the extracellular compartment. Thus the elimination of contrast from a liver lesion may differ slightly between CEUS and CT/MR. This may be seen in cholangiocarcinoma or desmoplastic metastases with sustained enhancement on CT/MR, mimicking a benign lesion. CEUS will show washout in these lesions, in keeping with malignancy. In addition, as CEUS operates in real time with a higher temporal and spatial resolution than CT and MR, fast changes during the arterial phase or late enhancement are captured that may be missed on the pre-determined timing of CECT or CEMR.

Benign Focal Liver Lesions

Hepatic Cysts

Simple hepatic cysts are extremely common benign lesions. These can usually be fully characterised on B-mode ultrasound, where they appear as well-defined, smooth-walled, anechoic lesions with through transmission of sound without Doppler-detected vascularity.

B-mode ultrasound can confidently diagnose a sub-centimetre simple cyst, which may not be possible on CT or MR because of the ultrasound's superior spatial resolution. Simple cysts demonstrate no enhancement on any phase of CEUS (Figure 5.1). CEUS is rarely required to characterise a simple hepatic cyst.

Complex cysts often need further characterisation with CEUS (Figure 5.2). There is overlap in appearances between haemorrhagic cysts, pyogenic abscesses, cystadenomas, and cystic metastases [12–14]. CEUS can demonstrate flow in the wall, septa, as well as internal masses and nodules, which can help to characterise lesions.

Haemangioma

Cavernous haemangiomas are the most common benign solid liver lesion, occurring in 7–20% of adults, with 10% being multiple. They are commoner in females and are usually an incidental finding. They range in size from a few mm to greater than 20 cm. Small haemangiomas (<2 cm) are known as capillary haemangiomas. Haemangiomas are typically seen on B-mode ultrasound as well-defined echogenic lesions <3 cm in size (60–70%) and are frequently sub-capsular/peripheral or adjacent to

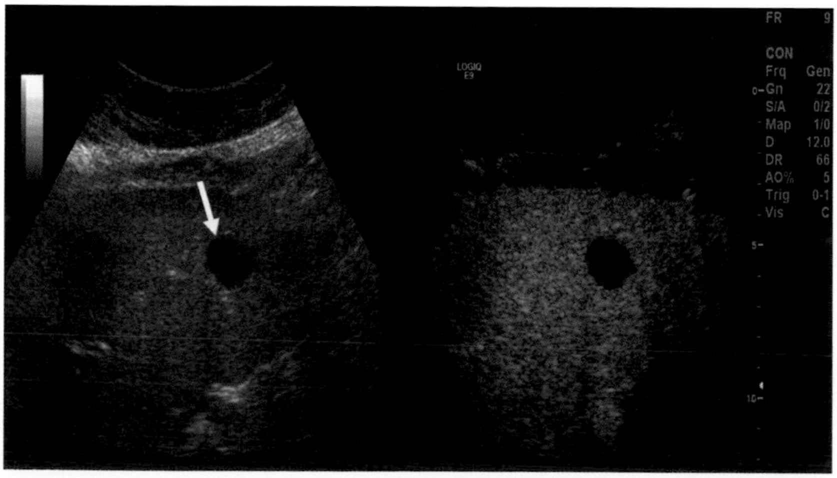

Figure 5.1 Simple cyst seen as a well-defined thin-walled anechoic lesion (arrow) on the B-mode (left screen) of a dual-display contrast-enhanced ultrasound (CEUS). No enhancement is seen in the cyst on CEUS (right screen).

Figure 5.2 Complex liver cyst (arrow) shows complex internal structure on the B-mode (left screen) but no enhancement of the septa or rim on contrast-enhanced ultrasound (right screen).

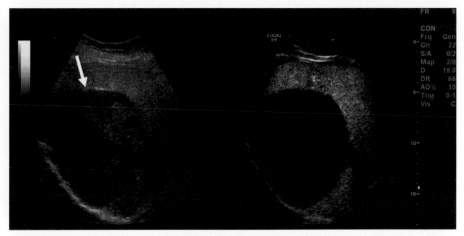

a hepatic vein. They may show posterior acoustic shadowing. Atypical features that usually occur in larger lesions include heterogeneity with echopoor areas due to haemorrhage, necrosis, or fibrosis. They may rarely show calcification. They are usually asymptomatic, although lesions >4 cm in size may exert mass effect. Large tumours may be pedunculated. They rarely bleed even after biopsy. They are composed of multiple endothelial-lined blood spaces separated by fibrous septa. Despite their vascular composition, blood flow is too slow to be detected by conventional Doppler.

On CEUS, haemangiomas typically demonstrate gradual peripheral nodular enhancement in the arterial and portal venous phases, with progressive centripetal fill-in, and become isoenhancing/hyperenhancing to liver parenchyma in the late phase (Figure 5.3) (Video 5.1). CEUS has

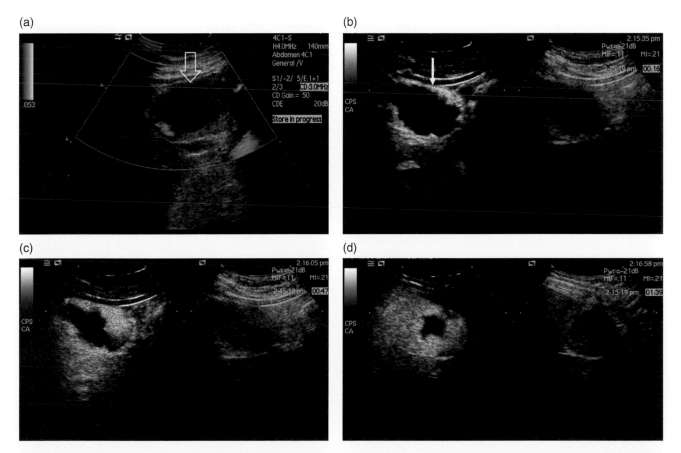

Figure 5.3 Haemangioma. (a) Baseline B-mode ultrasound shows an echopoor avascular solid lesion (open arrow). (b–d) Following intravenous SonoVue, the lesion exhibits classic peripheral globular enhancement (arrow in b) with progressive centripetal fill-in over time (16 seconds in b, 47 seconds in c and 99 seconds in d).

(a)   (b)

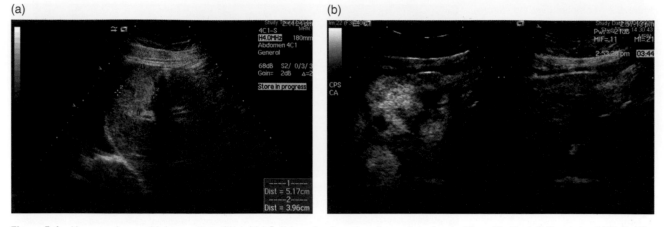

Figure 5.4 Haemangioma with incomplete 'fill-in'. (a) Solid predominantly echogenic lesion (callipers) in the left liver lobe. (b) Following intravenous SonoVue, the lesion shows partial fill-in but has pathognomonic peripheral globular enhancement, allowing a confident diagnosis of benign haemangioma.

significantly improved the accurate diagnosis of haemangioma, to over 95% of cases [15]. The combination of peripheral nodular enhancement with complete fill-in has 98% sensitivity for the diagnosis of a haemangioma [16]. In hepatic steatosis, haemangiomas may appear hypo- or isoechoic, becoming echogenic if the fatty changes resolve. Larger haemangiomas, which may have atypical appearances on B-mode, may not fully fill in on the delayed phase due to central thrombosis, necrosis or fibrosis, which leaves a central area of non-enhancement (Figure 5.4) (Videos 5.2 and 5.3). However, these lesions can be confidently diagnosed as haemangiomas by their characteristic centripetal nodular enhancement and by the fact that the lesions appear smaller on the late-phase CEUS images compared to the B-mode images [17].

Small 'flash' or 'high-flow' haemangiomas may show brief avid enhancement with rapid fill-in and then become isoechoic with adjacent liver.

Focal Nodular Hyperplasia

Focal nodular hyperplasia (FNH) is the second most common benign solid liver tumour and is more frequent in females (F : M 8 : 1). It is usually solitary, measuring <6 cm. Multiple lesions occur in 20% of cases. It is usually asymptomatic. FNH is composed of normal liver hepatocytes, bile ducts, and Kupffer cells and may be thought of as a

hamartomatous lesion. It lacks a true capsule. Its aetiology is uncertain, but it is thought to be due to a hyperplastic response to a pre-existing vascular malformation. The oral contraceptive pill (OCP) does not cause this lesion, but FNH may enlarge in response to hormonal stimulation. Usually FNH is a subtle lesion and even large ones may be missed. It is often isoechoic to liver parenchyma on B-mode ultrasound, but may be visible as a faintly echogenic lesion.

FNH typically demonstrates centrifugal enhancement in a 'spoke–wheel' pattern, arising from a central feeding vessel (Figure 5.5). These lesions show rapid hyperenhancement (in the arterial phase, and up to 50% may have a central non-enhancing 'scar' that does not appear until the late phase). The FNH then 'disappears' and becomes isoechoic to liver on the portal venous or late phase (Video 5.4).

The spoke–wheel sign with a central feeding artery is a very specific finding of FNH [18]. CEUS has a high specificity for the diagnosis of FNH (100%), but sensitivity varies based on lesion size (93% for lesions >3.5 cm and only 7.7% for lesions <3.5 cm) [19].

The key to diagnosing FNH is the early arterial enhancement, as it usually becomes invisible in the portal-venous and late phases and this often requires review of the stored cineloop. Similarly, FNH is often imperceptible on a portal-venous phase CT of the liver.

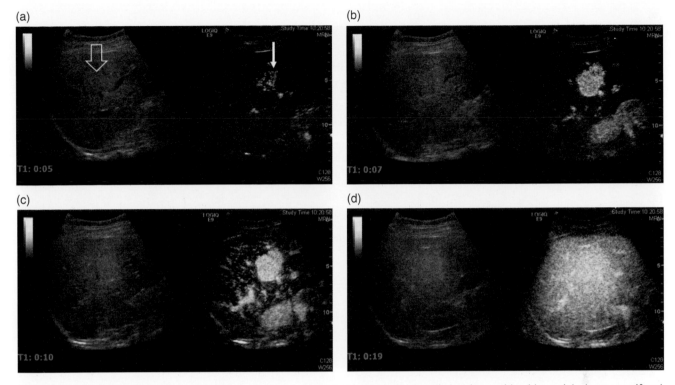

Figure 5.5 Focal nodular hyperplasia. (a–d) Dual-display contrast-enhanced ultrasound showing rapid avid arterial phase centrifugal enhancement of a subtle focal liver lesion (open arrow on B-mode in a) from a central feeding vessel in a spoke–wheel pattern (solid arrow on CEUS in a). The lesion becomes isoechoic with the rest of the liver by 19 seconds (d) and does not wash out in the late phase (not shown).

Hepatic Adenoma

Hepatic adenomas are usually solitary (70–80%), with varying sizes up to 8–10 cm. They may be multiple (>10 in hepatic adenomatosis). They are usually intraparenchymal in a sub-capsular site, but may be pedunculated (10%).

The four sub-types are inflammatory (50% – most prone to bleeding), HNF-1-α inactivated (35%, contain fat, associated with adenomatosis), β-catenin activated, and unclassified [20–22].

They are more common in females than males, particularly in young women who take OCPs. They are also increased in men on anabolic steroids, glycogen storage disease, and fatty liver disease.

While benign, these lesions often present with pain due to haemorrhage (the risk of which increases with the size of the adenoma) and a small proportion undergo malignant change to HCC, hence the recommendation for close surveillance or surgical excision.

On B-mode ultrasound, adenomas present as heterogeneous lesions within homogeneous liver parenchyma, containing anechoic components due to foci of haemorrhage, though they are sometimes difficult to discern and may only be evident by the mass effect they produce (capsular and vascular distortion). Some 30% are echogenic due to fat content. Calcification may be seen in 5–15%.

Adenomas demonstrate centripetal enhancement in the arterial phase, and usually become isoenhancing to liver parenchyma by the portal venous and late phases (Figure 5.6) (Video 5.5), although in some cases a variable washout in the late phase is described (Figure 5.7). The haemorrhagic components of an adenoma are avascular, and therefore do not enhance in any phase. Laumonier et al. [23] studied inflammatory and HNF-1-α inactivated sub-types. The inflammatory sub-type was more likely to show arterial enhancement with centripetal filling, a peripheral rim enhancement, and late washout. The HNF-1-α inactivated sub-type is echogenic on B-mode (due to fat), hypervascular to isoenhancing in the arterial phase, and isoenhancing in the late phase. No specific features were shown on the β-catenin and unclassified types. Manichon [24] showed that a minority of inflammatory and HNF-1-α inactivated sub-types demonstrated washout.

Focal Fatty Sparing and Focal Fatty Change

Fatty change in the liver can produce a wide range of patterns: diffuse, focal, geographical, and perivascular [25]. Areas of focal fatty sparing (FFS) and focal fatty change (FFC) within the liver appear on B-mode ultrasound as echopoor and echogenic areas, respectively, in comparison to background liver parenchyma [26, 27]. However, these lesions can be focal and can be mistaken for focal liver masses, and are particularly worrying in the context of a patient with a known malignancy.

FFS typically occurs in the gallbladder bed and adjacent to the falciform ligament and porta hepatis.

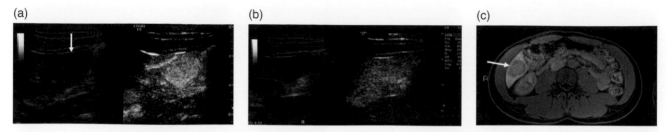

Figure 5.6 Adenoma. (a) Dual-display contrast-enhanced ultrasound showing enhancement of a focal liver lesion (arrow in B-mode [left screen]). (b) There is no washout in the late phase, indicating benignity. Biopsy revealed an adenoma. (c) Magnetic resonance imaging of liver with hepatocyte-specific contrast media shows a defect (arrow) consistent with an adenoma.

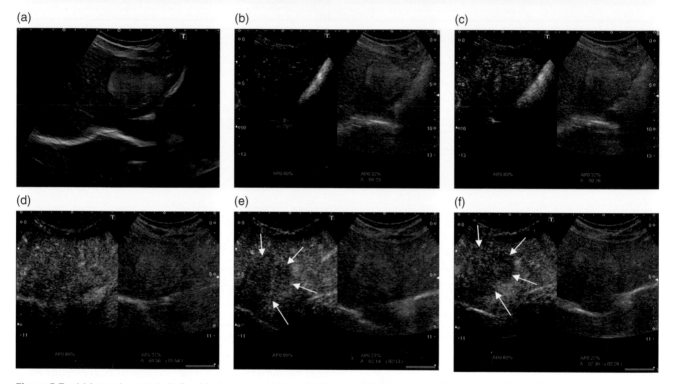

Figure 5.7 (a) Large hyperechoic focal lesion seen on B-mode that on contrast-enhanced ultrasound shows (b, c) homogeneous subtle arterial hyperenhancement, (d) portal venous isoenhancement and (e, f) delayed washout in the late vascular phase (arrows). Surgical exeresis revealed a hepatic fat-filled adenoma.

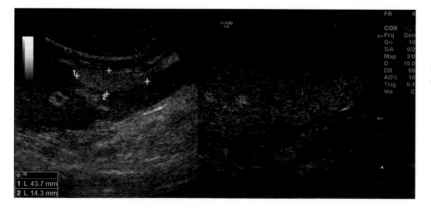

Figure 5.8 Focal fatty change. Echogenic focal liver lesion adjacent to the falciform ligament on baseline B-mode. Contrast-enhanced ultrasound showed homogeneous isoenhancement with the adjacent liver in all phases, consistent with focal fatty change.

FFC is less common than sparing and is classically found adjacent to the falciform ligament, but can occur at the same sites as FFS. It has no mass effect and vessels run through it undisplaced. FFS and FFC are areas of essentially normal hepatic parenchyma, and thus on CEUS demonstrate identical enhancement to the surrounding liver parenchyma in all phases (Figures 5.8 and 5.9) and 'disappear' on the CEUS images. In a study comparing B-mode ultrasound/Doppler with CEUS, the sensitivity, specificity, and accuracy increased from 44%, 97%, and 81% to 88%, 100%, and 96%, respectively [28].

Figure 5.9 Multiple focal fatty sparing. Patient with colon cancer who was referred for a contrast-enhanced ultrasound (CEUS) following the finding of echopoor liver lesions in an echogenic fatty liver and metastases were queried. CEUS (right screen) in the late phase shows no washout of the focal lesions, the largest of which has been arrowed on the B-mode image (left screen) consistent with multifocal fatty sparing.

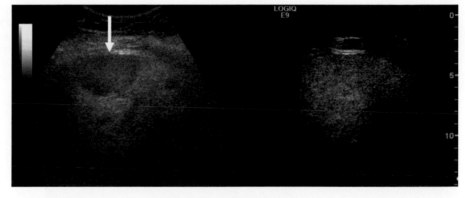

Regenerative and Dysplastic Nodules

These nodules occur in cirrhotic livers. The development of HCC is thought to follow a progression from benign regenerative nodules to low-grade dysplastic nodule to high-grade dysplastic nodule to HCC. During this carcinogenesis there is a change in blood supply of the nodule from predominantly portal venous in the regenerative nodule to arterial in HCC.

A regenerative nodule is an area of regenerative liver parenchyma within a cirrhotic liver. Histologically the nodule contains portal tracts surrounded by fibrous septa. These nodules are of variable echogenicity on B-mode imaging and may appear isoechoic to liver parenchyma (only being apparent due to the 'mass-like' appearance of the nodule). Like FFS and FFC, regenerative nodules demonstrate identical enhancement characteristics to adjacent liver parenchyma on all phases of CEUS (Figure 5.10).

Dysplastic nodules are similar to regenerative nodules, but contain dysplastic cells (which may be low or high grade, when examined histologically). Again, these demonstrate similar enhancement characteristics to the adjacent liver parenchyma on CEUS. High-grade dysplastic nodules and those with foci of HCC in them may show focal arterial enhancement ('nodule within a nodule' appearance) on CEUS [29]. Unfortunately, some well-differentiated HCCs have identical enhancement characteristics to regenerative or dysplastic nodules, but may exhibit delayed washout after 5 minutes. For suspicious lesions additional factors (such as serological tumour markers or lesion growth over serial ultrasound studies) must be taken into account or the lesion followed up at three-monthly intervals.

Infectious and Inflammatory Focal Lesions

A hepatic abscess is a focal area of infection within the liver, and the patient will usually display clinical signs and symptoms of sepsis and might have a clinical history of exposure to an infectious source. There are usually deranged liver function tests, increased inflammatory markers, and elevated white blood cell count. The most frequent causes are bacterial followed by parasitic and fungal infections. The route of infection is either haematogenous (via the portal vein in diverticulitis and appendicitis), biliary tract (ascending cholangitis, especially in obstructed systems), or direct inoculation (following interventional procedures). Diagnosis and treatment are ultrasound-guided aspiration and drainage, respectively, along with antibiotic therapy. On B-mode ultrasound, as a liver abscess matures, it progresses from an isoechoic (pre-liquefaction/necrosis) and thus subtle area to a necrotic, hypoechoic cyst-like lesion, sometimes accompanied by an acoustic posterior enhancement, which may or may not contain gas according to aetiology. The lesion might be single, multiple, or present as a

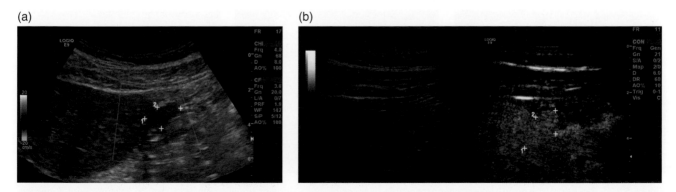

(a)

(b)

Figure 5.10 Regenerative nodule. (a) Pedunculated lesion in a cirrhotic liver on baseline B-mode (callipers). (b) Dual-display contrast-enhanced ultrasound showed homogeneous isoenhancement with the adjacent liver with no washout, consistent with a regenerative nodule.

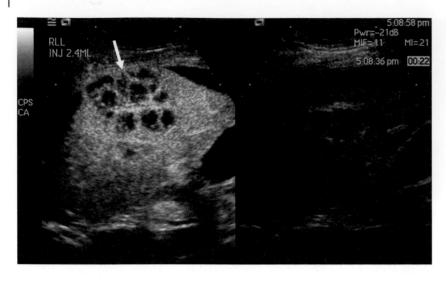

Figure 5.11 Liver abscess. Dual-display contrast-enhanced ultrasound shows enhancement of thickened septa in the abscess (arrow; not visible on B-mode) as well as increasing the conspicuity of two sub-capsular collections.

cluster of coalescent cyst-like lesions with a 'honeycomb' appearance. At CEUS, a hepatic abscess may demonstrate avid rim and internal septa enhancement (Figure 5.11) [30]. The central necrotic region does not enhance. CEUS can help in the characterisation of abscesses depicting the internal loculation and so ascertain whether they are amenable to drainage. It can also help differentiate abscesses, which have a sharp boundary to the necrotic centre and lack of internal enhancement, from hypovascular metastases, which have ill-defined margins, a variable amount of internal enhancement, and are less structurally complex [31].

However, while in the majority of cases the interpretation of the CEUS abscess pattern of enhancement is quite straightforward, in other cases the variability in the pattern of enhancement of the inflamed tissue adjacent to the necrotic core can make interpretation uncertain. A rim arterial hyperenhancement with subsequent isoenhancement or delayed vascular hypoenhancement is often described (Figure 5.12) (Video 5.6). Nevertheless, the inflammatory area involved in the infectious process, after arterial iso- or hyperenhancement, can show rapid hypoenhancement in the portal phase and complete washout in the late vascular phase (Figure 5.13) (Video 5.7) [1, 32].

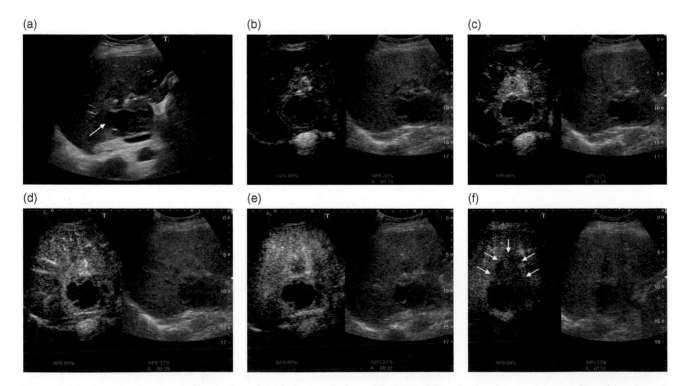

Figure 5.12 B-mode ultrasound shows a hypo/anechoic liver lesion with signs of liquefaction (a, arrow) in keeping with a hepatic abscess. (b–d) Contrast-enhanced ultrasound shows rapid arterial hyperenhancement of the parenchyma adjacent to a non-enhancing core with some internal enhancing septa. It is of note that the hyperenhancing area shows subsequent washout (e, f) more pronounced in the late vascular phase (f, arrows), as it is sometimes seen in tissue inflammation (Video 5.6).

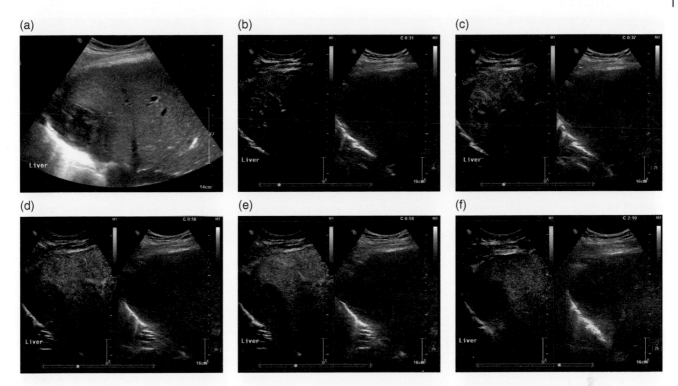

Figure 5.13   (a) An ill-defined heterogeneic focal lesion was identified in segment VII six days after endoscopic retrograde cholangio-pancreatography (ERCP) for choledocolithiasis. Contrast-enhanced ultrasound examination showed (b, c) arterial isoenhancement, except for an anechoic non-enhancing core. The enhancing area showed initial portal (d, e) and subsequent complete washout in the late vascular phase (f). The history of the patient, previous imaging, and improvement of the lesion with resolution at three months are all elements compatible with a hepatic abscess. The contrast pattern of enhancement raises concerns of underlying malignancy. Integration of clinical and biochemical information as well as follow-up are fundamental in this case (Video 5.7).

Caution should be used in differential diagnosis of liver abscesses from cyst-like metastasis found in gastrointestinal stromal tumours, pancreatic neuroendocrine tumours, and mucinous cystoadenocarcinoma as well as ovarian cystoadenocarcinoma. Large lesions that have outgrown the tumour blood supply can develop intralesional necrosis and eventually liquefaction, which may or may not present superimposed infection (Figure 5.14).

The clinical picture and biochemistry are important discriminants for the differential diagnosis in these cases. Nevertheless, sometimes biopsy of the enhancing tissue might be required and second-level imaging might be extremely useful to exclude a primary tumour or a source of infection, as especially seen in appendicitis or diverticular abscesses.

Inflammatory pseudotumours are a rare expression of an infectious or inflammatory process presenting as solitary or multiple focal lesions. They have a non-specific variable appearance, being either well defined or poorly defined, and they have a CEUS appearance with arterial enhancement and washout that mimics malignancy. Liver biopsy is usually required for a definitive diagnosis and appropriate treatment (Figure 5.15) [33].

The appearance of granulomas and liver tuberculosis (TB) on CEUS is often not conclusive and is very difficult to distinguish from malignancy (Figure 5.16) (Video 5.8). Although the most common finding is rim hyperenhancement with hypo- and non-enhancement of the centre, pathological studies confirmed that the different appearances of hepatic TB on CEUS were related to the different pathological stages of the lesions, for which again the background history, laboratory results, cross-sectional imaging, and eventually liver biopsy may be necessary [34].

Hepatic Trauma

Traditionally CT is the modality of choice for imaging abdominal trauma, but it has drawbacks in terms of ionising radiation, nephrotoxic contrast media, and accessibility. CEUS is more sensitive than conventional ultrasound and almost as sensitive as CT in the detection of solid organ injury in blunt abdominal trauma.

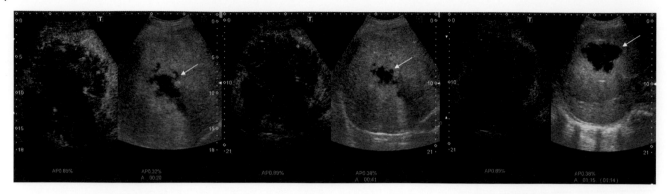

Figure 5.14 Dual display contrast enhanced ultrasound (CEUS) showing a large colorectal liver metastasis with central necrotic liquefaction (B-mode, white arrow). CEUS reveals hypo-enhancement of the lesion throughout all vascular phases compatible with diffuse hypovascularity and necrosis of the lesion.

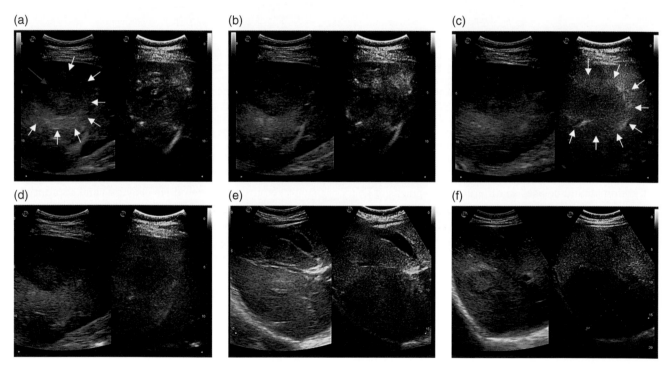

Figure 5.15 Dual display contrast enhanced ultrasound (CEUS) of a segment VI/VII target-like lesion with a hyperechoic centre (a, left side, red arrow) surrounded by an ill-defined hyperechoic halo (a, left side, white arrows). (a, b) CEUS shows peripheral heterogeneous arterial hyperenhancement and central hypoenhancement of the target-like lesion. (c, d) During the portal venous phase the lesion becomes hypoenhancing, while the surrounding hyperechoic halo seen on B-mode stands out as a subtle hyperenhancing area (arrows in c). In the late vascular phase, a large and well-defined hypoenhancing area, including both the target lesion and the surrounding hyperechoic ill-defined halo, appears, showing subsequent complete washout (area between calipers in e and f). A percutaneous liver biopsy was carried out, revealing a histology compatible with eosinophilic inflammatory pseudotumor. Of note is that inflamed liver parenchyma hyperenhances and may show complete washout in the late phase, as seen in this case. The washout of any lesion, however, makes it difficult to completely exclude malignancy and thus in these cases biopsy is warranted.

(a)

(b)

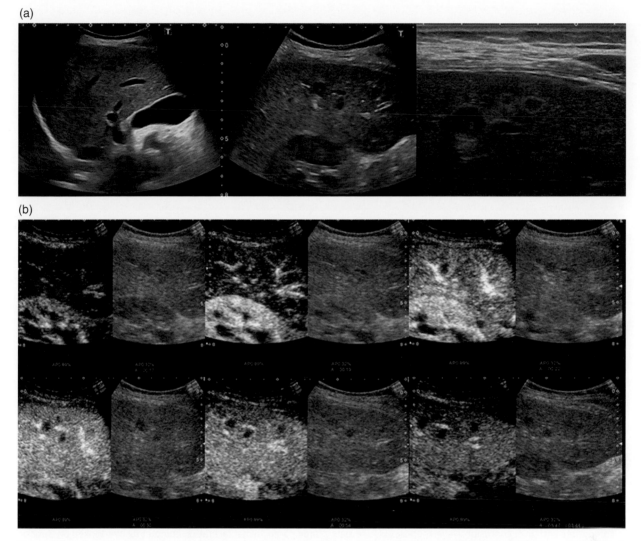

Figure 5.16 (a) Sub-centimetric hypoechoic focal lesions with hyperechoic outline are revealed by magnification with a high-frequency transducer in a patient with miliary tuberculosis. (b) At contrast-enhanced ultrasound the lesions show a subtle rim enhancement, while the central area remains hypo/non-enhancing in all vascular phases, although more pronounced in the delayed phase (Video 5.8).

Lacerations (Figure 5.17), haematomas, contusions, and infarcts are seen as non-enhancing areas surrounded by normal-enhancing parenchyma (Video 5.9). Pseudoaneurysms and active bleeding can also be diagnosed. Scanning CEUS protocols allow assessment of all the abdominal organs in the arterial phase for active bleeding and in the late phase for lacerations. CEUS has the advantages of being quick and allows repeated real-time examination of the solid organs for several minutes, without ionising radiation and nephrotoxic contrast. It can also be performed at the bedside in casualty and intensive care units. Current guidelines [8] recommend that CEUS may be used in isolated moderate-energy injuries in a haemodynamically stable patient (not high-energy injuries); where CT is not available, contraindicated, or inconclusive (due to artefacts); in minor trauma (especially children); and for follow-up of injuries and in renal impairment. CEUS can be added to a FAST (focused assessment and sonography in trauma) scan, which is primarily used for the detection of free abdominal fluid (see Chapter 12).

(a)

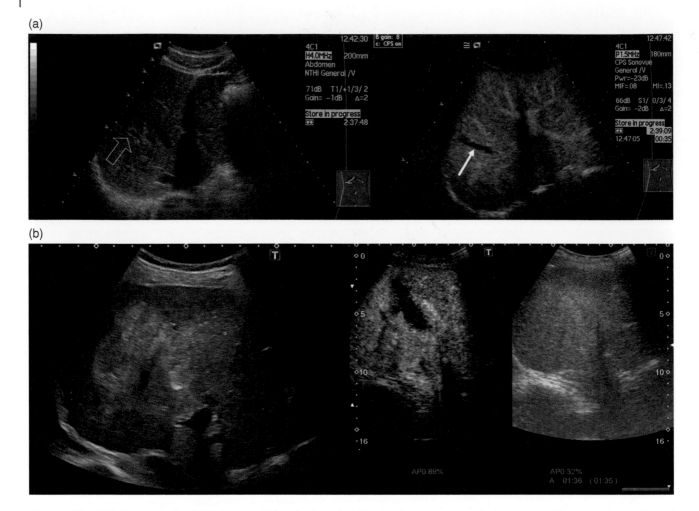

(b)

Figure 5.17 (a) A liver laceration following a stabbing. On B-mode it has a subtle appearance (open arrow), while on contrast-enhanced ultrasound (CEUS) it is more conspicuous (arrow). (b) Liver contusion following blunt trauma. An ill-defined hyperechoic area seen on B-mode is compatible with liver contusion. Nevertheless, CEUS reveals a large parenchymal laceration completely overlooked on B-mode (Video 5.9).

Malignant Focal Liver Lesions

Metastases

The liver is the commonest site of metastatic disease from gastrointestinal system cancers and carries a poor prognosis. Hepatic metastases have a varied appearance on B-mode ultrasound, ranging from hypoechoic (most common) to hyperechoic or heterogeneous. Some may assume a target morphology. Certain metastases may calcify, for example mucinous tumours from the gastrointestinal tract or ovary. Metastases from the same tumour can have different appearances. Some metastases such as in the ovary may be sub-capsular in site. On CEUS, hypervascular metastases (e.g. from neuroendocrine tumours, melanoma, renal, and thyroid cancers) typically demonstrate avid enhancement throughout the lesion in the arterial phase, with washout in the portal and late phases so that they become hypo/non-enhancing (Figure 5.18) (Video 5.10). A typical enhancement pattern of

(a)

(b)

(c)

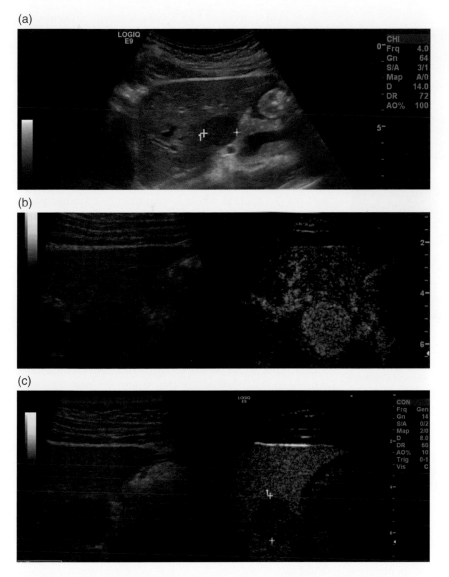

Figure 5.18 Hypervascular metastasis from a primary parathyroid cancer. (a) On B-mode the lesion is seen as a focal echopoor lesion (callipers). (b) Following intravenous SonoVue, arterial-phase imaging (20 seconds post injection) shows avid enhancement of the metastasis. (c) The metastasis appears as a defect in the late phase (callipers).

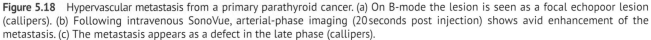

hypovascular metastases (e.g. from colon, pancreas, or lung cancers) is rim enhancement in the arterial phase (Figure 5.19), followed by hypo/non-enhancement in the portal venous and late phases (Videos 5.11 and 5.12). Metastases that contain cystic or necrotic components demonstrate no enhancement in these regions, while the solid component will follow the enhancement pattern described above (Video 5.13). CEUS significantly increases the conspicuity of metastases compared to B-mode ultrasound, allowing the detection of isoechoic and sub-centimetre lesions down to 3 mm. Conventional ultrasound has a false negative rate of up to 30% in the detection of liver metastases. CEUS increases the sensitivity and specificity of ultrasound in the detection of liver metastases to rival those of CECT and CEMR [35–37].

(a)

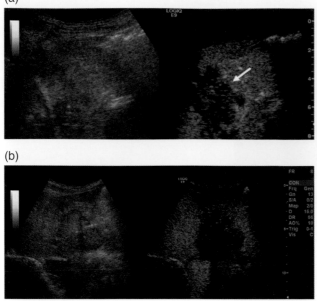

(b)

Figure 5.19 Hypovascular metastasis from colorectal cancer. (a) Dual-display contrast-enhanced ultrasound showing irregular rim enhancement (arrow on contrast-enhanced image) around the metastasis. (b) Washout of the lesion in the late phase, confirming malignancy. The conspicuity of the metastasis is significantly improved compared to B-mode.

Hepatocellular Carcinoma

HCC occurs most commonly in cirrhotic livers and is the commonest primary liver malignancy. There are three morphological presentations of HCC: (i) a single large mass with or without satellite nodules; (ii) nodular with multifocal nodules throughout the liver; and (iii) diffuse with multiple indistinct tiny nodules throughout the liver. Cirrhosis is a major risk factor, and such patients undergo regular six-monthly 'screening' ultrasound for HCC. HCCs typically appear as hypoechoic lesions on B-mode ultrasound, although they may be heterogeneous in echotexture due to necrosis, and more rarely hyperechoic. On CEUS, HCCs typically demonstrate hyperenhancement in the arterial phase, in a chaotic 'basket-weave' pattern, followed by hypoenhancement/non-enhancement (i.e. washout) in the portal venous and late phases. Nevertheless, it is important to bear in mind that a significant variability of HCC's enhancement pattern is described, including portal/venous phase isoenhancement or delayed, subtle washout of some well differentiated HCCs (Figures 5.20–5.26) (Videos 5.14–5.18) [8, 10, 38, 39].

Jang et al. compared CEUS enhancement patterns with the degree of differentiation [40]. They showed that 7/9 (78%) well-differentiated HCCs showed no washout up to 5 minutes. Also some of the well-differentiated HCCs showed arterial-phase hypovascularity or isovascularity as well as portal-phase isovascularity. The majority of poorly differentiated HCCs washed out by 90 seconds. The moderately differentiated tumours showed classic heterogeneous arterial hypervascularity with portal venous washout [40].

Because of the variable enhancement pattern of HCC and the fact that the whole liver cannot be adequately surveyed in the brief arterial phase to look for HCC enhancement, CEUS is not currently indicated for screening, but is employed in the assessment of focal lesions once detected. The European Association for the Study of the Liver (EASL) advocates imaging lesions of 1 cm or larger using CECT or CEMR, taking arterial-phase hyperenhancement with washout in the portal venous and delayed phases as diagnostic criteria [41]. CEUS can be used to diagnose HCC if either CECT or CEMR is not diagnostic. Lesions <1 cm should be followed up with ultrasound. The American Association for the Study of Liver Diseases (AASLD) uses the Liver Imaging Reporting and Data System (LI-RADS) criteria for the diagnosis of HCC [42–44].

For suspicious lesions additional factors (such as serological tumour markers or lesion growth over serial ultrasound studies) must be taken into account or the lesion followed up at three-monthly intervals.

Portal vein involvement is a poor prognostic sign. CEUS is very accurate at distinguishing tumour thrombus from bland thrombus, with enhancement in the thrombus equating to tumour infiltration (Figure 5.27) (Videos 5.19 and 5.20).

A rare kind of primary liver tumor is fibrolamellar HCC that differs from classic HCC in its morphology, behaviour, and prognosis. It occurs in younger patients (adolescents to a peak age of 25 years). It is usually a solitary, well-defined tumour. It is not associated with cirrhosis or viral hepatitis. The α-fetoprotein (AFP) is not elevated. It is often calcified (35–68%). There is typically a central scar (the central scar in fibrolamellar HCC is non-enhancing, whereas in FNH the scar does enhance – an important diagnostic feature). The rarity of the tumour does not allow accurate CEUS descriptions. It has a better prognosis compared to classic HCC (the five-year survival is double that of conventional HCC).

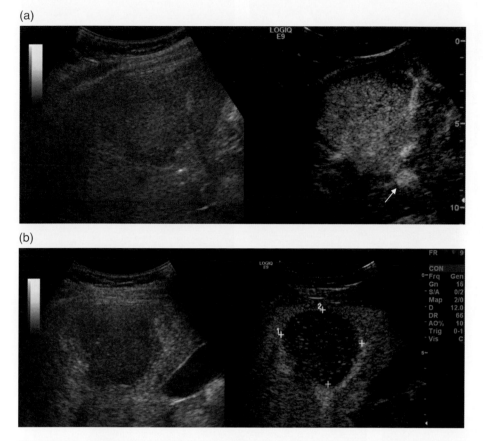

Figure 5.20 Hepatocellular carcinoma. (a) Dual-display contrast-enhanced ultrasound demonstrating avid enhancement from large feeding vessels (arrow) in the arterial phase. (b) Compete washout in the late phase (callipers).

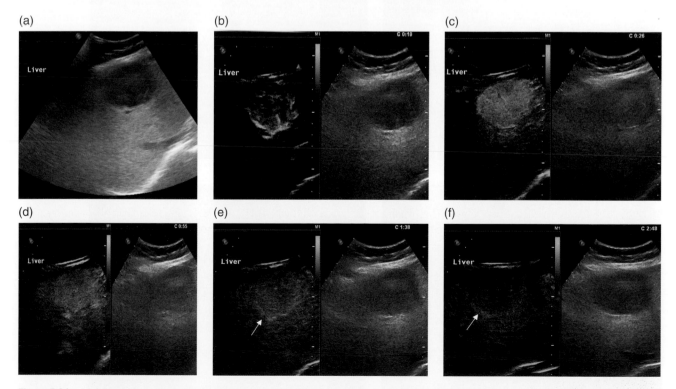

Figure 5.21 (a) A large hypoechoic focal lesion in a patient with recurrent cirrhosis in a transplanted liver. (b, c) Contrast-enhanced ultrasound reveals avid arterial hyperenhancement with (b) an initial 'basket-weave' pattern. (d) Persistence of hyperenhancement, although less pronounced, in the portal venous phase and subsequent homogeneous hypoenhancement with washout in the late vascular phases (e, f). Note is made of the mild persistence of enhancement of a pseudocapsule (e and f, arrows) (Video 5.14).

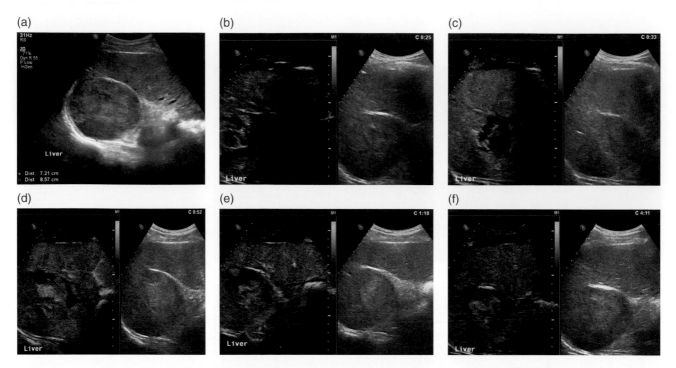

Figure 5.22 (a) On B-mode ultrasound a large right liver lobe heterogeneous focal lesion in a patient with hepatitis C cirrhosis. Contrast-enhanced ultrasound reveals (b, c) arterial disorganized hyperenhancement with non-enhancing areas compatible with intralesional necrosis. (d, e) Subsequent washout is observed in the portal venous and late vascular phases (f) compatible with hepatocellular carcinoma (confirmed on histology).

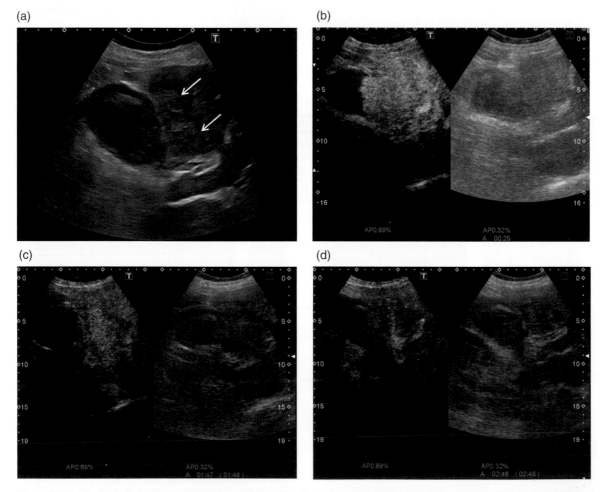

Figure 5.23 (a) Ill-defined heterogeneous area (arrows) adjacent to the gallbladder (GB), which is filled with echogenic content on a background of alcohol-related cirrhosis and known hepatocellular carcinoma (HCC). Contrast-enhanced ultrasound reveals simultaneous arterial hyperenhancement of both the ill-defined area and part of the GB content (b), with subsequent washout in the following vascular phases (c,d). Features in keeping with HCC invading the GB.

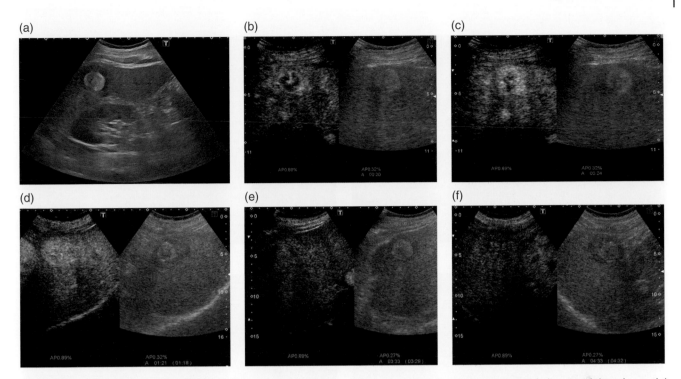

Figure 5.24 (a) A segment VI hyperechoic focal lesion with a subtle echopoor halo. (b, c) On contrast-enhanced ultrasound there is arterial centripetal hyperenhancement. However, (d) there is no washout in the portal phase and only (e, f) very subtle and incomplete washout in the late vascular phase. The patient underwent liver resection confirming a diagnosis of a well-differentiated hepatocellular carcinoma.

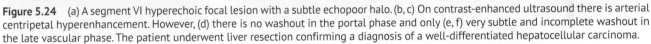

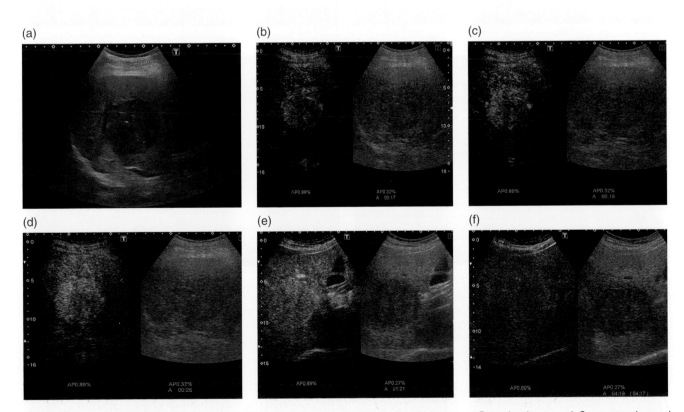

Figure 5.25 (a) A large hypoechoic and heterogeneous right liver lobe focal lesion seen on B-mode ultrasound. Contrast-enhanced ultrasound reveals (b–d) arterial hyperenhancement, (e) almost isoenhancement in the portal venous phase, and (f) subsequent subtle hypoenhancement in the late vascular phase at 4.18 minutes. Percutaneous liver biopsy was carried out revealing a well-differentiated hepatocellular carcinoma (Video 5.15).

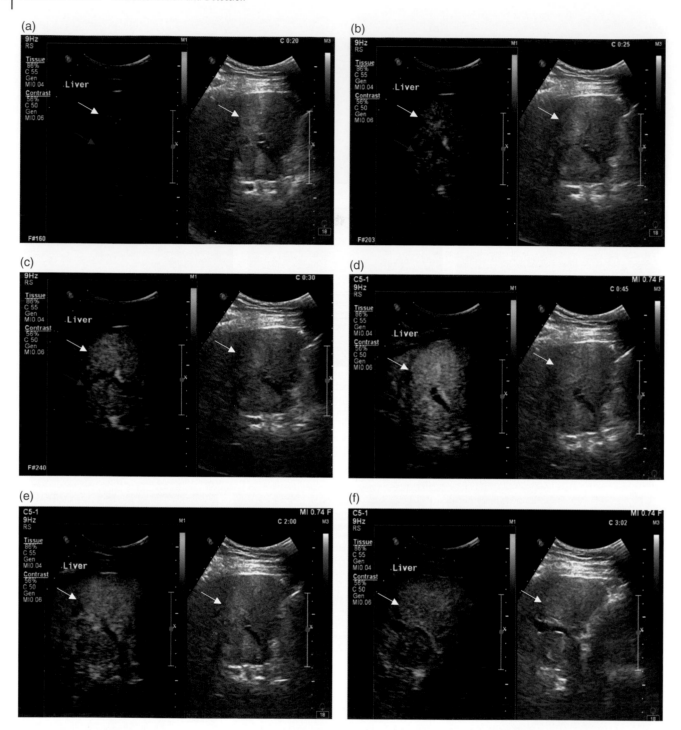

Figure 5.26 Dual-display contrast-enhanced ultrasound of two slightly hyperechoic focal liver lesions on a background of alcohol-related cirrhosis. (a–c) Contrast-enhanced ultrasound shows homogeneous arterial hyperenhancement of the lesions more pronounced in the anterior one (white arrow) compared to the posterior one (red arrow). The anterior lesion maintains its hyperenhancement in the portal venous phase (d) and becomes isoenhancing in the late vascular phase (e, f). The posterior lesion instead shows hypoenhancement in the portal phase (d) and complete washout in the late vascular phase (e, f). Biopsy was carried out on both lesions. The anterior lesion's histology corresponded with a well-differentiated hepatocellular carcinoma (HCC), while the posterior one corresponded to a poorly differentiated HCC (Video 5.18).

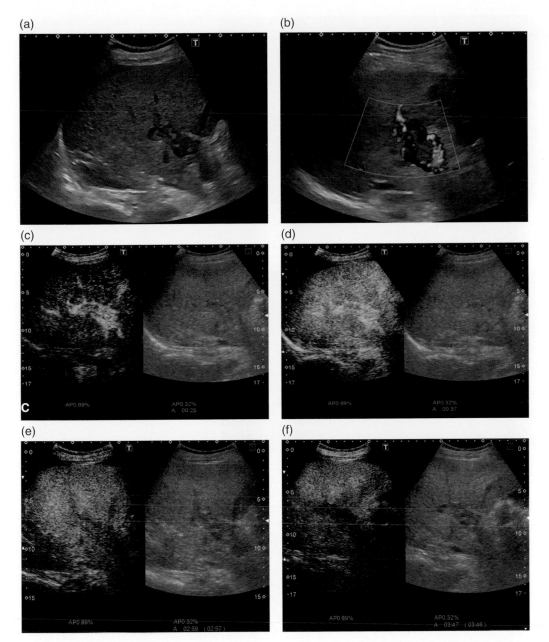

Figure 5.27 (a) Echogenic material fills and stretches the portal vein (PV). (b) Colour Doppler shows a clear vascular signal around and within the occluded PV. These features are highly suspicious for neoplastic tissue growing within the PV. Contrast-enhanced ultrasound more accurately confirms the presence of neoplastic thrombosis by showing arterial hyperenhancement (c, d) and subsequent washout of the thrombus in the late vascular phase (e, f).

Cholangiocarcinoma and Gallbladder Cancer

Cholangiocarcinomas are a form of adenocarcinoma arising from the bile ducts (intra- or extrahepatic). The intrahepatic tumours are further classified as peripheral or hilar (Klatskin) tumours (Figure 5.28). There are three distinct macroscopic growth patterns of the intrahepatic cholangiocarcinomas: (i) mass forming, which is the commonest type; (ii) periductal infiltrative; and (iii) intraductal growth. The appearance of cholangiocarcinomas on B-mode ultrasound is highly variable, although the parenchymal mass of peripheral tumours is most commonly hyperechoic. In some cases,

hilar cholangiocarcinomas may only be manifest as segmental dilatation of intrahepatic bile ducts without a perceptible mass. The enhancement pattern of cholangiocarcinomas in the arterial phase is also variable, in that some demonstrate avid arterial enhancement whereas others do not. The key characteristic (as with hepatic metastases) is washout of the contrast agent, with the lesion becoming hypo- or non-enhancing in the portal venous and late phases (Videos 5.21 and 5.22). There may be discordant findings with CECT, which can show iso- or hyperenhancement in the delayed phase not seen on CEUS. This is due to the fact that ultrasound agents are purely intravascular, whereas

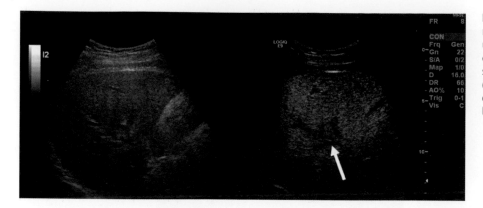

Figure 5.28 Klatskin cholangiocarcinoma. Dual-display contrast-enhanced ultrasound showing a defect on the contrast mode (arrow), which is inconspicuous on the co-registered B-mode (left screen). Note the dilated bile ducts characteristic of a central Klatskin tumour.

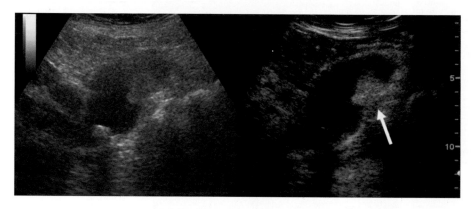

Figure 5.29 Gallbladder (GB) carcinoma. Dual-display contrast-enhanced ultrasound showing enhancement of a polypoid mass (arrow) with a thickened wall at its base, confirmed as a cancer on histology. Note the stone in the neck of the GB on the B-mode (left screen).

CT agents diffuse into the interstitium, enhancing the fibrous component, which appears hypoenhancing on CEUS. In some cases of cholangiocarcinoma, an enhancing intraductal component of the tumour may be seen at CEUS. Cholangiocarcinomas show marked fibrotic stroma, which can produce a classic overlying liver capsular retraction in a peripheral lesion.

Gallbladder cancer is a rarer form of adenocarcinoma. It may manifest as an intraluminal mass (Figure 5.29), diffuse mural thickening, or a mass replacing the gallbladder. The clinical presentation depends on its direction of growth: spread into the bowel may cause obstruction and extension into the liver may produce obstructive jaundice. CEUS may show variable enhancement in the arterial phase, with hypoenhancement/ non-enhancement in the portal venous phase and late phase.

Lymphoma

The liver is usually affected by secondary hepatic lymphoma as part of a systemic process in Hodgkin's or non-Hodgkin's lymphoma. Risk factors include human immunodeficiency virus (HIV), hepatitis C, organ transplantation, and immunosuppression. Liver involvement may occur in post-transplant lymphoproliferative disorder (PTLD). Primary hepatic lymphoma is very rare. Typical patterns of liver involvement are (i) solitary mass; (ii) multifocal nodules; and (iii) diffuse infiltrative disease.

On B-mode ultrasound, lymphomatous deposits within the liver typically appear as hypoechoic masses, which may have posterior acoustic shadowing giving a 'pseudocystic' sign. On CEUS, these lesions show variable enhancement in the arterial phase, but show the typical 'malignant' appearance of 'washout' in the portal venous and late phases (Figure 5.30) (Video 5.23).

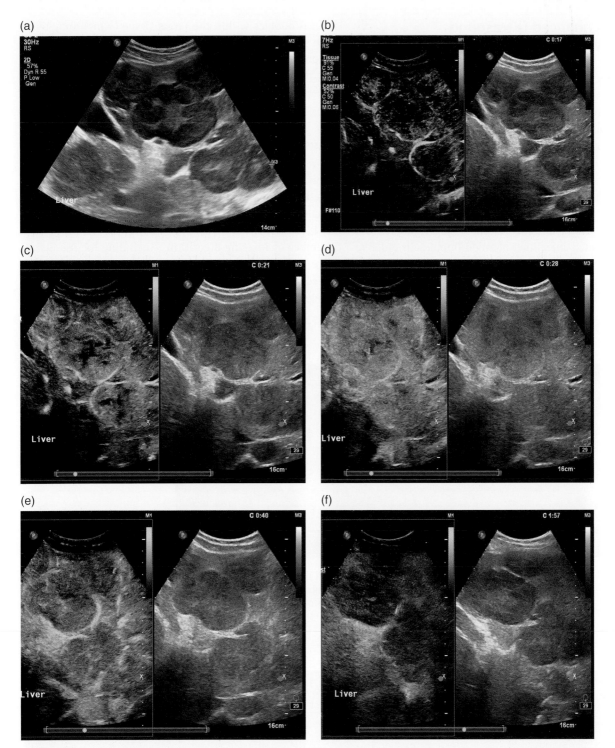

Figure 5.30 (a) Multiple liver target-like lesions with a hyperechoic spiculated center on the background of common variable immu-nodeficiency and granulomatous liver disease. Contrast-enhanced ultrasound shows (b–d) arterial hyperenhancement followed by subsequent washout at 40 seconds (e, early portal phase), more pronounced at 117 seconds (f, late portal venous phase). Biopsy revealed a diagnosis of non-Hodgkin's lymphoma (Video 5.23).

Contrast-Enhanced Ultrasound and Intervention

Occasionally a focal liver lesion (e.g. one that may have been diagnosed on CECT or CEMR) will not be clearly visible on B-mode ultrasound. The use of CEUS may allow better visualisation of the lesion on ultrasound and facilitate a targeted ultrasound-guided biopsy. Even if such a procedure requires more than one bolus of contrast agent, microbubbles have no nephrotoxicity and patients can safely receive multiple doses.

CEUS may also be used before and after interstitial ablation of a focal malignant liver lesion. The operator is able to perform repeated injections of microbubbles in order to establish whether viable (enhancing) tumour remains, and whether further on-table ablative therapy is required. However, ablation therapy usually results in the formation

of gas bubbles within the target tissue (which may block the ultrasound beam), although these usually resolve shortly. CEUS following tumour embolization can also yield important information on the presence of residual neoplastic tissue (Figures 5.31 and 5.32).

Liver Imaging Reporting and Data System

This system was created by the American College of Radiology in 2011 to guide and increase consistency and quality assurance of imaging and reporting of HCC in at-risk patient groups [43–45]. This guidance provides a number of imaging algorithms, including for the definitive diagnosis of HCC on CT/MR imaging without the need for histopathological confirmation. The LI-RADS diagnostic criteria range from LR-1 (definitely benign) to

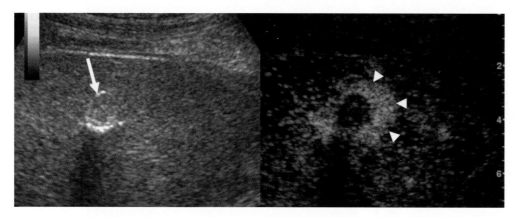

Figure 5.31 Local recurrence in a treated hepatocellular carcinoma (HCC). Dual-display contrast-enhanced ultrasound showing a crescent of viable tumour in the arterial phase (arrowheads on contrast-enhanced image, right screen) following previous transarterial chemoembolization treatment of an HCC. On B-mode (left image) the lesion is echogenic (arrow).

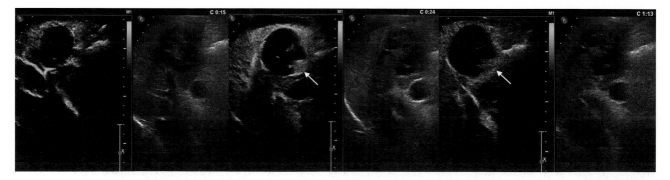

Figure 5.32 Contrast-enhanced ultrasound follow-up in a hepatocellular carcinoma treated with transcatheter arterial chemoembolization. There is a well-defined non-enhancing rounded area as a result of post-embolic tumor necrosis. However, note is made of a small peripheral enhancing area in keeping with residual active neoplastic tissue (arrows).

LR-5 (definitely HCC). In 2016 a version of LI-RADS that applies to CEUS was published: CEUS LR-1 to LR-5 as well as LR-M (metastatic but not specific for HCC). The most recent update was 2018 [43].

It is important to note that LI-RADS and CEUS LI-RADS criteria apply to patients at high risk for HCC. This includes cirrhosis, chronic hepatitis-B infection with or without cirrhosis, and current or prior HCC. Major features used for lesion assessment on CEUS are (i) arterial phase hyperenhancement; (ii) timing of washout; (iii) washout degree; and (iv) size.

Conclusion

Ultrasound is the initial modality of choice used in the imaging of liver conditions and therefore the majority of focal liver lesions are usually detected by ultrasound.

Unfortunately, conventional B-mode and Doppler ultrasound may not allow an accurate diagnosis to be reached, necessitating further imaging with CT or MR. Following the introduction of ultrasound contrast agents, the sensitivity and specificity of ultrasound have significantly improved to rival those of CT and MR, allowing accurate detection and characterisation of focal lesions. The superior spatial and temporal resolution of ultrasound along with real-time imaging of the microcirculation of focal lesions has dramatically expanded the role and applications of liver ultrasound.

Videos

Videos for this chapter can be accessed via the companion website: www.wiley.com/go/LiverUltrasound.

References

1 Anderson, S., Kruskal, J., and Kane, R. (2009). Benign hepatic tumors and iatrogenic pseudotumors. *Radiographics* 29 (1): 211–229.

2 Low, G. and Leen, E. (2011). Focal liver lesions/echo enhancing agents and the liver. In: *Diagnostic Ultrasound*, 3e (ed. P. Allan, G. Baxter and M. Weston), 138–166. London: Churchill Livingstone Elsevier.

3 Wilson, S. and Burns, P. (2010). Microbubble-enhanced US in body imaging: what role? *Radiology* 257: 24–39.

4 Burrowes, D., Medellin, A., Harris, A. et al. (2017). Contrast-enhanced US approach to the diagnosis of focal liver masses. *Radiographics* 37 (5): 1388–1400.

5 Cosgrove, D.O. (2010). Contrast-enhanced ultrasound of liver lesions. *Ultrasound Med. Biol.* 36: 2146.

6 Quaia, E., Calliada, F., Bertolotto, M. et al. (2004). Characterization of focal liver lesions with contrast-specific US modes and a sulfur hexafluoride-filled microbubble contrast agent: diagnostic performance and confidence. *Radiology* 2004 (232): 420–430.

7 Durot, I., Wilson, S., and Willmann, J. (2018). Contrast-enhanced ultrasound of malignant liver lesions. *Abdom. Radiol. (NY)* 43 (4): 819–847.

8 Claudon, M., Dietrich, C.F., Choi, B.I. et al. (2013). Guidelines and good clinical practice recommendations for contrast enhanced ultrasound (CEUS) in the liver--update 2012: a WFUMB-EFSUMB initiative in cooperation with representatives of AFSUMB, AIUM, ASUM, FLAUS and ICUS. *Ultrasound Med. Biol.* 39 (2): 187–210.

9 National Institute for Health and Clinical Excellence (2012). SonoVue (Sulphur Hexafluoride Microbubbles) – Contrast Agent for Contrast-Enhanced Ultrasound Imaging of the Liver. Diagnostic Guidance [DG5]. www.nice.org.uk/dg5.

10 Morin, S.H.X., Lim, A.K.P., Cobbold, J., and Taylor-Robinson, S. (2007). Use of second generation contrast-enhanced ultrasound in the assessment of focal liver lesions. *World J. Gastroenterol.* 13: 5963–5970.

11 Zarzour, J.G., Porter, K.K., Tchelepi, H., and Robbin, M.L. (2018). Contrast-enhanced ultrasound of benign liver lesions. *Abdom. Radiol. (NY)* 43: 848–860.

12 Lin, M.X., Xu, H.X., Lu, M.D. et al. (2009). Diagnostic performance of contrast-enhanced ultrasound for complex cystic focal liver lesions: blinded reader study. *Eur. Radiol.* 19 (2): 358–369.

13 Corvino, A., Catalano, O., Setola, S.V. et al. (2015). Contrast-enhanced ultrasound in the characterization of complex cystic focal liver lesions. *Ultrasound Med. Biol.* 41 (5): 1301–1310. https://doi.org/10.1016/j.ultrasmedbio.2014.12.667 11.

14 Lantinga, M.A., Gevers, T.J., and Drenth, J.P. (2013). Evaluation of hepatic cystic lesions. *World J. Gastroenterol.* 19 (23): 3543–3554.

15 Strobel, D., Seitz, K., Blank, W. et al. (2008). Contrast-enhanced ultrasound for the characterization of focal liver lesions–diagnostic accuracy in clinical practice (DEGUM multicenter trial). *Ultraschall Med.* 29: 499–505.

16 Dietrich, C.F., Mertens, J.C., Braden, B. et al. (2007). Contrast-enhanced ultrasound of histologically proven haemangiomas. *Hepatology* 45: 1139–1145.

17 Sirli, R.S.I., Popescu, A., Danila, M. et al. (2011). Contrast enhanced ultrasound for the diagnosis of liver haemangiomas in clinical practice. *Med. Ultrason.* 13 (2): 95–101.

18 Yen, Y.H., Wang, J.H., Lu, S.N. et al. (2006). Contrast-enhanced ultrasonographic spoke-wheel sign in hepatic focal nodular hyperplasia. *Eur. J. Radiol.* 60 (3): 439–444.

19 Roche, V., Pigneur, F., Tselikas, L. et al. (2015). Differentiation of focal nodular hyperplasia from hepatocellular adenomas with low mechanical-index contrast-enhanced sonography (CEUS): effect of size on diagnostic confidence. *Eur. Radiol.* 25 (1): 186–195.

20 Torbenson, M. (2018). Hepatic adenomas: classification, controversies, and consensus. *Surg. Pathol. Clin.* 11: 351–366.

21 Bioulac-Sage, P., Sempoux, C., and Balabaud, C. (2017). Hepatocellular adenomas: morphology and genomics. *Gastroenterol. Clin. North Am.* 46: 253–272.

22 Katabathina, V.S., Menias, C.O., Shanbhogue, A.K. et al. (2011). Genetics and imaging of hepatocellular adenomas: 2011 update. *Radiographics* 31 (6): 1529–1543.

23 Laumonier, H., Cailliez, H., Balabaud, C. et al. (2012). Role of contrast-enhanced sonography in differentiation of subtypes of hepatocellular adenoma: correlation with MRI findings. *Am. J. Roentgenol.* 199 (2): 341–348. https://doi.org/10.2214/ajr.11.7046.

24 Manichon, A.F., Bancel, B., Durieux-Millon, M. et al. (2012). Hepatocellular adenoma: evaluation with contrast-enhanced ultrasound and MRI and correlation with pathologic and phenotypic classification in 26 lesions. *HPB Surg.* 2012: 418745.

25 Bhatnagar, G., Sidhu, H.S., Vardhanabhuti, V. et al. (2012). The varied sonographic appearances of focal fatty liver disease: review and diagnostic algorithm. *Clin. Rad.* 67: 372–379.

26 Décarie, P.O., Lepanto, L., Billiard, J.S. et al. (2011). Fatty liver deposition and sparing: a pictorial review. *Insights Imaging* 2: 533–538.

27 Jang, J.K., Jang, H.-J., Kim, J.S., and Kim, T.K. (2017). Focal fat deposition in the liver: diagnostic challenges on imaging. *Abdom. Radiol.* 42 (6): 1667–1678.

28 Liu, L.P., Dong, B.W., Yu, X.L. et al. (2008). Evaluation of focal fatty infiltration of the liver using color doppler and contrast-enhanced sonography. *J. Clin. Ultrasound* 36 (9): 560–566.

29 Quaia, E., D'Onofrio, M., Cabassa, P. et al. (2007). Diagnostic value of hepatocellular nodule vascularity after microbubble injection for characterising malignancy in patients with cirrhosis. *Am. J. Roentgenol.* 189: 1474–1483.

30 Catalano, O., Sandomenico, F., Raso, M.M., and Siani, A. (2004). Low mechanical index contrast-enhanced sonographic findings of pyogenic hepatic abscesses. *Am. J. Roentgenol.* 182 (2): 447–450.

31 Kim, K.W., Choi, B.I., Park, S.H. et al. (2004). Pyogenic hepatic abscesses: distinctive features from hypovascular liver malignancies on contrast-enhanced ultrasound with SHU 508A; early experience. *Ultrasound Med. Biol.* 30 (6): 725–733.

32 Dietrich, C.F., Nolsøe, C.P., Barr, R.G. et al. (2020). Guidelines and good clinical practice recommendations for contrast-enhanced ultrasound (CEUS) in the liver-update 2020 WFUMB in cooperation with EFSUMB, AFSUMB, AIUM, and FLAUS. *Ultrasound Med. Biol.* 46 (10): 2579–2604.

33 Patnana, M., Sevrukov, A.B., Elsayes, K.M. et al. (2012). Inflammatory pseudotumours: the great mimicker. *Am. J. Roentgenol.* 198: W217–W227.

34 Cao, B.-S., Li, X.-L., Li, N., and Wang, Z.-Y. (2010). The nodular form of hepatic tuberculosis. Contrast-enhanced ultrasonographic findings with pathologic correlation. *J. Ultrasound Med.* 29 (6): 881–888.

35 Harvey, C.J., Blomley, M., Eckersley, R. et al. (2000). Hepatic malignancies: improved detection with pulse inversion US in the late phase of enhancement with SH U508A – early experience. *Radiology* 216: 903–908.

36 Harvey, C.J., Blomley, M., Eckersley, R. et al. (2000). Pulse-inversion mode imaging of liver specific microbubbles: improved detection of subcentimetre metastases. *Lancet* 355: 807–808.

37 Seitz, K., Strobel, D., Bernatik, T. et al. (2009). Contrast-enhanced ultrasound (CEUS) for the characterization of focal liver lesions – prospective comparison in clinical practice: CEUS vs. CT (DEGUM multicenter trial). *Ultraschall Med.* 30 (4): 383–389.

38 Ayuso, C., Rimola, J., Vilana, R. et al. (2018). Diagnosis and staging of hepatocellular carcinoma (HCC): current guidelines. *Eur. J. Radiol.* 101: 72–81.

39 Navin, P.J. and Venkatesh, S.K. (2019). Hepatocellular carcinoma: state of the art imaging and recent advances. *J. Clin. Transl. Hepatol.* 7 (1): 1–14.

40 Jang, H.J., Kim, T.K., Burns, P.N., and Wilson, S.R. (2007). Enhancement patterns of hepatocellular carcinoma at contrast US: comparison with histologic differentiation. *Radiology* 244: 898–906.

41 Galle, P., Forner, A., Llovet, J. et al. (2018). EASL clinical practice guidelines: management of hepatocellular carcinoma. *J. Hepatol.* 69 (1): 182–236.

42 Marrero, J.A., Kulik, L.M., Sirlin, C.B. et al. (2018). Diagnosis, staging, and management of hepatocellular carcinoma: 2018 practice guidance by the American association for the study of liver diseases. *Hepatol.* 68 (2): 723–750.

43 Chernyak, V., Fowler, K., Kamaya, A. et al. (2018). Liver imaging reporting and data system (LI-RADS) version 2018: imaging of hepatocellular carcinoma in at-risk patients. *Radiology* 289 (3): 816–830.

44 Tang, A., Bashir, M.R., Corwin, M.T. et al. (2018). Evidence supporting LI-RADS major features for CT- and MR imaging-based diagnosis of hepatocellular carcinoma: a systematic review. *Radiology* 286 (1): 29–48.

45 Wilson, S.R., Lyshchik, A., Piscaglia, F. et al. (2018). CEUS LI-RADS: algorithm, implementation, and key differences from CT/MRI. *Abdom. Radiol. (NY)* 43: 127–142.

6

Ultrasound of the Biliary System

Matteo Rosselli[1,2], Maija Radzina[3,4,5], and Adrian K.P. Lim[6,7]

[1] *Department of Internal Medicine, San Giuseppe Hospital, USL Toscana Centro, Empoli, Italy*
[2] *Division of Medicine, Institute for Liver and Digestive Health, University College London, Royal Free Hospital, London, UK*
[3] *Radiology Research laboratory, Riga Stradins University, Riga, Latvia*
[4] *Diagnostic Radiology Institute, Paula Stradins University Hospital, Riga, Latvia*
[5] *Medical Faculty, University of Latvia, Riga, Latvia*
[6] *Department of Imaging, Imperial College Healthcare NHS Trust, London, UK*
[7] *Department of Metabolism, Digestion and Reproduction, Imperial College London, UK*

Biliary disorders include a variety of congenital and acquired pathological conditions that might be asymptomatic or present clinically with jaundice, abdominal pain, and fever in the case of biliary obstruction and superimposed infection. Ultrasound is the imaging modality of choice for a first differential diagnosis of jaundice in order to determine the presence, level, and cause of biliary obstruction. This chapter provides a brief introduction to the normal anatomy and topography of the biliary system, describing congenital abnormalities and anatomical variants, with a subsequent focus on benign and malignant pathologies.

Anatomy and Topography of the Gallbladder and Biliary Tree

The gallbladder (GB) is a pear-shaped structure, composed of a fundus, body, infundibulum, and neck (Figure 6.1). It is usually located on the visceral surface of the liver, along the major interlobar fissure between the right hepatic lobe and the medial part of the left one. In normal fasting conditions it is usually distended, thin walled (≤3 mm), and the lumen can clearly be visualised since it is filled with anechoic bile. When scanning the GB it is very important to keep in mind that its development might be affected by anatomical variants, resulting in a different size, number, shape, or location. Some malformations can lead to misdiagnosis and it is important to be aware of their presence in order to avoid incorrect clinical judgement and management. GB agenesis and hypoplasia [1] are rare congenital findings due to failure or incomplete development during morphogenesis. Agenesis is the complete absence of the GB, which is sometimes associated with other gastrointestinal and cardiovascular malformations and can manifest with right upper quadrant pain, often misinterpreted/misdiagnosed as biliary cholic secondary to cholelithiasis [2]. Hypoplasia is an incomplete development of the GB bud. When present it is often associated with other pathological conditions such as cystic fibrosis and biliary atresia [3]. Ectopic GB is a variation of its normal anatomical location. The most frequent positions are under the left lobe, intrahepatic, transverse, and retrohepatic [4]. It is important to bear in mind the possibility of an ectopic GB, since its unusual position can be mistaken for agenesis. In addition inflammation/infection of an ectopic GB can mimic different conditions. If surgery is indicated, this information is important because different GB locations may require different technical approaches.

Phrygian cap GB is the most common anatomical variant, characterised by folding of the fundus on the body (Figure 6.2). The GB might present with septations, which can be partial or complete (Figure 6.3), leading to bile stasis, sludge, and stone formation (Figure 6.4). Multiseptate GB is a rare condition that leads to a multiloculated or honeycomb appearance [4]. Double or duplicated GB is also a rare congenital malformation. There are two main types of duplicated GB. The first corresponds to a bilobated GB with one common cystic duct that enters the common bile duct (CBD). The second is a true duplication that is also further classified into a first subtype in which two separate GBs have separate cystic ducts that independently enter the CBD; and a second subtype where two separate GBs have separate cystic ducts that join before entering the CBD. Ultrasound findings usually show two adjacent 'cystic-like' structures within the GB fossa. However, ultrasound may not completely differentiate this from other conditions such as phrygian cap,

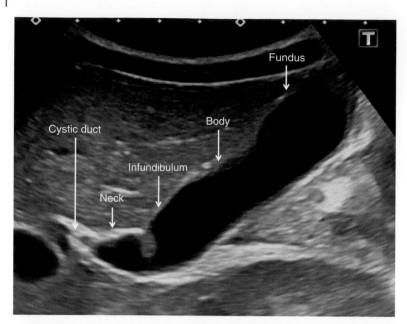

Figure 6.1 The gallbladder is composed of a fundus, body, infundibulum, and neck.

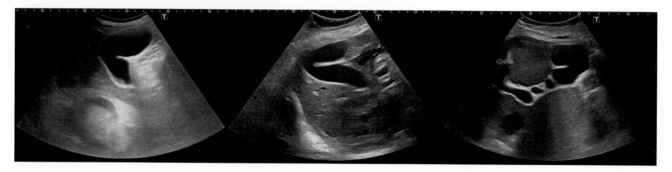

Figure 6.2 Examples of a 'phrygian cap' of the gallbladder, which is characterised by folding of the fundus over the body.

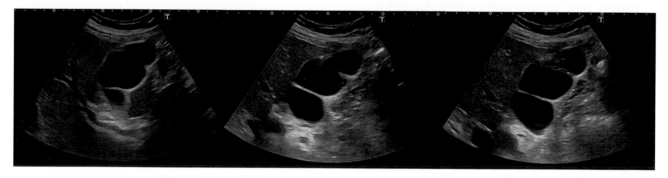

Figure 6.3 Septated gallbladder.

choledochal cyst, folded GB, GB diverticulum, Ladd's bands (intraperitoneal fibrous bands), and dilated cystic duct remnant. In addition, ultrasound may not be able to differentiate between the three variants and second-level imaging such as magnetic resonance cholangiopancreatography (MRCP) is especially recommended if the patient needs to undergo cholecystectomy [5].

The biliary tree is divided into intrahepatic and extrahepatic segments. The intrahepatic biliary tree is characterised by a canalicular network, interlobular ducts and main hepatic duct. The cystic duct originates as a direct continuation of the neck of the GB and joins the main hepatic duct to form the intrahepatic CBD. After a short tract, the CBD exits the liver (extrahepatic CBD), ending with the pancreatic duct in the ampulla of Vater at the level of the second part of the duodenum. The biliary ducts run across the liver together with the portal vein and hepatic artery from the periphery to the liver hilum, where they are enveloped in the

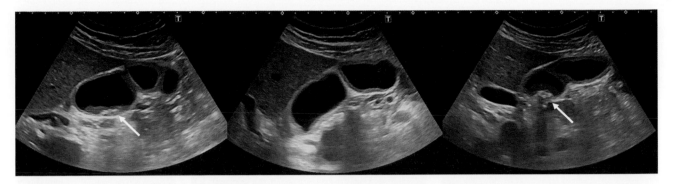

Figure 6.4 Septated thickened gallbladder containing sludge and stones (arrows).

hepatoduodenal ligament. The anatomical relationship of the hepatic artery and portal vein is important and must be kept in mind when considering and interpreting different causes of liver disease, as will be highlighted in the following sections.

Gallbladder Pathology

Cholelithiasis

Cholelithiasis can be found on ultrasound as an incidental finding in asymptomatic patients or in those who typically present with right upper quadrant pain, associated or not with jaundice or fever in the case of biliary duct obstruction and infection. It is reported that the accuracy of ultrasound in diagnosing gallstones is almost 100%, with them appearing as highly reflective, well-defined mobile structures of different shape and size that cast a posterior acoustic shadow (Figure 6.5) [6]. Nevertheless, it is important to bear in mind potential pitfalls, especially in symptomatic patients, since missed pathology and inappropriate management of cholelithiasis can lead to severe complications. False-negative results more frequently occur when the stone size is very small (1–2 mm), when the stone calcium content is low or absent with significant reduction or no posterior acoustic shadowing (Figure 6.6), or in cases in which the stone is lodged in the neck of the GB or in the cystic duct. Changing the patient's position can be very useful to improve visualisation of small or distal stones that might have been difficult to visualise because of overlying bowel gas. Alternatively, false-positive results can be a consequence of side lobe and partial volume artefacts [7]. When a large stone or multiple stones completely fill the GB, the ultrasound image can be that of a wall-echo-shadow sign, characterised by a curvilinear or straight hyperechogenic line representing the GB wall, a thin hypoechoic space representing a small amount of bile, and a hyperechogenic line corresponding to the close surface of the gallstones with posterior acoustic shadowing [8]. The wall-echo-shadow sign needs to be differentiated from porcelain GB, in which complete or partial calcification of the wall occurs. In this case, the acoustic shadowing arises directly from the GB wall with no interposition (Figure 6.7).

(a) (b) (c)

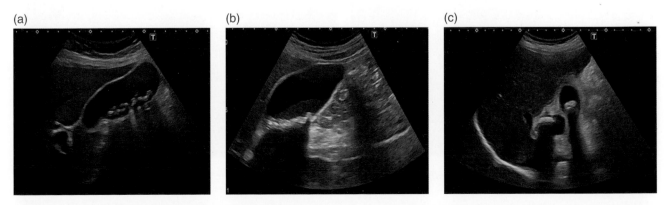

Figure 6.5 (a–c) Different examples of gallstones with typical posterior acoustic shadowing. In (b) a subtle layer of mobile sludge can be observed covering small stones accumulating in the infundibulum.

(a)

(b)

(c)

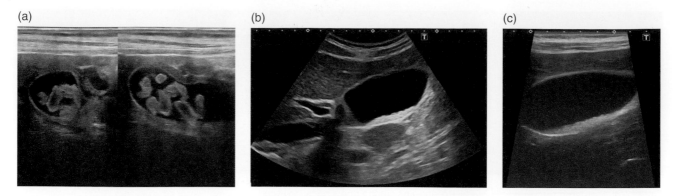

Figure 6.6 (a) The gallbladder (GB) is filled with cholesterol stones with no acoustic shadowing. (b, c) A layer of small stones without acoustic shadowing accumulates along the posterior wall of the GB.

(a)

(b)

(c)

(d)

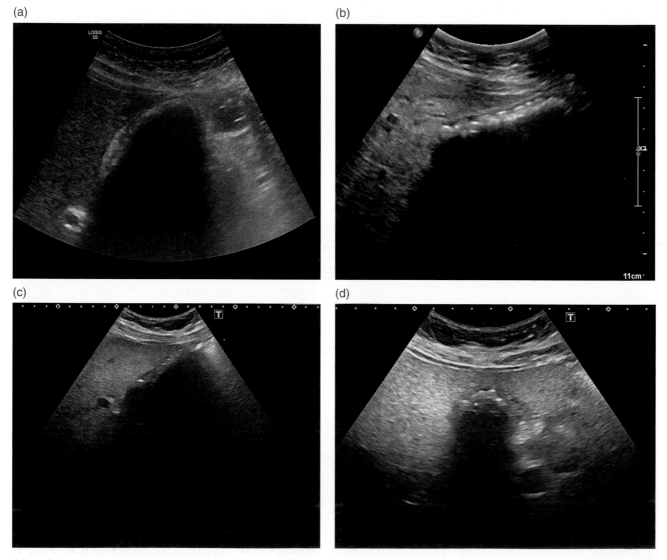

Figure 6.7 (a) Porcelain gallbladder (GB). (b–d) Two examples of the wall-echo-shadow (WES) sign. In both cases, the GB is contracted and packed with stones. (d) reveals the appearance of the WES sign on a transverse scan view.

Biliary Sludge

Sludge refers to a bile precipitate with a sonographic appearance of echogenic homogeneous material without acoustic shadowing, which usually is mobile and accumulates in the most dependent portion of the GB following gravity. It can be a precursor of gallstones and it might present as isolated or mixed with gallstones (Figure 6.8). It can accumulate in the GB as a consequence of prolonged fasting and is often seen after prolonged total parenteral nutrition, or it might be associated with increased cholesterol levels, diabetes and haemolysis. Even in the absence of stones, biliary sludge can cause biliary obstruction, although the biliary system is usually not particularly dilated. Nevertheless, it can be responsible for cholecystitis, cholangitis, as well as pancreatitis. In the majority of cases biliary sludge is fluid and mobile and ultrasound can identify a clear interface between the sludge level and the 'normal bile'. Alternatively it can completely fill the GB (Figure 6.8). Nevertheless, in other circumstances biliary sludge can solidify (Figure 6.8), appearing as a GB mass or pseudopolyp for which contrast-enhanced ultrasound (CEUS) has high accuracy in differential diagnosis (Figure 6.9).

Cholecystitis

Gallstones can impact the neck of the GB, causing obstruction and an inflammatory reaction with possible superimposed infection. The sonographic signs of lythiasic cholecystitis are GB wall thickening >3 mm, cholecystolithiasis, and a positive Murphy sign that refers to maximal tenderness, exacerbated by the pressure of the transducer over the GB (Figure 6.10) [6]. Hyperaemia on colour Doppler and pericholecystic fluid are reported as additional findings. Overdistension of the GB resulting in a longitudinal diameter >10 cm and a transverse diameter >4 cm can also be observed [6]. Nevertheless, increased GB size is not pathological per se and might be a physiological finding.

Gangrenous Cholecystitis

In up to 15–20% of cases acute cholecystitis may be complicated by a gangrenous process, with a high probability of perforation and sepsis [9]. Ultrasound features are not specific but the clinical picture together with sonographic findings increases the diagnostic accuracy. In gangrenous cholecystitis, the GB wall has a striated and

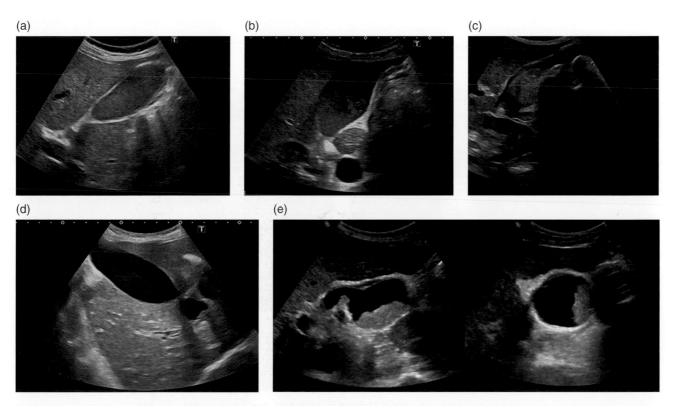

(a) (b) (c)

(d) (e)

Figure 6.8   (a, b) The gallbladder (GB) is filled with sludge. (c) Sludge-filled GB with large stones casting a typical acoustic shadow. (d) A clear interface is seen between sludge and anechoic bile. (e) Solidified sludge can be slightly mobile but is mostly adherent to the GB wall.

(a)

(b)

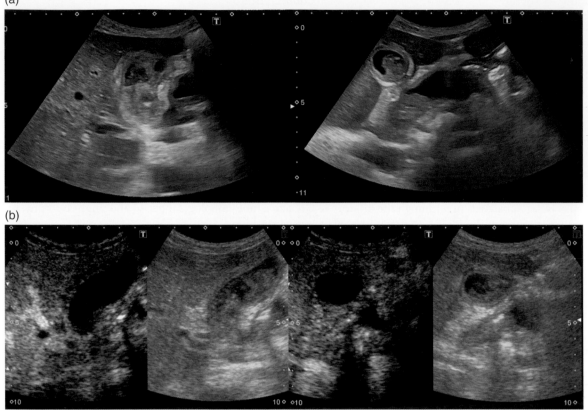

Figure 6.9 The gallbladder (GB) lumen is filled with heterogeneous material that seems in direct continuity with the GB wall, suggesting a possible neoplastic growth (a). However, on contrast-enhanced ultrasound the GB content does not show any enhancement thus excluding a neoplastic growth and steering the diagnosis towards solidified sludge (b).

(a)   (b)

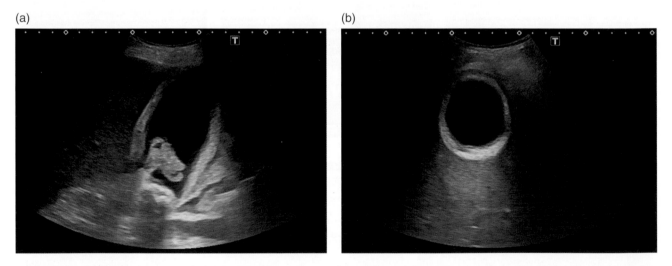

Figure 6.10 (a, b) A patient was admitted with right upper quadrant pain and fever. Ultrasound confirmed the diagnosis of acute gallstone cholecystitis based on the presenting symptoms and sonographic findings of gallbladder (GB) wall thickening and evidence of solidified sludge and stones accumulating in the GB neck, causing its obstruction. Both longitudinal and transverse planes show marked thickening of the GB wall compatible with the inflammatory process.

thickened appearance and intraluminal membranes can be observed as a consequence of wall detachment (Figure 6.11) [9, 10]. Moreover, marked asymmetry of the GB wall can often be seen, as well as echogenic debris within the GB lumen, together with pericholecystic collections (Figure 6.12). It is of note that frequently in the presence of gangrenous cholecystitis, Murphy's sign can be negative, as a consequence of reduced GB intraluminal

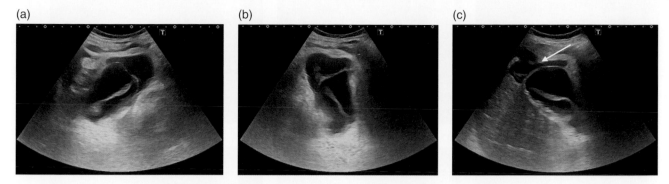

Figure 6.11   (a–c) Ultrasound reveals detachment of the gallbladder walls, visualised as floating intraluminal 'membranes' and a discontinuity at the level of the fundus communicating with a collection (c, arrow), in keeping with gangrenous cholecystitis.

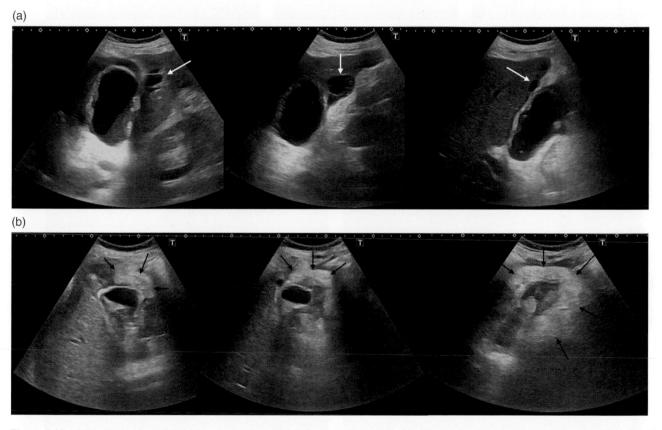

Figure 6.12   (a) Acute cholecystitis in a septic patient presenting with right upper quadrant pain. Ultrasound highlights the intraluminal sludge, a thickened gallbladder (GB) wall, and a loculated pericholecystic collection (white arrows), orienting the diagnosis towards gangrenous cholecystitis with initial perforation. (b) The second sequence of images, taken after sudden hypotension and haemoglobin drop, revealed heterogeneous material almost filling completely the GB lumen, as well as thick, ill-defined hyperechoic material surrounding the GB wall (black arrows). The features are in keeping with intraluminal and pericholecystic haemorrhage, likely caused by severe thrombocytopenia on a background of known myelodysplastic syndrome.

pressure. When perforation occurs, a defect in the GB wall is always present, although owing to the heterogeneous echogenicity of the inflammatory reaction and surrounding tissues, it can be difficult to delineate. An indirect sign can be the presence of loculated fluid collections surrounding the GB and liver. In cases of doubt, CEUS is extremely accurate in highlighting even small defects in the GB wall as a sign of perforation (Figures 6.13 and 6.14) (Videos 6.1 and 6.2).

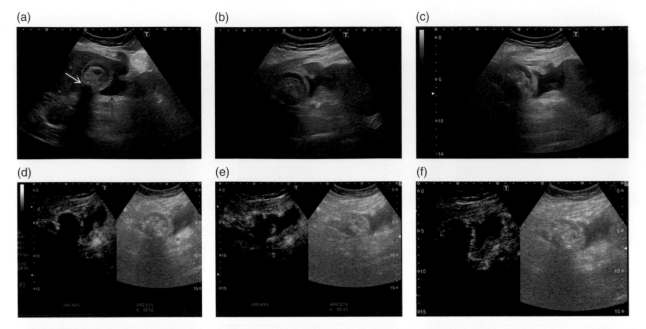

Figure 6.13 (a–c) The gallbladder (GB) wall is thickened and the lumen is filled with heterogeneous material and a stone with clear posterior acoustic shadowing (white arrow). There is a pericholecystic collection adjacent to the left liver lobe (red arrow). However, while B-mode ultrasound shows apparent integrity of the GB wall, contrast-enhanced ultrasound (d–f) reveals a clear discontinuity, with leakage of the GB content in keeping with a perforated gangrenous cholecystitis (Video 6.1).

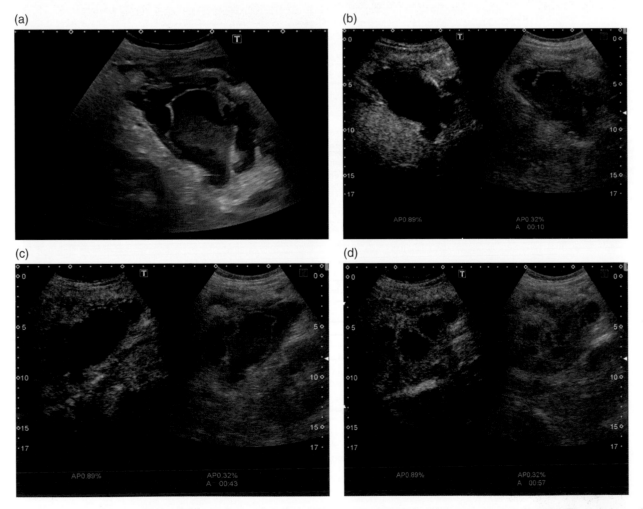

Figure 6.14 Gangrenous cholecystitis. (a) The gallbladder (GB) lumen is replaced with heterogeneous material. There is loss of the normal GB wall that appears as a thin layer between the lumen and a circumferential collection. (b, c) Contrast-enhanced ultrasound (CEUS) reveals that there is almost no enhancement of the GB wall, suggesting that it is likely necrotic. (d) CEUS helps to define the boundaries of the resulting collection that has a more loculated appearance at the level of the fundus (Video 6.2).

Emphysematous Cholecystitis

Emphysematous cholecystitis is a severe complication of acute cholecystitis secondary to gas- forming bacteria. It may be associated with cholelithiasis, but also with acalculous cholecystitis and is more commonly associated with diabetes mellitus [9]. It is typically characterised by air in the GB lumen, wall or in an adjacent hepatic collection, in cases of perforation. Air in the GB can be seen on ultrasound as a curvilinear hyperechoic band with reverberation artefacts that accumulate anteriorly just below the GB wall (Figure 6.15) (Video 6.3). If there has been a perforation, gas-related artefacts can be identified within the wall. Alternatively, comet-tail artefacts related to gas bubbles with the tendency to accumulate in the anterior space of the GB lumen can be seen scattered within echogenic suppurative material. Emphysematous cholecystitis can easily be complicated by perforation and has a higher mortality rate, hence its recognition and correct management are crucial [11].

Biloma

A biloma is an intra- or extrahepatic bile collection secondary to a GB or biliary duct leak. Bilomas can be caused by perforation as a consequence of acute cholecystitis (Figure 6.16) or as a complication of severe abdominal trauma involving the liver and biliary structures. Alternatively, a biloma may be a consequence of biliary and GB damage secondary to interventional procedures such as liver biopsy, endoscopic retrograde cholangiopancreatography (ERCP), or surgical intervention [12, 13].

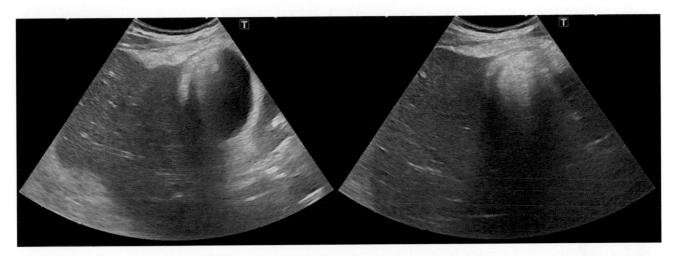

Figure 6.15 There is thickening of the gallbladder (GB) wall and evidence of reverberation artefacts rising from the GB wall and the fundus, in keeping with an emphysematous cholecystitis (Video 6.3).

(a)   (b)   (c)

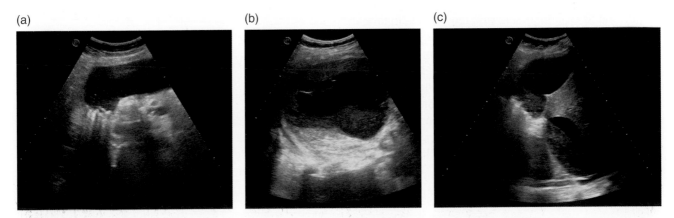

Figure 6.16 (a) Multiple small stones accumulate in the gallbladder (GB) neck. (b) There is evidence of a large heterogeneous hepatic collection with both anechoic and echogenic content and debris. (c) The collection is aligned and in direct continuity with the GB neck, revealing a similar content, hence suggesting the diagnosis of GB perforation and biloma.

In liver transplantation direct damage of the biliary tree can occur, most commonly at the site of the CBD anastomosis, or as a consequence of biliary ischaemia because of hepatic artery thrombosis, or in cadaveric ischaemic grafts (see Chapter 13). The sonographic appearance of a biloma is a well-defined anechoic collection proximal to the biliary system or GB. Most commonly bilomas are at high risk of infection and can easily evolve into biliary abscesses. In this case the collection might have a more complex appearance and a heterogeneous echogenic content as well as gas, depending on the aetiology of the infection. According to the cause and size of the biloma, its management will be conservative, require percutaneous drainage, endoscopic management with bile duct stenting, or surgical intervention.

Acalculous Cholecystitis

Acalculous cholecystitis refers to GB inflammation without signs of obstruction. This is a relatively rare condition accounting for 5–10% of the causes of cholecystitis. It is described in trauma, extensive burns injury [14], inflammatory as well as infectious diseases such as human immunodeficiency virus (HIV), although rarely reported. It is of note that the risk of perforation and complication is higher than in cholecystolithiasis [9].

Mimics of Cholecystitis

GB wall thickening is described as one of the main features of cholecystitis. However, it can also be found in several paraphysiological or pathophysiological conditions that should always be kept in mind to avoid a misleading diagnosis. Physiologically the GB contracts after food intake and this is one of the main reasons why an upper abdominal ultrasound examination always requires fasting for at least six hours, especially if the aim is to assess the GB. In cirrhotic and non-cirrhotic clinically significant portal hypertension, splanchnic venous congestion occurs and GB wall thickening is a common finding (Figure 6.17). In non-cirrhotic portal hypertension secondary to portal vein thrombosis with cavernous transformation, GB thickening can also be associated with pericholecystic varices (Figure 6.17). Right-sided heart failure is a common cause of congestive GB thickening (Figure 6.17).

Acute hepatitis (especially viral) can lead to a pericholecystic reaction with thickening of the GB wall. Often these patients complain of right upper quadrant pain and have a positive Murphy sign due to Glisson's capsule distension, making the differential diagnosis with acalculous cholecystitis particularly challenging. In some inflammatory diseases and pathological conditions such as severe malabsorption or nephrotic syndrome, low protein levels can cause pronounced GB thickening with a stratified appearance (Figure 6.17). Finally, cystic formations (liver, kidney, pancreas) or other adjacent fluid-filled organs such as the stomach or duodenum can sometimes be mistaken for the GB. It is therefore always important to perform a careful scan of the GB, or what is thought to be the GB, in all planes to avoid misinterpretation, keeping in mind the anatomical landmarks and the possibility of different phenotypes.

Chronic Cholecystitis

Chronic cholecystitis is most typically characterised by a thick-walled GB filled with debris, sludge, and stones. Often the GB is chronically contracted and it can be extremely difficult to visualise its content, a condition that should be considered carefully since it can potentially hide underlying malignant pathology. However, despite these general features chronic cholecystitis can have different appearances and characteristics, such as wall-echo-sign complexes, porcelain GB, and xanthogranulomatous cholecystitis [6]. Of note is that ongoing inflammation may lead to chronic perforation and formation of a cholecystoenteric fistula, allowing the passage of stones directly into the bowel lumen and eventually causing mechanical obstruction, usually at the level of the ileum or duodenum (Bouveret's syndrome) [11, 15].

Gallbladder Wall Pathology

Adenomyomatosis

Adenomyomatosis is a benign condition characterised by excessive GB wall epithelial proliferation leading to infoldings in the underlying muscular layer and subsequent formation of diverticular cyst-like pouches known as

(a)

(d)

(b)

(e)

(c)

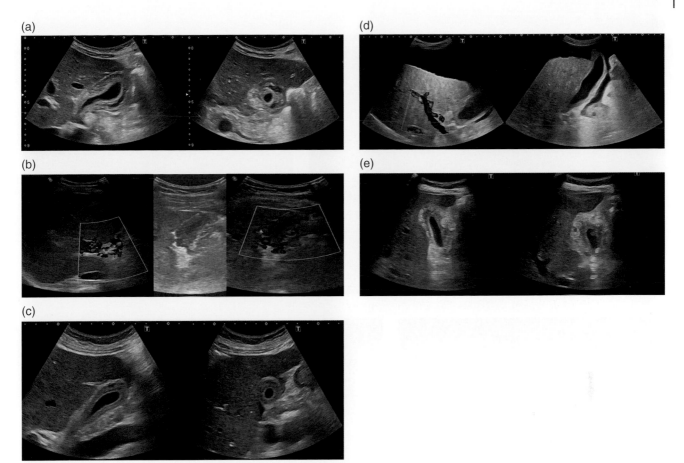

Figure 6.17 Mimics of cholecystitis. (a) Stratified thickening of the gallbladder (GB) secondary to severe hypoalbuminaemia in a patient with nephrotic syndrome. (b) Diffuse GB thickening with small pericholecystic varices in a patient with portal venous cavernoma and pre-hepatic portal hypertension (PH). (c) Diffuse GB thickening in a patient with hypoalbuminaemia and right-sided heart failure. (d) GB wall thickening in a patient with cirrhosis and severe PH, as shown by the presence of complete inversion of portal venous flow. (e) Diffuse thickening of the GB wall in acute hepatitis.

Rokitansky–Aschoff sinuses [16]. These spaces can be filled with cholesteric material with intraparietal crystals (depicted as small comet-tail artefacts) or small stones with or without acoustic shadowing or reverberations, according to their composition. Depending on its extent, GB adenomyomatosis can be focal, annular, segmental, or diffuse. Annular adenomyomatosis is a morphological variant characterised by a ring-shaped thickening of the GB wall that sometimes is so pronounced as to develop an 'hourglass' appearance and even have two separate compartments, with consequent accumulation of sludge and stones in the fundal compartment, while normal bile drains physiologically through the neck and cystic duct. Diffuse adenomyomatosis involves the whole GB wall, which appears diffusely thickened with small anechoic cystic spaces, while segmental and focal variants have a more limited extension (Figure 6.18). When a diagnosis of adenomyomatosis is suspected it is important that the outer layer of the GB is sharp, with a clear cleavage plane with the liver [16]. There should be no sign of pericholecystic fluid or collections. Exophytic growths are usually secondary to cholesteric polyps and not to adenomyomatosis. However, sometimes polyps and adenomyomatosis can coexist. The use of high-frequency transducers is of help as

(a)

(b)

(c)

(d)

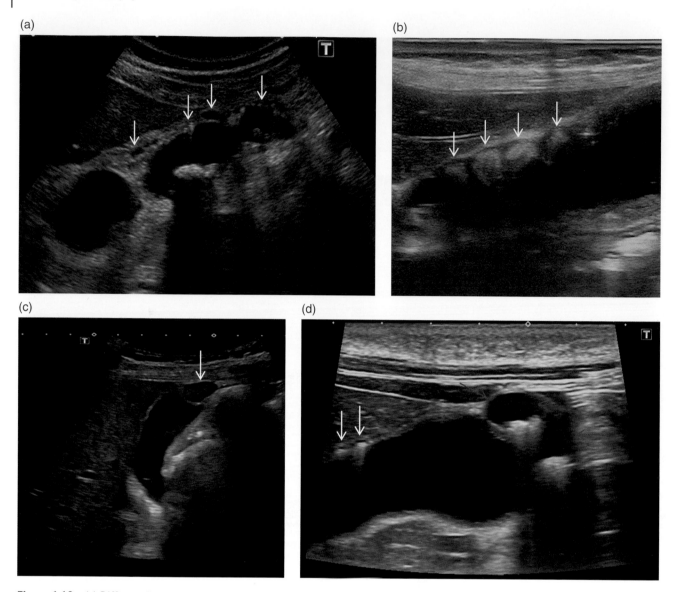

Figure 6.18 (a) Diffuse adenomyomatosis in a thick-walled gallbladder (GB) and cholelithiasis. Note is made of Rokitansky-Aschoff sinuses (white arrows) some of which are filled with cholesterol crystals (highlighted by ring-down artefacts) and small lithiasic aggregates. (b) Diffuse adenomyomatosis with intraparietal stone formation (white arrows). (c) Anular adenomyiomatosis (white arrow). (d) Another example of focal adenomyomathosis of the anterior GB wall (white arrows) and anular adenomyomatosis of the fundus containing lithiasic material (red arrows).

well as CEUS in highlighting the details of the GB wall abnormalities, leaving the use of magnetic resonance imaging (MRI) to those cases in which ultrasound imaging is inconclusive [16].

Gallbladder Polyps

GB polyps are defined as growths of tissue that protrude from the wall into the lumen.

On ultrasound they appear as elevation of the GB wall that is not mobile and does not present posterior acoustic shadowing or comet-tail artefact (Figure 6.19).

It is important to distinguish polyps from pseudopolyps, since the latter are more common and do not have malignant potential, requiring no follow-up. Pseudopolyps are most commonly cholesterol pseudopolyps, but also include inflammatory pseudopolyps and focal adenomyomatosis. True polyps can be benign or malignant. While benign polyps are most commonly

(a)

(b)

(c)

(d)

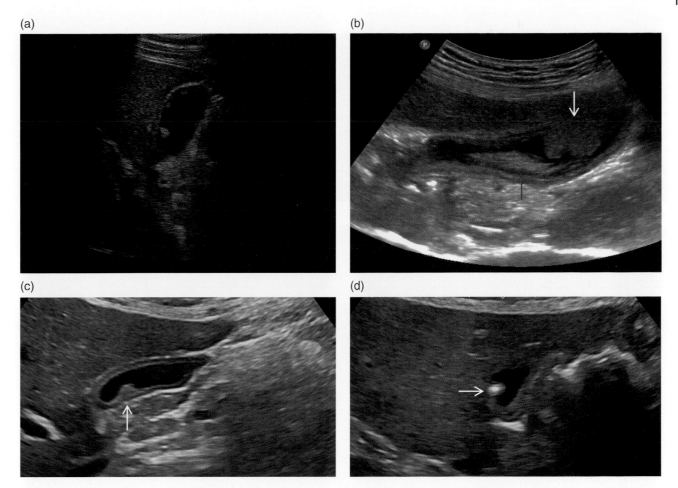

Figure 6.19 Different examples of gallbladder (GB) polyps. (a) Multiple polyps in a distended GB; (b) Large lobulated polypoid lesion in a contracted GB (white arrow), a layer of solidified sludge can also be visualised along the poterior wall (red arrow); (c) small sessile polyp in a small contracted GB; (d) small cholesterol pseudopolyp in a contracted GB.

adenomas or leiomyomas and lipomas, malignant polyps are adenocarcinomas and more rarely polypoid metastases or lymphomas [17]. Although GB cancer is rare, the presence of cancer in a polyp cannot be detected on imaging, especially in the early stages. Therefore appropriate stratification is crucial for correct management.

It is generally advised that in the case of multiple polyps, management should refer to the larger polyp, and in the presence of GB polyps ≥10 mm patients should undergo cholecystectomy because of the recognised independent risk of malignancy. Nevertheless, surveillance strategies for smaller polyps are uncertain and may vary among different countries and centres, although caution is always advocated in the presence of individual risk factors such as age >50, a diagnosis of primary sclerosing cholangitis, Indian or South American ethnicity, possible related symptoms, co-existence of gallstones, and growth rate [18].

Gallbladder Tumours

Malignant tumours of the GB are rare neoplasms of which adenocarcinomas are the most frequent, followed by mesenchymal tumours, metastases, and lymphomas [17]. GB carcinoma is almost always associated with age (>60 years) and a history of chronic cholecystitis and cholelithiasis. In the majority of cases diagnosis unfortunately is delayed, since GB tumours are often asymptomatic until obstructive jaundice appears as a clear sign of direct compression of the primary expanding mass at the level of the hepatic hilum. The most common finding is a mass completely replacing the GB, sometimes with the loss of clear demarcation between the mass and the adjacent hepatic parenchyma (Figure 6.20) (Video 6.4). Other findings include an intraluminal polypoid mass or an intramural heterogeneous thickening that extends beyond the GB wall and infiltrates the liver (Figure 6.21). The presence of a polypoid mass resulting in the concealment of the normal

(a)

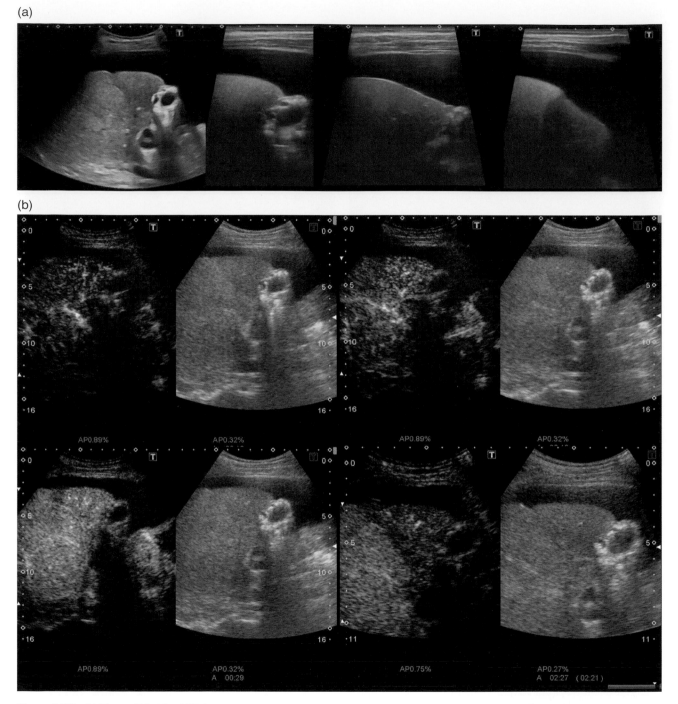

(b)

Figure 6.20 (a) The gallbladder (GB) has a contracted appearance with thickened walls, containing small pseudocystic areas. A liver ill-defined hypoechoic wedge-shaped area with capsule retraction is seen adjacent to the GB. (b) Contrast-enhanced ultrasound shows arterial isoenhancement with subtle portal venous phase washout that is clearer in the late vascular phase. These features are suggestive of malignancy and histology revealed a GB carcinoma (Video 6.4).

stratification of layers of the GB wall, a vascularised mass protruding in the lumen, and stones encased in a solid vascularised mass are all signs that orient diagnosis towards GB cancer [17]. Differential diagnosis is more difficult and requires extreme caution in the early stages of cancer development where it might be confounded with solidified

motionless sludge, segmental adenomyomatosis, or adenomas. CEUS has shown very high accuracy, especially in the differential diagnosis between solidified sludge, polypoid lesions or in general vascularised lesions protruding in the GB lumen (Videos 6.5–6.7). However, CEUS may not be able to differentiate a large benign adenoma and a dysplastic

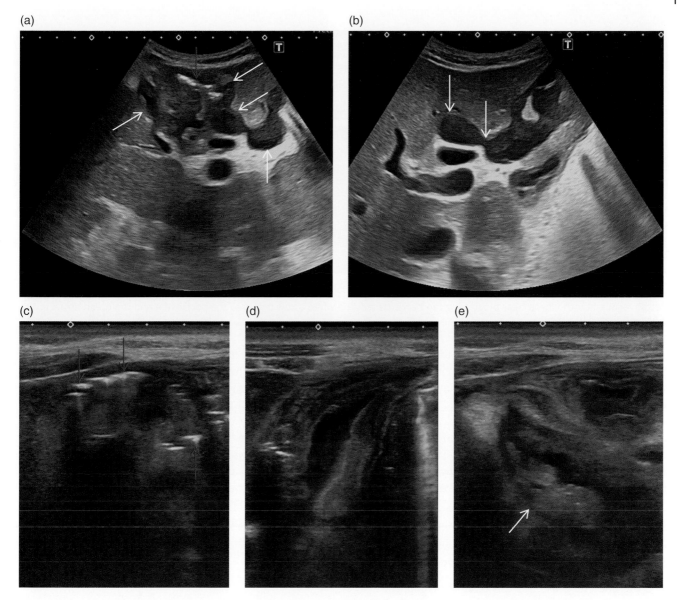

Figure 6.21 (a, b) The gallbladder (GB) is completely substituted by an ill-defined mass in connection with hypoechoic collections (white arrows). Note is also made of air within the collection/mass (a, red arrow) more clearly visible at higher magnification and using a high frequency transducer (c). On closer observation, the remnant of the GB lumen is identified (d) and a pseudopolypoid growth can be seen along its posterior wall (e, white arrow). The overall findings are in keeping with a GB malignancy.

lesion, for which management usually requires prompt cholecystectomy [18].

Biliary Duct Dilatation

Biliary duct dilatation can be functional or structural, when an intraluminal, parietal, or extrinsic cause determines outflow bile obstruction. Ultrasound is the first imaging modality used to identify the pattern and extension of biliary tree involvement, which is correlated to both the site and cause of the obstruction. As previously described in Chapter 3, the calibre of the CBD is measured from the anterior to the posterior inner wall, at the level of the porta hepatis [9]. In general its calibre measures about 4–5 mm, while the upper normal Iimit is considered to be 6–7 mm. A CBD functional dilatation up to 10–12 mm after cholecystectomy is instead considered a normal finding. Usually distal intrahepatic bile ducts are considered dilated if they measure >2 mm or >40% of the calibre of the adjacent portal vein [9]. Often biliary dilatation is described as irregular angular branching of dilated ducts with a 'double-barrel shotgun appearance'.

(a) (b)

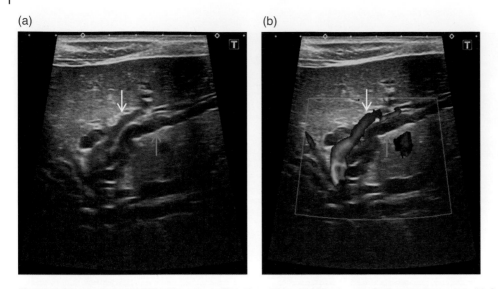

Figure 6.22 (a) Pronounced biliary duct dilatation with a double barrel shotgun appearance. (b) Colour Doppler helps to identify the portal venous branch where clear blood flow can be visualised. The white arrow points to the portal vein and the green arrow to the adjacent dilated bile duct.

This aspect is in line with the 'two tubes' that run across the hepatic parenchyma, where one 'tube' refers to the portal vein branch and the other 'tube' corresponds to the dilated duct (Figure 6.22). In advanced cirrhosis, when the portal venous flow is severely reduced or inverted, arterial buffering takes place with pronounced hypertrophy of the hepatic artery. Since the hepatic artery runs parallel to the portal vein and bile ducts (portal triad), its hypertrophy can be mistaken for dilated ducts. In case of doubt, the use of colour Doppler can be very useful to distinguish dilated bile ducts from vessels.

Biliary Obstruction Secondary to Choledocolithiasis

The presence of gallstones can often be complicated by migration through the CBD with choledocolithiasis and biliary obstruction (Figure 6.23). A proximal obstruction of the CBD will lead to obstruction of the whole biliary tree, but a distal obstruction with a stone lodged near the ampulla will lead also to pancreatitis. Choledocolithiasis of the distal CBD can be very challenging to identify with ultrasound because of overlying gas in the duodenum. However, the presence of intra- and extrahepatic biliary dilatation with a biochemical cholestatic picture associated with biliary colic is highly suspicious and diagnosis can eventually be confirmed by MRCP and ERCP. More rarely, stones can form directly within the biliary tree without migrating from the GB, as can sometimes be observed in patients who have undergone previous cholecystectomy but who have maintained a clear tendency for biliary stone formation (Figure 6.24). A rare cause of lithiasic biliary obstruction is Mirizzi syndrome, which is characterised by the presence of

a stone impacted in the cystic duct or neck of the GB, with compression of the hepatic duct and CBD and subsequent obstructive jaundice (Figure 6.25) (Video 6.8). In some circumstances chronic compression might take place, leading to fibrosis or necrosis and the formation of a fistula with the common hepatic duct or CBD.

It should always be kept in mind that stones can be present in the biliary tree even in the absence of biliary dilatation and they can lead to superimposed infection or intermittent outflow obstruction [7]. However, repeated episodes of intermittent obstruction might lead to fibrotic stricturing of the ampulla, with increased risk of distal stenosis and chronic outflow obstruction requiring sphincterotomy.

Non-lithiatic Causes of Biliary Obstruction

The presence of biliary obstruction and dilatation in the absence of cholelithiasis can be secondary to malignant and non-malignant pathology. From a clinical point of view, the most important difference is that obstructive cholelithiasis is always associated with acute right upper quadrant or epigastric pain, while other causes including malignancies are often associated with painless jaundice or a duller kind of pain. Benign pathology includes large simple cysts, which can be solitary or multiple, as found in polycystic liver disease and hydatid disease. A pseudocyst of the head of the pancreas or a large suprarenal aortic aneurysm, especially in a lean subject, might cause displacement of the duodenum or ampulla and hence biliary dilatation (Figure 6.26). In the latter case, it is usually a chronic condition more associated with asymptomatic

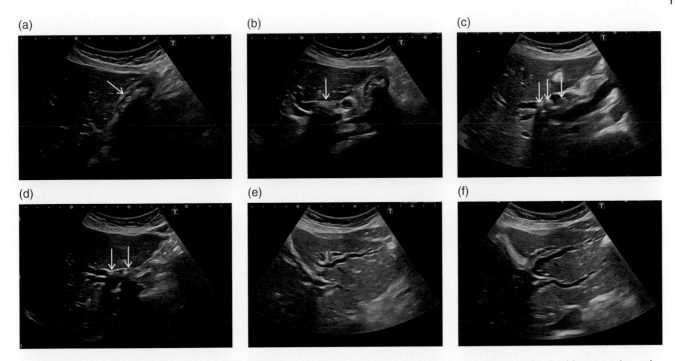

Figure 6.23 Cholecystolithiasis (a, white arrow) with gallstones migration into the common bile duct (b–d, white arrows) causing biliary obstruction and dilatation (e–f).

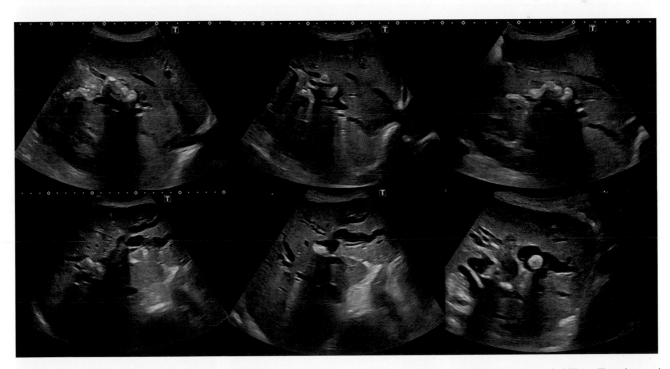

Figure 6.24 Diffuse intrahepatic biliary dilatation with multiple intrahepatic stones. Note is made of intrahepatic biliary dilatation and the clear presence of intrahepatic stones with posterior acoustic shadowing.

biliary dilatation than clear obstructive jaundice. Other benign large focal lesions include haemangiomas, focal nodular hyperplasia, or adenomas that, according to their location, can displace biliary ducts, leading to focal or more diffuse biliary dilatation.

Primary malignant liver lesions such as hepatocellular carcinoma and cholangiocarcinoma, may cause right, left, or bilateral biliary dilatation, according to their location. A Klatzkin tumour, which is a cholangiocarcinoma developing at the confluence of the right and left biliary ducts, leads to

(a)

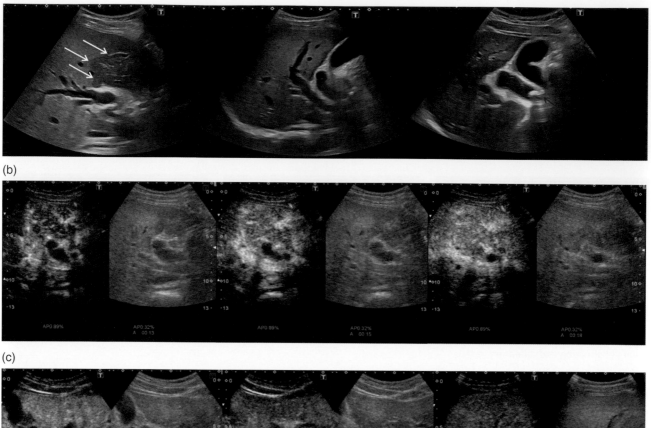

(b)

(c)

Figure 6.25 (a) On B-mode ultrasound there is evidence of an ill-defined hypoechoic area at the liver hilum (white arrows), intrahepatic biliary dilatation and a stone stuck in the cystic duct (red arrow). (b) Contrast enhanced ultrasound (CEUS) reveals isoenhancement of the hypoechoic area that is therefore compatible with focal fatty sparing. (c) The intrahepatic biliary dilatation is highlighted on CEUS. Endoscopic retrograde cholangiopancreatography (ERCP) was subsequently carried out highlighting compression of the intrahepatic common bile duct by the cystic duct stone in keeping with Mirizzi's syndrome (Video 6.8).

(a)   (b)   (c)

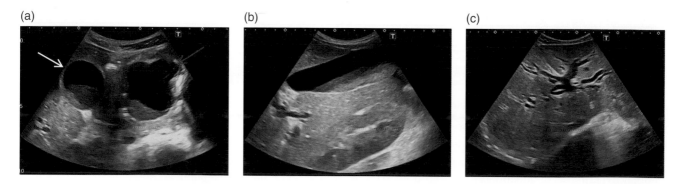

Figure 6.26 Large pseudocyst of the head of the pancreas causing compression of the common bile duct and diffuse biliary dilatation in a patient with recurrent pancreatitis secondary to biliary sludge. (a) Gallbaldder (GB) (white arrow) and pancreatic pseudocyst (red arrow). (b) GB with stratified sludge. (c) Diffuse intrahepatic biliary duct dilatation.

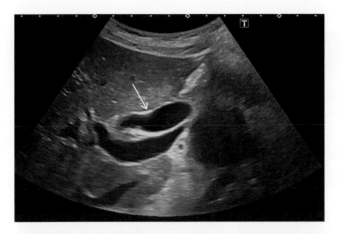

Figure 6.27 Common bile duct dilatation (white arrow) secondary to compression exerted by a large pancreatic mass (red arrow).

diffuse and pronounced intrahepatic biliary dilatation. Periampullary tumours will cause intra- and extrahepatic biliary dilatation, while liver metastasis can lead to focal or more diffuse biliary dilatation when occurring respectively at the periphery of the biliary tree or at the hepatic hilum. Pancreatic tumour, especially of the head of the pancreas,

can cause obstructive jaundice, compressing usually the distal CBD (Figure 6.27). Hilar pathological lymphadenopathies can compress the CBD leading to obstructive jaundice.

A relatively rare cause of biliary obstruction is portal biliopathy, a condition found as a complication of portal vein thrombosis with cavernous transformation. In this case portal venous collaterals develop around the thrombosed portal vein, compressing the adjacent CBD and leading to obstructive jaundice, requiring cautious stenting.

Haemobilia is bleeding that occurs within the biliary tree. It can be a consequence of cholangitis, biliary duct neoplasm, or trauma, although the most frequent cause is iatrogenic as a consequence of ERCP or biopsies. On ultrasound it appears as moderate distension of the biliary tract involved, associated with echogenic content related to blood and clots [19].

Biliary Stent Function

Despite recent advances in stent technology, many complications can still occur, including stent dysfunction, clogging, tissue ingrowth, and overgrowth, as well as stent migration with bile outflow obstruction (Figure 6.28). Ultrasound

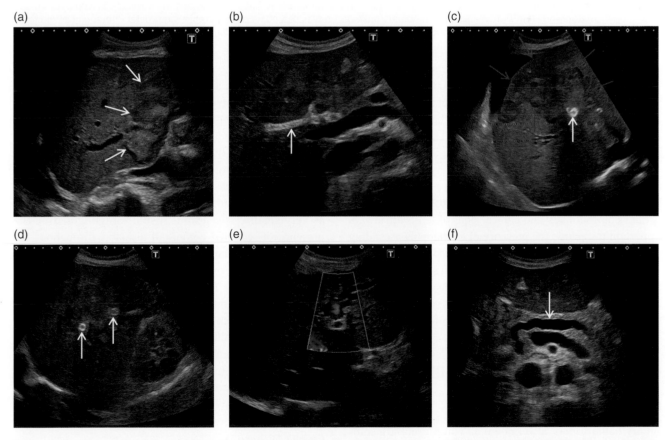

Figure 6.28 The galldbladder has been substituted by an ill-defined echogenic mass (a, white arrows) causing obstructive jaundice for which a metal stent was positioned (b, white arrow). However, with disease progression the stent (c, d white arrows) was completely encased within the expanding lesion (c, red arrows). This led to recurrent biliary obstruction as evidenced by persistent dilatation of the biliary tree (e) and pancreatic duct (f, white arrow).

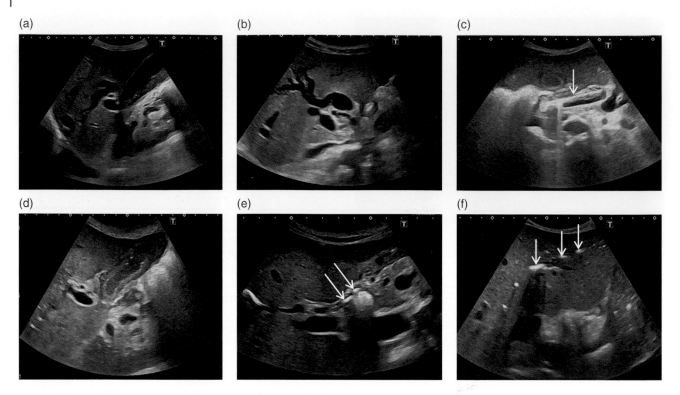

Figure 6.29 (a, b) Pronounced intrahepatic biliary dilatation. The gallbladder is filled with sludge. However, endoscopic retrograde colangiopancreatography (ERCP) revealed that the biliary obstruction was secondary to inoperable intraductal cholangiocarcinoma of the common bile duct. (c) A metal stent was positioned (white arrow) with resolution of the biliary dilatation (d, e). The presence of aerobilia is an indirect sign of stent patency and good function (e, f white arrows).

imaging is the first-line approach to evaluate stent position and obstruction by assessing the presence of biliary dilatation, mass compression, tissue ingrowth, and the visualisation or not of the stent that might be dislodged. It should be kept in mind that a functioning choledochal stent usually causes air to pass from the duodenum into the biliary tree. Therefore acrobilia (or pneumobilia) can be interpreted as proof of good stent patency and function (Figure 6.29), although the patient's biochemistry and clinical signs of sepsis are always important to exclude the presence of overlapping ascending cholangitis, which can also be associated with aerobilia. The absence of aerobilia after ERCP with stent positioning and sphincterotomy with no or very little improvement of obstructive jaundice must be carefully evaluated, since it can suggest early stent obstruction or malfunction.

Congenital Pathologies of the Biliary Tree

Biliary Hamartomas

Biliary hamartomas, also known as Von Meyenburg complexes, are congenital remnants secondary to ductal plate malformations composed of cystic dilated bile ducts embedded in fibrous stroma [20, 21]. In the majority of cases hamartomas are small, ranging from 0.5 to 1.5 cm, although larger findings are also described. In view of their common embryological defect, they may or may not be associated with other conditions such as congenital hepatic fibrosis, polycystic liver, or kidney disease.

The diagnosis is often incidental during imaging carried out for different reasons or on histopathological examination. On ultrasound, biliary hamartomatosis may appear as very small cystic lesions, usually highlighted by the presence of scattered comet-tail artefacts throughout the hepatic parenchyma. In other conditions they might appear as multiple hyper- or hypoechoic lesions, with or without comet-tail artefact (Figure 6.30). Magnification with a high-frequency transducer is usually helpful for highlighting cystic areas with reverberation artefact or hyperechoic smaller round focalities, compatible with small cysts with an undetectable lumen. When biliary hamartomatosis is very diffuse it can mimic chronic liver disease, metastatic disease [22], or microangiomatosis. If inconclusive, MRCP is the gold standard for a definitive diagnosis [23].

Caroli's Disease

Caroli's disease is a rare inherited disorder caused by plate duct malformation leading to multifocal, segmental, lobar,

(a) (b) (c)

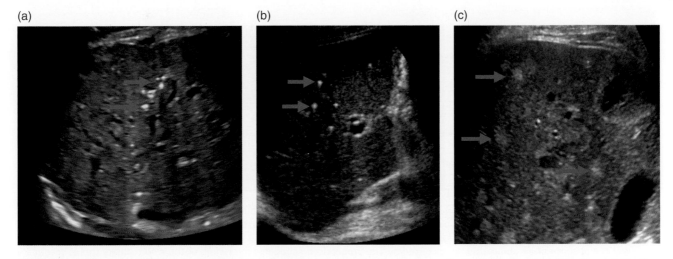

Figure 6.30 Biliary hamartomas (von Meyenburg complexes; arrows) appear as small, focal developmental lesions of the liver composed of groups of dilated intrahepatic bile ducts. On ultrasound they appear as scattered hyperechoic foci with ring-down artefact (a, b). At higher magnification they appear as echogenic small rounded areas (c).

or diffuse dilatation of the large intrahepatic bile ducts [24]. Its genetic background is shared with other conditions with which it may be associated, such as congenital fibrosis, polycystic liver, and kidney disease. Typical imaging findings include bile duct ectasia and irregular cystic dilatation of the proximal intrahepatic ducts with sparing of the CBD, or intraluminal portal vein sign characterised by saccular dilated ducts surrounding the portal vein [25, 26]. Rarely intraductal calculi can be observed, as well as intraductal bridging that can be visualised as echogenic septa crossing the dilated bile duct lumen [26]. When plate duct malformation is associated with congenital hepatic fibrosis, the condition is named Caroli's syndrome rather than disease, and it is characterised by more distal involvement and periportal fibrosis leading to biliary stasis, cirrhosis, and portal hypertension [26].

Biliary Atresia

Biliary atresia is the most common cause of paediatric chronic liver disease and the first indication for liver transplantation in the paediatric population. A detailed description of this condition with its sonographic findings is outlined in Chapter 10.

Cholangitis

Cholangitis is an inflammatory disorder of the biliary ducts. It is caused by acute, chronic, or acute-on-chronic pathological processes. Acute cholangitis is usually secondary to biliary duct obstruction complicated by superimposed bacterial infection. Cholelithiasis is the most

common cause, although any condition leading to bile outflow obstruction can cause cholangitis, including parietal stricturing or extrinsic compression by primary or secondary neoplastic growth [27]. More rarely, cholangitis can be caused by recurrent pyogenic cholangiohepatitis [28] and parasitic infections that typically colonise the hepatobiliary system (see Chapter 7) [27]. Finally, recurrent acute ascending cholangitis can also occur in patients who have undergone hepaticojejunostomies or malfunction of a biliary stent previously positioned for obstructive jaundice.

The typical sonographic features of acute cholangitis are diffuse thickening of the biliary duct walls and the presence of echogenic bile, which might be secondary to sludge or purulent material and debris (Figures 6.31 and 6.32). Gas-producing bacteria can also lead to aerobilia. However, aerobilia is most commonly found as a consequence of procedures such as ERCP, an incompetent sphincter of Oddi (most commonly after sphincterotomy), Whipple's procedure, cholecystoenterostomy, or biliary enteric fistula, as found in Bouveret's syndrome or gallstone ileus. On ultrasound aerobilia appears as bright echogenicity with prominent reverberation artefacts that follows the branching of the biliary tree. Depending on the cause it can be localised or more diffuse and also involve the GB (Figures 6.29 and 6.33). It typically moves in accordance with the patient's position and it is more concentrated in the left biliary tree when supine, owing to the left lobe of the liver being more anterior than the right.

Chronic cholangitis is secondary to sclerosing processes that can be distinguished between primary and secondary. Primary sclerosing cholangitis (PSC) is a chronic inflammatory disease of unknown cause. It affects the biliary tree causing epithelial inflammation, fibrosis, and focal and segmental stricturing of the intra- or extrahepatic bile ducts

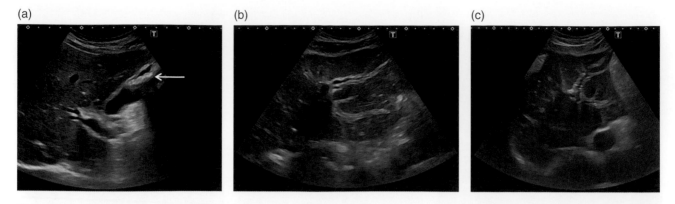

Figure 6.31 Diffuse thickening of the biliary tree in a patient with cholecystolithiasis and choledocholithiasis who recently underwent endoscopic retrograde cholangiopancreatography (ERCP). (a) There is persistence of gallstones (arrow) and evidence of persistent biliary duct thickening and mild dilatation (b,c). Nevertheless, what is striking in this patient who developed post-procedural sepsis was the absence of aerobilia after sphincterotomy. The pronounced echogenic thickening of the whole biliary tree is secondary to a cholangitis, ongoing obstruction and superimposed infection.

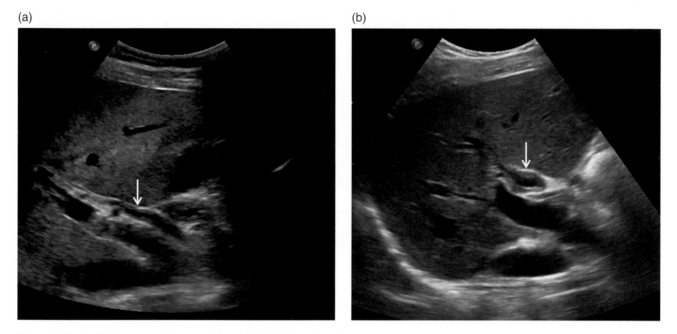

Figure 6.32 (a, b) Two cases of acute cholangitis highlighted by diffuse thickening of the common bile duct (arrows).

(Figures 6.34 and 6.35), eventually leading to cirrhosis, portal hypertension, and liver failure. Its natural history is also characterised by predisposition to the development of cholangiocarcinoma (Figure 6.36) and more rarely hepatocellular carcinoma. The typical features of PSC are the segmental distribution and the irregular pattern of inflammation that affects the biliary system (see Chapter 8). Nevertheless, its natural history, especially in those who develop dominant strictures, is often characterised by biliary stasis and pyogenic cholangitis.

Secondary causes of sclerosing cholangitis include HIV-related cholangiopathy, a condition characterised by biliary duct infection from opportunistic microorganisms that lead to fibro-inflammatory changes and stricturing of the biliary of the

biliary tree (See Chapter 7). On imaging, HIV cholangiopathy is almost indistinguishable from PSC [29]. Critically ill patients can be affected by a rare form of sclerosing cholangitis likely secondary to ischaemia of the intrahepatic biliary epithelium, as a consequence of direct ischaemia, hypoxia, or sepsis. Sclerosing cholangitis in the critically ill is a progressive disease that never affects the extrahepatic biliary system, leading eventually to biliary cirrhosis and liver failure and for which liver transplantation remains the only curative option [30].

Biliary ischaemia occurring as a consequence of hepatic artery thrombosis secondary to trauma, liver transplant, or coagulopathies can lead to severe damage of the biliary epithelium, with inflammation, thickening, and often

(a)

(b)

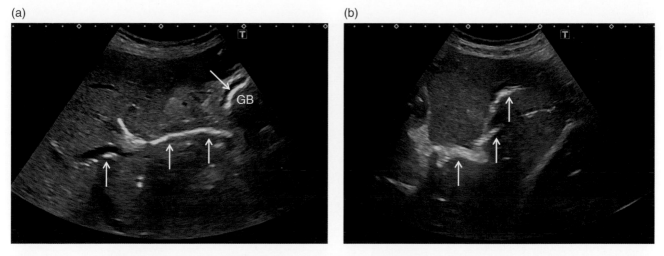

Figure 6.33 Aerobilia after endoscopic retrograde cholangiopancreatography (ERCP) and stent placement in a patient with obstructive jaundice. In these images, the stent is not visualised, but there is extensive aerobilia at the level of the common bile duct, right intrahepatic ducts, and gallbladder (arrows, a), as well as in the left biliary ducts (arrows, b).

(a)

(b)

(c)

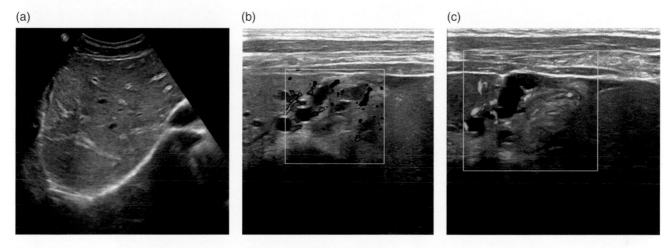

Figure 6.34 Primary sclerosing cholangitis. (a) Pronounced thickening of the biliary ducts. (b, c) Distal focal bile duct dilatation.

superimposed infection that can be typically complicated by infective cholangitis and the formation of biliary abscesses. Another rare form of secondary sclerosing cholangitis is immunoglobulin IgG4 related cholangitis, which can lead to inflammatory thickening of the biliary epithelium and stricturing. The sonographic features of sclerosing cholangitis are thickening, stricturing, and upstream dilatation of the biliary tree. Debris, sludge, and intraductal calcification are common findings and might be indistinguishable from PSC on imaging.

Contrast-Enhanced Ultrasound in Biliary Disorders

The utility of CEUS in the diagnosis of liver tumours is widely accepted. However, it can also be useful in biliary disorders, as stated in the most recent update of European Federation for Ultrasound in Medicine (EFSUMB) guidelines on the

non-hepatic use of CEUS [31]. In this context CEUS is able to increase ultrasound diagnostic accuracy by differentiating benign from malignant causes of obstructive jaundice. It also can improve the detection of bile duct invasion of hepatic malignancies, allowing a better evaluation of intra- and extraductal extension of hilar hepatobiliary tumours [32].

In addition, by enhancing the background hepatic parenchyma, CEUS improves the visualisation of intrahepatic bile duct dilatation (Figure 6.25) (Video 6.8) and helps detect and clarify the cause of intraluminal obstruction, whether secondary to a vascularised lesion or solidified biliary sludge and stones. It is also extremely accurate in differentiating solidified sludge from a noplastic growth protruding in the GB lumen (Figure 6.9) (Videos 6.5–6.7). Finally, CEUS is also an excellent tool for detecting even small enhancement defects of the GB wall during cholecystitis compatible with necrosis and perforation (Figures 6.13 and 6.14) (Video 6.1 and 6.2).

(a)

(b)

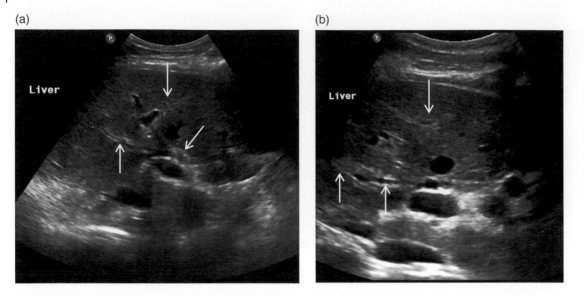

Figure 6.35 (a, b) Diffuse thickening of both proximal and more distal biliary ducts (arrows) can be observed in this patient with primary sclerosing cholangitis.

(a)

(b)

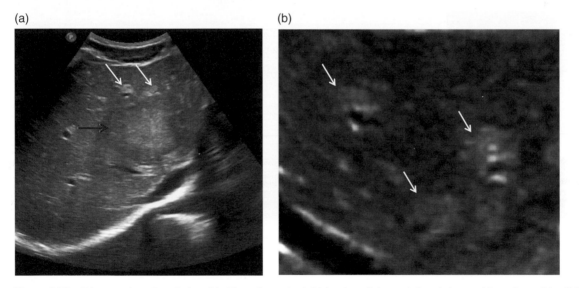

Figure 6.36 Primary sclerosing cholangitis. There is marked thickening of the peripheral ducts with periportal/peribiliary fibrosis (a, b, white arrows). Note is made of a large isoechoic focal lesion compatible with peripheral cholangiocarcinoma (a, red arrow).

Videos

Videos for this chapter can be accessed via the companion website: www.wiley.com/go/LiverUltrasound.

References

1 Praseedom, R.K. and Mohammed, R. (1998). Two cases of gall bladder agenesis and review of the literature. *Hepatogastroenterology* 45 (22): 954–955.

2 Peloponissios, N., Gillet, M., Cavin, R., and Halkic, R. (2005). Agenesis of the gallbladder: a dangerously misdiagnosed malformation. *World J. Gastroenterol.* 11 (39): 6228–6231.

3 Kosmidis, C.S., Koimtzis, G.D., Kosmidou, M.S. et al. (2017). Gallbladder hypoplasia, a congenital abnormality of the gallbladder: a case report. *Am. J. Case Rep.* 18: 1320–1324.

4 Jenssen, C., Bridson, J.-M., Barreiros, A.P. et al. (2012). Ultrasound of the biliary system. In: *EFSUMB Course Book*, 2e (ed. C.F. Dietrich), 105–140. EFSUMB.

5 Apolo Romero, E.X., Gálvez Salazar, P.F., Estrada Chandi, J.A. et al. (2018). Gallbladder duplication and cholecystitis. *J. Surg. Case Rep.* 7: 1–3.

6 Rubens, D.J. (2007). Ultrasound imaging of the biliary tract. *Ultrasound Clin.* 2: 391–413.

7 Laing, F.C. (1998). The gallbladder and bile ducts. In: *Diagnostic Ultrasound*, 2e, vol. 1 (ed. C.M. Rumack, S.R. Wilson and J.W. Charboneau), 175–223. St. Louis: Mosby Year Book.

8 Datta, A., Garg, N., and Lema, P.C. (2010). The significance of the wall echo shadow triad on ultrasonography: a case series. *Crit. Ultrasound J.* 2: 107–108.

9 Rubens, D.J. (2004). Hepatobiliary imaging and pitfalls. *Radiol. Clin. North Am.* 42: 257–278.

10 Teefey, S.A., Baron, R.L., Radke, H.M. et al. (1991). Gangrenous cholecystitis: new observations on sonography. *J. Ultrasound Med.* 10: 603–606.

11 Oppenheimer, D.C. and Rubens, D.J. (2019). Sonography of acute cholecystitis and its mimics. *Radiol. Clin. North Am.* 57: 535–548.

12 Lee, C.M., Stewart, L., and Way, L.W. (2000). Postcholecystectomy abdominal bile collections. *Arch. Surg.* 135: 538–542.

13 Yousaf, M.N., D'Souza, R.G., Chaudhary, F. et al. (2020). Biloma: a rare manifestation of spontaneous bile leak. *Cureus* 12 (5): e8116.

14 Cornwell, E.E., Rodriguez, A., Mirvis, S.E. et al. (1989). Acute acalculous cholecystitis in critically injured patients. *Ann. Surg.* 219 (1): 52–55.

15 Hanbidge, A.E., Buckler, P.M., O'Malley, M.E. et al. (2004). From the RSNA refresher courses: imaging evaluation for acute pain in the right upper quadrant. *Radiographics* 24 (4): 1117–1135.

16 Bonatti, M., Vezzali, N., Lombardo, F. et al. (2017). Gallbladder adenomyomatosis:imaging findings, tricks and pitfalls. *Insights Imaging* 8: 243–253.

17 Sandrasegaran, K. and Menias, C.O. (2017). Imaging and screening of cancer of the gallbladder and bile ducts. *Radiol. Clin. North Am.* 55: 1211–1222.

18 Wiles, R., Thoeni, R.F., Barbu, S.T. et al. (2017). Management and follow up of gallbladder polyps. Joint guidelines between the European Society of Gastrointestinal and Abdominal Radiology (ESGAR), European Association for Endoscopic Surgery and other Interventional Techniques (EAES), International Society of Digestive Surgery – European Federation (EFISDS) and European Society of Gastrointestinal Endoscopy (ESGE). *Eur. Radiol.* 27 (6): 3856–3866.

19 Badea, R., Zaro, R., Tantău, M., and Chiorean, L. (2015). Ultrasonography of the biliary tract – up to date. The importance of correlation between imaging methods and patients' signs and symptoms. *Med. Ultrason.* 17 (3): 383–391.

20 Zheng, R., Zhang, B., Kudo, M. et al. (2005). Imaging findings of biliary hamartomas. *World J. Gastroenterol.* 11 (40): 6354–6359.

21 Lev-Toaff, A.S., Bach, A.M., Wechsler, R.J. et al. (1995). The radiologic and pathologic spectrum of biliary hamartomas. *Am. J. Roentgenol.* 165: 309–313.

22 Cooke, J.C. and Cooke, D.A. (1987). The appearances of multiple biliary hamartomas of the liver (von Meyenberg complexes) on computed tomography. *Clin. Radiol.* 38: 101–102.

23 Mortelé, B., Mortelé Seynaeve, P., Vandevelde, D. et al. (2002). Hepatic bile duct hamartomas (von Meyenburg complexes): MR and MR cholangiography findings. *J. Comput. Assist. Tomogr.* 26: 438–443.

24 Summerfiled, J.A., Nagafuchi, Y., Sherlock, S. et al. (1986). Hepatobiliary fibropolycystic disease. A clinical and histological review of 51 patients. *J. Hepatol.* 2: 141.

25 Brancatelli, G., Federle, M.P., Vilgrain, V. et al. (2005). Fibropolycystic liver disease: CT and MR imaging findings. *RadioGraphics* 25: 659–670.

26 Marchal, G.J., Desmet, V.J., Proesmans, W.C. et al. (1986). Caroli disease: high-frequency US and pathologic findings. *Radiology* 158: 507–511.

27 Lim, J.H., Kim, S.Y., and Park, C.M. (2007). Parasitic diseases of the biliary tract. *Am. J. Roentgenol.* 188: 1596–1560.

28 Ahmed, M. (2018). Acute cholangitis – an update. *World J. Gastrointest. Pathophysiol.* 9 (1): 1–7.

29 Baron, R.L., Tublin, M.E., and Peterson, M.S. (2002). Imaging the spectrum of biliary tract disease. *Radiol. Clin. North Am.* 40 (6): 1325–1354.

30 Gudnason, H.O. and Björnsson, E.S. (2017). Secondary sclerosing cholangitis in critically ill patients: current perspectives. *Clin. Exp. Gastroenterol.* 10: 105–111.

31 Piscaglia, F., Nolsøe, C., Dietrich, C.F. et al. (2012). The EFSUMB guidelines and recommendations on the clinical practice of contrast enhanced ultrasound (CEUS): update 2011 on non-hepatic applications. *Ultraschall Med.* 33: 33–59.

32 Fontán, F.J., Reboredo, A.R., and Siso, A.R. (2015). Accuracy of contrast-enhanced ultrasound in the diagnosis of bile duct obstruction. *Ultrasound Int. Open* 1 (1): E12–E18.

7

Tropical Infections of the Liver

Tom Heller[1,2], Michaëla A.M. Huson[3], and Francesca Tamarozzi[4]

[1] *Lighthouse Clinic, Lilongwe, Malawi*
[2] *International Training and Education Center for Health, University of Washington, Seattle, WA, United States*
[3] *Radboud University Medical Center, Department of Internal Medicine and Radboud Center of Infectious Diseases (RCI), Nijmegen, The Netherlands*
[4] *Department of Infectious Tropical Diseases and Microbiology, WHO Collaborating Centre on Strongyloidiasis and other Neglected Tropical Diseases, IRCCS Sacro Cuore Don Calabria Hospital, Negrar di Valpolicella, Verona, Italy*

Ultrasound plays a key role in the diagnosis and management of hepatic infections. It is particularly helpful in resource-limited, mainly tropical, settings where ultrasound is usually the first tool to screen, diagnose, guide treatment, and follow up cases, as it is often the only imaging modality available besides chest X-ray [1]. Ultrasound is sensitive in the detection of many infections. However, it lacks specificity, particularly in necrotic abscess-like infections, which can mimic benign (e.g. haemorrhagic cysts) or malignant (e.g. necrotic tumours) conditions. Like any diagnostic test, it is important to interpret it in the context of epidemiological and clinical details such as age, sex, and area of residence, exposure, presenting history, symptoms, and current immune status to achieve an accurate presumptive diagnosis. Often this needs to be narrowed down further by employing laboratory tests, for instance serology, or by using other diagnostic imaging modalities. Aspiration and biopsy are frequently required to conclude the final diagnosis and ultrasound is an ideal modality to guide this process.

In this chapter, we will summarise the most important infections of the liver, their sonographic presentations, further tests that may be utilised, and potential treatment options. Infections of the liver will be categorised as parasitic, bacterial, fungal, and viral. Viral hepatitis, although prevalent in many tropical areas and probably the most frequent liver infection worldwide, is not included in this chapter as it is discussed in more detail in Chapter 8.

Parasitic Infections of the Liver

Ultrasound can help with the detection of numerous parasitic diseases endemic in tropical regions. As ultrasound is the imaging mode of choice in echinococcosis and plays a key role in amoebic liver abscess (ALA), these topics will be described in more detail. Schistosomiasis is an important cause of portal hypertension in tropical settings and will also be addressed in detail. Other parasitic infections that can be detected by ultrasound will be described briefly, including *Fasciola, Toxocara, Opisthorchis, Clonorchis,* and *Ascaris.*

Cystic Echinococcosis

Introduction and Clinical Picture

Cystic echinococcosis (CE) is caused by the larval stage of the tapeworm *Echinococcus granulosus sensu lato.* CE has a worldwide distribution, and is especially prevalent in livestock-raising areas. The natural cycle of the parasite develops between dogs and livestock. In humans, after accidental ingestion of parasite eggs from the environment, CE cysts may develop in any organ or tissue, most commonly in the liver (approximately 80% of cases) followed by the lungs (approximately 20% of cases). CE cysts evolve through stages, either spontaneously or as a consequence of treatment. When symptoms occur, they are due either to the growth of the cyst(s) exerting pressure on neighbouring structures, or to the loss of cyst integrity or its rupture, causing local and/or systemic manifestations. Symptoms are non-specific and depend on the organ affected. For those in the liver, these include poor appetite, right upper quadrant pain, and jaundice. The most common complication is rupture, which can cause jaundice in case of communication with the biliary tree, anaphylactic reaction, or may be further complicated by superinfection or dissemination (secondary echinococcosis).

Ultrasound Features

Ultrasound is the examination of choice for the diagnosis and staging of abdominal CE cysts. The currently accepted international classification of CE cysts, based on hepatic ultrasound features, is the World Health Organization Informal Working Group on Echinococcosis (WHO-IWGE) classification [2]. This includes six stages, each characterised by a pathognomonic sign that, when clearly visible, allows the diagnosis of CE (Figure 7.1):

- **CE1 'double-wall sign'**: univesicular cyst with anechoic content, with or without low-intensity floating echoes on decubitus change and with a visible 'double-wall sign' consisting of an inner hyperechoic and outer hypoechoic wall. *Pathognomonic sign*: double-wall sign.
- **CE2 'honeycomb sign'**: multivesicular cyst with one or more daughter cysts filling the cyst in part or completely, causing a 'honeycomb' appearance. *Pathognomonic sign*: the adjacent walls of juxtaposed daughter cysts are clearly distinguishable, thin, regular, continuous, and avascular.
- **CE3a** 'water lily sign': univesicular cyst with partial or complete detachment of the inner parasitic layers,

visible as a hyperechoic thin and folded membrane floating in the anechoic cyst content. *Pathognomonic sign*: the whole membrane must be identified as a continuous, regular, hyperechogenic structure.
- **CE3b 'Swiss cheese sign'**: multivesicular cyst with heterogeneous structure, encompassing (i) avascular solid components and hypoechoic folded structures deriving from degenerating membranes, and (ii) one or more daughter cysts with anechoic content. *Pathognomonic sign*: heterogeneous cyst containing daughter cysts and hypoechoic folded structures.
- **CE4 'ball of wool sign'**: mass with heterogeneous avascular solid content containing hypoechoic folded structures. *Pathognomonic sign*: hypoechoic folded structures deriving from degenerating membranes visible in the solid heterogeneous matrix.
- **CE5 'eggshell pattern'**: a CE4 stage CE cyst (with its visible pathognomonic sign) with complete or nearly complete eggshell-like peripherally calcified wall.

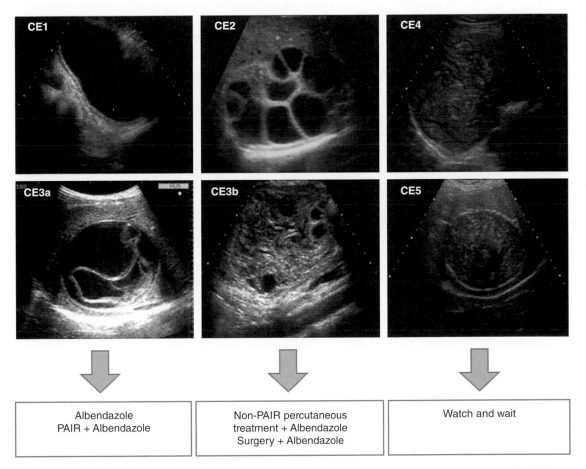

Figure 7.1   CE cyst stages and suggested stage-specific clinical management of cystic echinococcosis (CE). PAIR = puncture, aspiration, injection of a scolicidal agent, and re-aspiration. Non-PAIR percutaneous treatments include several percutaneous techniques using cutting instruments and large-bore catheters to evacuate the entire cyst content. *Source:* Bélard S et al. (2016), The American Society of Tropical Medicine and Hygiene.

It is important to remember that some calcification in CE cysts can occur at any stage (i.e. presence of calcification alone does not classify a CE cyst as CE5 stage), but these calcifications are always peripheral. CE cysts are also always avascular, therefore the presence of Doppler signal within the cyst excludes the diagnosis of CE.

Further Investigations

Rule-in/rule-out diagnosis in case of suspected CE can be achieved by the following:

- Serology is not standardised and is characterised by false-positive and false -negative results. In general, CE can be confirmed by two concordant positive first-line tests performed in parallel or at least one positive West Blot test. A negative serology does not rule out CE. Generally, patients with extrahepatic cysts and with single, small hepatic CE1 cysts or CE4–5 cysts are seronegative in a large percentage of cases. Particular care must be taken when interpreting serology for CE in co-endemic areas for both cystic and alveolar echinococcosis (AE; see the section on AE).
- Albendazole as a treatment trial (*ex juvantibus*): in the presence of liquid-content lesions, albendazole intake for one month followed by visualisation of a response on ultrasound (e.g. CE1 developing into CE3a stage) and/or seroconversion (if previously seronegative).
- Presence of contrast enhancement rules out CE: CE intracystic components do not enhance, although slight enhancement of the cyst wall may be observed.
- Diagnostic percutaneous puncture followed by microscopy of the cyst content or polymerase chain reaction (PCR).

Magnetic resonance imaging (MRI) performs better than computed tomography (CT) in defining the pathognomonic features of CE cysts; these techniques are mainly required pre-operatively to define the relation of the cyst with neighbouring structures.

Treatment and Follow-Up

Asymptomatic hepatic CE should be managed using a stage-specific approach:

- CE1 and CE3a: especially if <5 cm, albendazole for 3–6 months continuously; for larger cysts, percutaneous treatment, if available, associated with albendazole prophylaxis for 1–3 months to prevent dissemination. Surgery associated with albendazole prophylaxis may be indicated for very large or superficial cysts.
- CE2 and CE3b: surgery associated with albendazole prophylaxis. Medical therapy with albendazole may be attempted, especially if cysts are small, but there is a high recurrence rate. If available, modified percutaneous techniques associated with albendazole prophylaxis may also be envisaged.
- CE4 and CE5: watch-and-wait approach, with only regular follow-up every 6–12 months by ultrasound imaging to detect possible reactivations. These are rare if the CE4–5 stage was reached spontaneously.

Symptomatic CE should be treated surgically. Some experts also add peri-operative praziquantel to albendazole in cases of invasive procedures. An alternative, less effective drug than albendazole is mebendazole. During albendazole intake, regular (e.g. monthly) monitoring of blood cell counts and liver enzymes is recommended. Ultrasound follow-up is indicated yearly for a minimum of five years.

Alveolar Echinococcosis

Introduction and Clinical Picture

AE is caused by the larval stage of the tapeworm *Echinococcus multilocularis*. Similar to CE, humans acquire infection through accidental ingestion of parasite eggs, but AE infection is much less frequent than CE, it only occurs in the Northern Hemisphere, and its cycle is sylvatic. The natural cycle of the parasite develops between wild canids (especially foxes) and different species of small rodents. AE lesions are infiltrative and metastasising tumour-like lesions, cholangiocarcinoma being the main differential diagnosis. The primary organ affected is almost invariably the liver. AE lesions grow slowly and the asymptomatic period may last 5–15 years or longer; many infections are diagnosed at a late stage. Jaundice is the most common presenting symptom, often associated with itching, right upper quadrant pain, and fever in case of cholangitis or superinfection of the necrotic centre of the lesion. Loco-regional extension and distant metastases may cause a variety of symptoms. The WHO-IWGE classifies AE by PNM staging (P = extent and location of the parasitic lesion; N = invasion of neighbouring organs; M = presence of metastases).

Ultrasound Features

According to ultrasound appearance different AE's sonographic patterns are described [2, 3] (Figure 7.2):

- The hailstorm pattern is the most frequent, being observed in approximately half of AE patients. It is characterised by an irregular border and heterogeneous content, often with scattered hyperechoic formations with or without posterior acoustic shadowing.
- The pseudocystic pattern is characterised by a hyperechoic, irregular and non-homogeneous rim, with no sign of vascularity at color Doppler or CEUS.
- The ossification pattern is characterised by solitary or grouped, mostly sharply delineated lesions with posterior acoustic shadowing.
- The haemangioma-like pattern is characterised by a relatively clearly demarcated heterogeneous hyperecoic

lesion that may be difficult to distinguish from a typical haemangioma.

- The metastases-like pattern is mostly characterised by hypoechoic lesion or lesions with a central non-homogeneous hyperechoic scar. They are very difficult to distinguish from some liver neoplastic metastasis that show a hypoechoic halo.

In comparison to CE, no pathognomonic imaging signs of AE exist and especially the haemangioma- and metastasis-like patterns may pose a diagnostic challenge. However, the presence of calcifications and the pattern of contrast enhancement may suggest the diagnosis of AE.

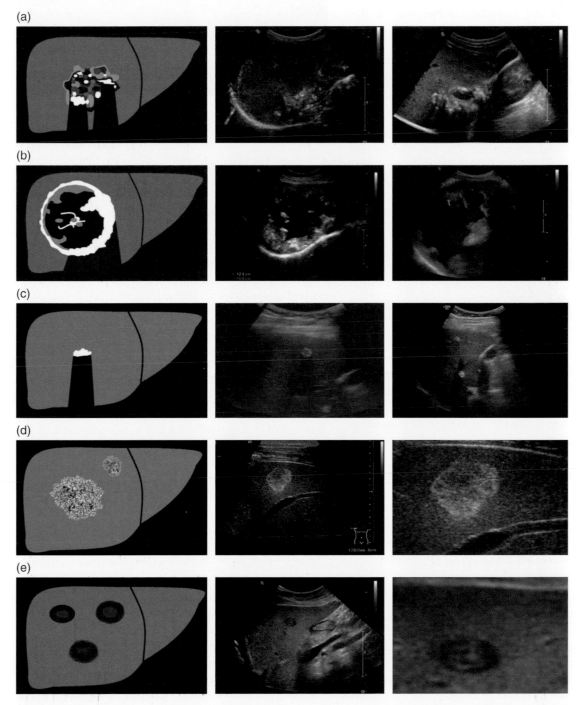

Figure 7.2 Sonographic patterns of E. multilocularis (a) 'Hailstorm', (b) 'pseudocystic', (c) 'ossification', (d) 'hemangioma-like' and (e) 'metastais like' appearance of alveolar echinococcosis lesions. *Source:* Courtesy of Dr Claudia Wallrauch.

Further Investigations

Serology is almost invariably positive; however, high cross-reactivity exists with CE, which makes the differential diagnosis between the two infections at times difficult, especially in co-endemic areas. Definitive diagnosis may be achieved by biopsy followed by histology or PCR. If untreated, the prognosis of AE is poor.

Treatment and Follow-Up

After assessment of the extension of the disease, the options may be curative resection (partial debulking should be avoided) followed by two years of albendazole, or prolonged, often life-long, albendazole administration, with interventional radiology or endoscopic procedures if complications occur. In some cases, liver transplant followed by albendazole may be an option. Regular follow-up with serology, imaging, and monitoring of blood cell counts, aminotransferases, and albendazole-sulfoxide blood levels is required. Discontinuation of albendazole treatment may be possible in case of seronegativity and negative fluorodeoxyglucose–positron emission tomography (FDG-PET; delayed imaging acquisition).

Amoebic Liver Abscess

Introduction and Clinical Picture

Amoebic liver abscess (ALA) is the most common extraintestinal manifestation of *Entamoeba histolytica* infections and around 8% of patients with intestinal amoebiasis develop hepatic abscesses. In tropical settings they are far more common than bacterial abscesses. After ingestion of the amoebic cysts through contaminated food or water, amoeba trophozoites develop in the bowel and cause amoebic colitis, although the infection is often asymptomatic. In some cases the parasites invade the mucosa and travel via the mesenteric and portal veins to the liver. Here substantial liquefaction necrosis of hepatocytes is induced 5–7 days after arrival of the amoeba in the liver, explaining the abrupt clinical onset with fever, right upper quadrant pain, and leucocytosis in previously healthy individuals. For unknown reasons ALAs are more frequent in adults than in children and more frequent in male than in female patients.

Ultrasound Features

ALAs are more frequently seen in the right liver lobe (77%); the most common location is the posterior segment of the right lobe. In the majority of patients a single lesion is found; nevertheless, about 40% of patients have two or more lesions. On ultrasound, typically a hypoechoic lesion measuring about 4–10 cm is seen (Figure 7.3). Inside the lesion there are often fine internal echoes. The shape is round and regular; due to the reduced echogenicity, mild

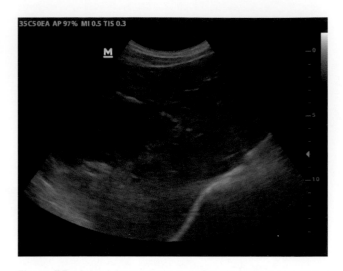

Figure 7.3 Round hypoechoic amoebic liver abscess without significant wall in the dorsal segments of the right lobe.

distal acoustic enhancement is seen. The lesion usually lacks significant wall echoes. All of these features may also occur in pyogenic abscesses and are thus not sufficient to make a distinction between the two.

Rarely, ALAs can present with atypical patterns like echogenic nodules, thick echogenic walls, mural nodules, and septations, causing difficulties in the differential diagnosis of solid masses and other lesions.

Further Investigations

Sonographic findings need to be combined with clinical information and serological results to reach the correct diagnosis. Diagnostic aspiration is an option and produces an 'anchovy sauce'–like product, but it is rarely indicated. Serology for anti-amoebic antibodies will be positive in more than 90% of patients with ALA and in combination with the history and the ultrasound findings it is usually diagnostic.

Treatment and Follow-Up

The treatment of choice is metronidazole. Usually a very rapid clinical response is seen within days – sonographically lesions shrink far more slowly. Initially the lesions tend to lose echogenicity with effective treatment and can become anechoic. For uncomplicated ALA there is no strong evidence for percutaneous aspiration or drainage over medical treatment only. Indications for percutaneous drainage are lack of response to metronidazole therapy, multiple or very large lesions, and continuing diagnostic uncertainty. ALAs may rupture into the pericardium, pleural cavity, or peritoneal cavity if they are located superficially. Prevention of these complications is another reason for initial drainage.

Time to complete resolution depends on the initial size of the lesion; it may take up to 3–6 months. In approximately 5% of ALA patients the resolution is not complete and post-ALA residual lesions may be found. These are usually hypo- to isoechoic compared to liver tissue and show a hyperechoic wall. The residual lesions were found to persist for more than a decade and may pose differential diagnostic problems.

Liver Schistosomiasis

Introduction and Clinical Picture

While genito-urinary schistosomiasis is caused by infection with the trematode *Schistosoma haematobium*, all other *Schistosoma* species affecting humans, mainly *S. mansoni* and less frequently *S. japonicum* and other species, cause intestinal and hepato-splenic schistosomiasis. *S. mansoni* occurs in Latin America, sub-Saharan Africa, and the Middle East, while other species have more localised geographical distributions in Africa, the Middle East, or Asia. Humans get infected percutaneously upon contact with freshwater contaminated with the infective larval stage of the parasite (cercariae), released in the water by a snail intermediate host. Mature adult worms live in the mesenteric venules, where females produce eggs that pass through the intestinal wall and are eliminated with faeces. In freshwater, eggs hatch ciliated miracidia that infect a competent snail, perpetuating the cycle. Acute infection with juvenile worms and early production of eggs may be clinically accompanied by a febrile systemic syndrome known as Katayama syndrome, characterised by fever, malaise, urticarial rash, abdominal pain, and respiratory symptoms. Chronic hepato-splenic disease results from prolonged release of eggs. Many eggs are not excreted and granuloma form around eggs trapped in the intestine and the liver, inducing a chronic inflammation that leads to disease manifestations. In the liver, chronic pathology is characterised by periportal fibrosis, also known as Symmer's pipe-stem fibrosis. Periportal fibrosis eventually leads to portal hypertension and collateral circulation, with variceal bleeding being the most dangerous complication of the disease. Clinical manifestations include hepatomegaly, splenomegaly, abdominal discomfort, and, in advanced cases, ascites and hematemesis. Pulmonary hypertension may also occur due to pulmonary arteritis from hematogenous spread of eggs.

Ultrasound Features

The typical ultrasound features of Symmer's fibrosis have been described and graded in WHO image patterns [4]. These include normal liver (pattern A), starry sky (pattern B), and thickening of the peripheral portal branches (pattern C), and progress to pathognomonic patterns: central portal wall thickening (pattern D), echogenic patches protruding in the parenchyma from the thickened central portal wall (pattern E), and fibrotic streaks reaching and retracting the liver capsule (pattern F) (Figure 7.4). Combinations of image patterns as well as thickening of

(a)

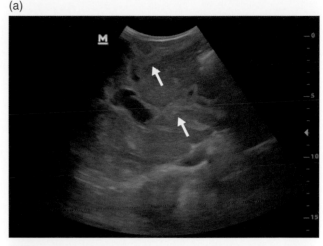

(b)

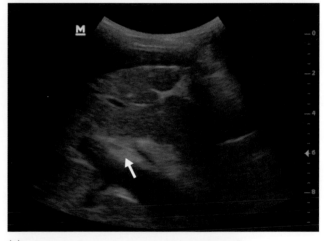

(c)

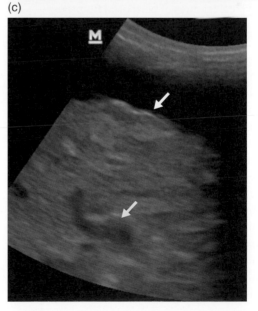

Figure 7.4 (a) Thickening of the peripheral portal branches (arrows), (b) echogenic patch and thickened central portal wall (arrow), as well as (c) retracted, nodular liver capsule (white arrow) in a Malawian patient with *Schistosoma mansoni* infection. The portal vein is dilated as a sign of portal hypertension (yellow arrow).

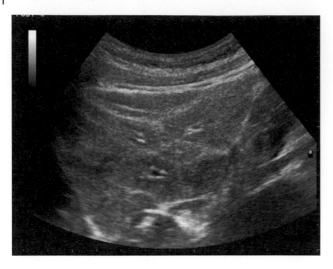

Figure 7.5 Criss-cross fibrotic septae of the tortoise-back pattern in a Filipino patient with *Schistosoma japonicum* infection. *Source:* Courtesy of Dr Axel Hempfling.

the gallbladder wall may also occur. Portal hypertension is indicated by portal dilatation, often with retained hepatopetal flow, and by collaterals. Splenomegaly and starry sky appearance of the spleen parenchyma are well described.

S. japonicum may cause a different pattern of fibrosis visualised as a 'meshwork' or 'tortoise-back' pattern (Figure 7.5).

Further Investigations

Patients with periportal fibrosis due to schistosomiasis retain normal liver function, different from other causes of chronic liver disease. Liver biopsy is not indicated in the presence of typical features of periportal fibrosis.

The diagnosis of schistosomiasis may be achieved by stool microscopy with identification of parasite eggs or PCR. Serology may be useful to diagnose *S. mansoni* schistosomiasis in travellers, but may be less useful in patients from endemic areas as antibodies persist for a long time even after therapy. Assays detecting parasite antigens in urine (e.g. circulating cationic antigen, CCA) are available, but their performance have been variable. Detection of CAA in serum or urine has much better performance but is not widely available at the time of writing.

Oesophageal varices require further investigation and potentially treatment by endoscopy. Ultrasound may be useful to stratify the risk of variceal bleeding: advanced periportal fibrosis (pattern E and even more pattern F) and portal vein size normalised by the height of the patient – portal vein diameter (mm)/height (m) >7.5 and even more >10 – are associated with increased bleeding risk.

Treatment and Follow-Up

Praziquantel is the drug of choice for the treatment of schistosomiasis. Regimens are not standardised and courses range from one to three days, repeated after one month as

praziquantel is not effective on juvenile flukes. Dividing the daily dosing in two administrations and administering the drug with food ameliorate the side effects, which include headache, dizziness, abdominal pain, nausea, and vomiting. A degree of amelioration of periportal fibrosis may be observed after several months from treatment, especially in children.

Clinical decision making for the management of portal hypertension requires expert consultation; options include surgical porto-systemic shunts, typically splenectomy with oesophagogastric devascularisation, and implantation of TIPS.

Fascioliasis

Fascioliasis is a foodborne infection caused by the trematodes *Fasciola hepatica*, the common liver fluke, and *F. gigantica*, the giant liver fluke. Humans get infected through ingestion of the larval stage of the parasite encysted on wild plants growing close to fresh water, such as watercress. Upon ingestion, the larvae migrate through the intestine into the peritoneal cavity and through the liver capsule. The juvenile flukes then migrate through the liver parenchyma until they reach the biliary tract and the gallbladder, where they develop into adults. During the larval migration (acute fascioliasis), symptoms include fever, abdominal pain, hepatosplenomegaly, and eosinophilia. On imaging, the acute phase may be characterised by abscess-like lesions or ill-defined hypoechoic lesions (Figure 7.6), which depart from the liver capsule and may change in number and location over time (*larva migrans*) [5]. Chronic fascioliasis with adult flukes is generally asymptomatic or pauci-symptomatic with malaise,

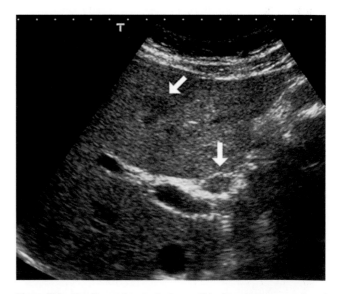

Figure 7.6 Confluent, hypoechoic small lesions (upper arrow) and periportal lymphadenopathy (lower arrow) in a Turkish patient with fascioliasis. *Source:* Courtesy of Prof Adnan Kabaalioğlu.

biliary colic, positive Murphy sign, and eosinophilia. On ultrasound, the most common finding is the dilatation of the common bile duct; sometimes the adult parasites may be observed as leaf-like floating structures in the gallbladder or in the common bile duct [5]. Positive serology in a patient with suggestive epidemiology and signs/symptoms is usually sufficient for diagnosis; however, hepatic biopsy in the acute stage will often be considered to rule out other diagnoses, especially malignancy. During the chronic phase, stool microscopy may allow the visualisation of parasite eggs. Triclabendazole is the drug of choice to treat fascioliasis. Triclabendazole is used at 10 mg/kg one daily for two days and the dose can be doubled in case of suspect resistance. Corticosteroids can be added when there are acute symptoms. Bithionol, nitazoxanide, and combination treatment of triclabendazole plus ivermectin or an artemisinin drug are possible second-line options. Praziquantel is not effective on *Fasciola*.

Toxocariasis

The abortive migration of the larvae of the dog parasite *Toxocara canis*, and less commonly of the cat parasite *Toxocara cati*, in the human body causes the syndrome known as 'visceral *larva migrans*', which involves the lungs, the liver, and occasionally other tissues such as the eye. In humans, infection is mainly acquired through accidental ingestion of parasite eggs dispersed in the environment. Most infections are asymptomatic. Vague abdominal pain, hepatomegaly, fever, and/or cough and wheeze may occur during acute infection, accompanied by eosinophilia. Liver lesions on ultrasound appear small, hypoechoic, and ill-defined, sometimes coalesce, and may change in number and place over time [6]. The pattern of contrast enhancement on CT or MRI allows differentiation with metastases. On histology, lesions are described as eosinophilic granulomas. Similar lesions may also be caused by other migrating larvae, such as those of *Ascaris*, *Ancylostoma*, and *Fasciola*. A positive serology supports the diagnosis. Symptomatic toxocariasis is treated with albendazole, associated with corticosteroids if required. Before treatment is started, eye examination is needed to ascertain the absence of eye involvement. This requires a different approach, primarily with steroids.

Opistorchiasis and Clonorchiasis

Small liver flukes encompass the trematodes *Clonorchis sinensis* (prevalent in China and far eastern Russia), *Opisthorchis viverrini* (prevalent in South East Asia), and *Opisthorchis felineus* (prevalent in Central Asia and eastern Europe). Humans, as well as several fish-eating mammals, get infected through ingestion of raw or poorly cooked fish

containing the parasite larvae. These ascend the biliary tree, where adult flukes develop and reside. Most infections are asymptomatic or pauci-symptomatic. Acute infection may present with fever, abdominal pain, nausea, hepatomegaly, jaundice, and allergic manifestations, accompanied by eosinophilia. Symptomatic chronic infection derives from cumulative infections with high parasite load, causing chronic biliary inflammation and fibrosis. Symptoms may include poor appetite, dyspepsia, weight loss, diarrhoea, and jaundice, as well as those caused by complications such as the formation of calculi, cholangitis, abscesses, and pancreatitis. *O. viverrini* and *C. sinensis* are International Agency for Research on Cancer (IARC) class 1 carcinogens, associated with the development of cholangiocarcinoma. On imaging, typical but non-specific findings are heterogeneous liver parenchyma, peripheral intrahepatic duct strictures, and dilatations, with hypoechoic periductal halo due to oedema and hyperechoic biliary walls due to fibrosis. Hyperechoic material, possibly calcified, may be visible in the dilated biliary ducts. The diagnosis of small liver fluke infection may be achieved by detection of eggs in faeces; in-house serological assays exist but are poorly specific; eosinophilia is present in only a minority of patients chronically infected. Praziquantel is the drug of choice to treat small liver fluke infection; alternative drugs include benzimidazoles.

Ascariasis

Ascaris lumbricoides, the round worm, is estimated to infect 1.2 billion people worldwide. Although the vast majority of infections are asymptomatic, pathology can be associated with the migration of the worms through the duodenal papilla into the biliary system or the pancreatic duct causing obstruction, cholangitis, or pancreatitis. Ultrasound can detect the worms (or worm fragments) in the biliary tract. The adult worms are 20 cm long and 5 mm in diameter, with a peculiar sonographic appearance. In high-resolution longitudinal sections, the worm appears as four parallel lines separated by three anechoic bands: the outer echogenic lines are the exterior cuticle of the worm, the two interior lines the lining of the worm's alimentary tract. This gives a 'strip sign' appearance, sometimes also called 'spaghetti sign' (especially when multiple worms are present; Figure 7.7) [7]. Diagnosis of ascariasis is usually achieved by stool examinations with visualisation of the eggs or, occasionally, by identification of worms passed with faeces. In most cases oral administration of albendazole is sufficient treatment. Endoscopic intervention with extraction of the worm across the papilla is indicated in cases of acute severe pyogenic cholangitis, recurrent biliary colic, and when worms persist in the bile duct for longer than two weeks.

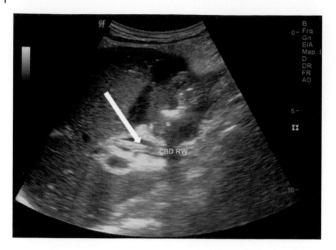

Figure 7.7 A patient with acute epigastric pain, common bile duct (CBD) showing double linear echogenic wall, indicating ascariasis 'strip sign' (arrow). *Source:* Lynser, D., Handique, A., Daniala, C. et al. (2015). Sonographic images of hepato-pancreatico-biliary and intestinal ascariasis: A pictorial review. *Insights Imaging.* 6(6): 641–646. doi:10.1007/s13244-015-0428-7. Creative Commons Attribution 4.0 International License (http://creativecommons.org/licenses/by/4.0).

Bacterial Infections of the Liver

Ultrasound has a primary role in diagnosis and follow-up of pyogenic liver abscesses, so this topic will be discussed in detail. Mycobacterial infections may involve the liver and will be considered briefly. Focal liver lesions are observed in some cases of melioidosis, syphilis, and brucellosis, so these topics will be touched on as well. Finally, leptospirosis is discussed briefly as it may present with acute acalculous cholecystitis.

Pyogenic Liver Abscess

Introduction and Clinical Picture
Pyogenic liver abscesses are the most common form of liver abscess in Europe. Most patients have an underlying condition predisposing them to the development of pyogenic liver abscesses. The most common source of the infection is extension from the biliary tract in patients with bacterial cholangitis or cholecystitis. Frequently patients have a history of surgery or intervention of the biliary system. Involvement of the liver is also seen due to spread via the portal vein from appendicitis, diverticulitis, or other inflammatory bowel disease. Hematogenous spread from bacterial endocarditis or osteomyelitis and penetrating injury from trauma are possible but less frequent underlying causes. The clinical presentation can be similar to ALA, with fever, anorexia, and right upper quadrant pain, although the clinical onset is often slower than in amoebic

disease. Most patients will have a leukocytosis and elevated gamma-glutamyltransferase and alkaline phosphatase.

Liver abscesses are mainly caused by Gram-negative bacteria and *Escherichia coli* has traditionally been the most commonly isolated organism. Often the infection is polymicrobial. Anaerobic bacteria species like *Clostridium* and *Bacteroides* are typically present, although less often isolated when no anaerobic cultures are performed.

Since the mid-1980s, a hypervirulent strain of *Klebsiella pneumoniae* (mostly serotype K1 or K2) has been increasingly identified as an important cause of mono-microbial community-acquired liver abscesses in Asians, particularly in patients from Taiwan and Korea. Diabetes mellitus is a predisposing condition, but a large proportion of patients are previously healthy. Metastatic infections, such as septic emboli in the lung, endophthalmitis, and meningitis, are frequently observed.

Ultrasound Features
The sensitivity of ultrasound for liver abscess detection is highly dependent on the localisation of the abscess. In subphrenic areas lesions may be missed, therefore CT may be required for additional imaging. Owing to the varied appearance the differential diagnosis of liver abscesses is wide, including haemorrhagic simple cysts, focal hematoma, as well as benign or malignant tumours.

Pyogenic liver abscesses are variable in shape and size and the echogenicity can range from almost anechoic cysts to echogenic masses (Figure 7.8). With liquefaction the majority of abscesses become less echogenic than liver; they are often increasingly heterogeneous and may show central necrotic cystic areas. Septations or floating fine echogenic debris may be seen. The hypo- to anechoic lesions can have distal acoustic enhancement. The abscess walls vary from indistinct to thick and are often irregular. When gas-forming bacteria cause the abscess, gas bubbles may be seen as highly reflective foci, possibly with acoustic 'dirty' shadows. The finding of gas in an abscess is characteristic of pyogenic lesions and helps to differentiate it from ALAs, which never contain gas (unless gas entered during diagnostic aspiration).

K. pneumoniae liver abscesses are predominantly single lesions, and have a solid, echogenic appearance on ultrasound. They have irregular or indistinct lesion margins and often only small quantities of pus (<2 mL) can be aspirated due to high viscosity.

Further Investigations
Ultrasound-guided needle aspiration confirms the diagnosis. The bacteriological yield from pus cultures is far higher than from blood cultures taken at the same time. Moreover, while blood cultures often demonstrate only a single agent,

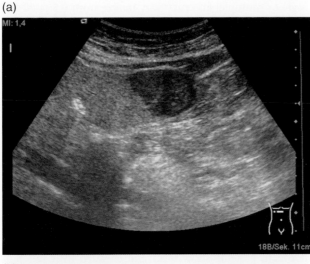

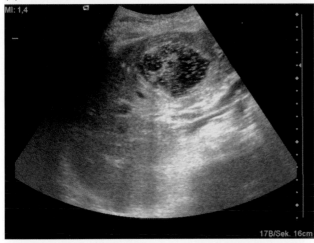

Figure 7.8 Pyogenic liver abscesses. (a) Abscess in the left liver lobe with an almost 'solid' appearance. (b) Larger abscess with echogenic floating debris, in the ventral area; gas bubbles create 'dirty shadows'. (c) Almost anechoic abscess with puncture needle in situ.

pus cultures more frequently reveal the polymicrobial nature of the abscess.

Treatment and Follow-Up

The main treatment for pyogenic liver abscesses is systemic antibiotics and drainage for larger lesions. Surgical drainage is usually not required and aspiration or drainage under ultrasound guidance is a good alternative. Percutaneous aspiration using an 18G needle can be used, depending on the size of the liver abscess. In case of multiple abscesses, the deepest is targeted first to avoid overlying artefacts from introduced gas bubbles. Repeated aspirations may be required depending on the clinical course. Percutaneous drainage is performed using Seldinger technique to place an 8–10F pigtail catheter. This is fixed and left for free drainage; additionally intermittent lavage with normal saline is possible. The drain is removed when the patient improves clinically or when the catheter fails to drain significant amounts of pus. Whether needle aspiration or catheter drainage is superior as first-line treatment is still open to debate; probably intermittent needle aspiration is as effective as continuous catheter drainage for the treatment of pyogenic liver abscess. Owing to the additional advantages of procedure simplicity, reduced price, and fewer in-hospital complications with staff unfamiliar with how to handle the drain, needle aspiration is often considered as a first-line approach, especially for smaller (<5 cm) abscesses.

On ultrasound follow-up, the resolution of treated lesions are significantly slower than the resolution of the clinical findings. The majority will resolve to sonographically normal liver parenchyma, but some lesions may show persisting cystic cavities or focal areas of calcification.

Tuberculosis and Other Mycobacteria

Primary infection with *Mycobacterium tuberculosis* of the liver is rare, but should be considered in patients with lung tuberculosis (TB) or TB in other locations. In these patients concomitant involvement of the liver is common (up to 80% in disseminated TB), but often without clinical manifestations. Patients show the non-specific systemic symptoms of fever, weight loss, and night sweats, and may additionally complain of abdominal pain (usually mild) and present abnormal liver function tests. Sonographically, mainly two forms of liver involvement in TB are seen. An enlarged liver with a homogeneous bright echo pattern points to diffuse hepatic granulomatous disease. Focal tuberculomas present as 'abscess-like' masses (Figure 7.9); this nodular hepatic disease is more often seen in immunocompromised individuals, especially HIV patients. On ultrasound the masses are usually hypoechoic or of mixed echogenicity, may be

(a)

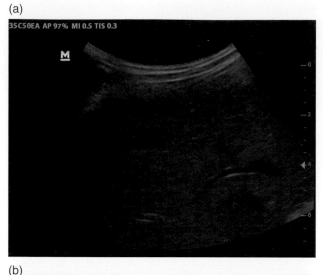

(b)

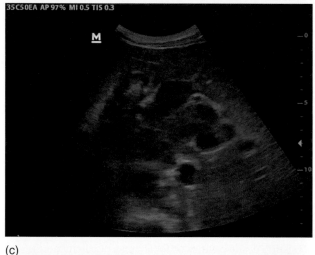

(c)

Figure 7.9 Disseminated tuberculosis in an HIV patient. (a) Hypoechoic focal lesions in the liver. (b) Abdominal lymphadenopathy. (c) Multiple 'miliary' focal spleen lesions.

single or multiple, and may vary in size from 0.5 to 12 cm. Additional ultrasound findings such as ascites, abdominal lymphadenopathy, and co-existing hypoechoic splenic lesions may suggest tuberculosis as the underlying diagnosis [8]. Diagnostic aspiration can be necessary if organisms cannot be isolated from other specimens. For treatment a combination of four anti-TB drugs is used. It should be noted that the hepatic lesions (as with all tuberculous lesions in general) during successful treatment initially may increase in size as the improved immunological response increases the inflammatory reaction. This does not point to treatment failure and it should be followed up.

Mycobacterium avium complex is a common opportunistic infection found in liver biopsies in HIV patients with CD4 <50/mm^3. It is usually widely disseminated throughout the abdomen; patients show fever and elevated liver function tests, in particular the alkaline phosphatase, possibly due to granulomatous obstruction of small biliary radices.

The most common reported ultrasound pattern is hepatomegaly, often with diffuse increased echogenicity similar to the diffuse disease seen in TB.

Melioidosis

Melioidosis is an infection caused by *Burkholderia pseudomallei*, prevalent in South East Asia and usually occurring in patients with underlying predisposing diseases such as diabetes mellitus, chronic renal failure, alcoholism, or malignancy. Exposure to water and soil, for instance in rice paddies, is an important risk factor. The clinical manifestations of melioidosis range from asymptomatic and subclinical to localised forms and acute septicaemia. Mortality from acute septicaemia exceeds 80% if not treated adequately. While any organ system can be affected by melioidosis, lung, spleen, and liver are the most commonly involved organs. Visceral organ abscesses appear on ultrasound as multiple, small, hypoechoic lesions. Melioid liver abscesses can show different ultrasound features. In abscesses larger than 2 cm, the lesion may have a multiloculated appearance with the locules corresponding to small abscesses at various stages of coalescence ('honeycomb sign') (Figure 7.10). In abscesses larger than 5 cm, smaller abscesses can be observed surrounding the primary honeycomb abscess ('necklace sign'). The larger abscess can be accompanied by secondary hypoechoic lesions representing 'satellite abscesses' [9]. Abscesses are most frequently located in the right lobe (about 80%), vary in size from 2 to 15 cm, and do not show calcification. Ruptures into neighbouring structures are reported. While in most other types of bacterial infection splenic abscesses are unusual, the detection of concomitant splenic abscesses is highly suggestive in

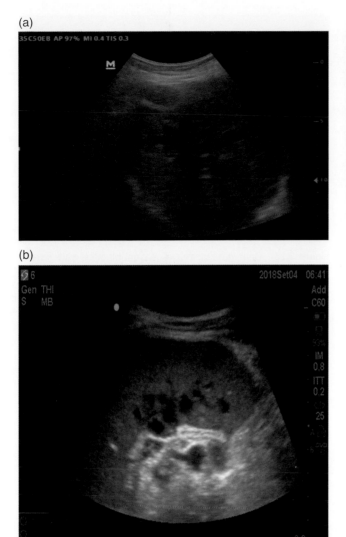

Figure 7.10 Multiple clustered hypoechoic lesions in diabetic patients from Laos with culture-proven melioidosis. (a) Liver; (b) spleen.

Figure 7.11 Hypoechoic liver lesion due to syphilis in an HIV-positive patient. Histology revealed a granulomatous inflammation, syphilis serology was positive, and the lesions disappeared after treatment with penicillin. *Source:* Courtesy of Dr Francesco Taccari.

melioidosis. The definite diagnosis is made by positive culture of the organism from the blood or infected organs. The recommended treatment is ceftazidime 3×2 g for 10 days followed by co-trimoxazole for 20 weeks.

Syphilis

Syphilis can affect the liver during the secondary stage of the disease as syphilitic hepatitis and during the tertiary stage as gummata. Syphilitic hepatitis, characterised by a high alkaline phosphatase relative to transaminases, is relatively frequent and the liver is sonographically normal.

Gummata, which can be seen as focal liver lesions, are rarely reported. Abdominal ultrasonography shows heterogeneous hypoechoic masses (Figure 7.11); hepatic and portal veins are normal. Typically multiple lesions are scattered through both hepatic lobes, simulating malignant lesions. Upon biopsy histological analysis usually shows an inflammatory infiltrate with multiple granulomas (and possibly multinucleated giant cells). As non-treponemal tests like the Venereal Disease Research Laboratory (VDRL) test are less sensitive in tertiary syphilis, it is important to obtain a treponemal test (such as fluorescent treponemal antibody absorption [FTA-Abs] or treponema pallidum haemagglutination [TPHA]) to serologically support the suspected diagnosis. Treatment of choice is penicillin.

Brucellosis

Brucellosis is the most common zoonosis worldwide affecting people in contact with cattle. It is endemic in the Mediterranean, Mongolia, India, Mexico, and Central America, with more than 500 000 new cases annually. It commonly presents with fever and systemic symptoms like anorexia and night sweats. Focal infection with *Brucella abortus* can involve any organ, with by far the most common localisation being osteoarticular sites. Abscesses in the liver and the spleen are well described, although they occur in only approximately 1% of brucellosis patients, mostly in adults. On ultrasound these abscesses appear as hypoechoic, usually single masses (75% of reported cases), more frequently located in the right lobe (74%) with central areas of liquefaction, and the majority show an area of focal central calcification (78%) (Figure 7.12) [10]. A different and less frequent pattern shows multiple hypoechoic,

(a)

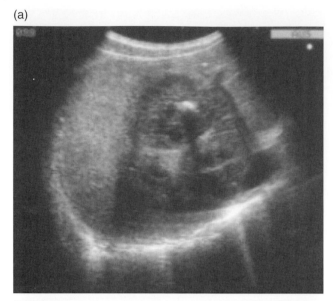

(b)

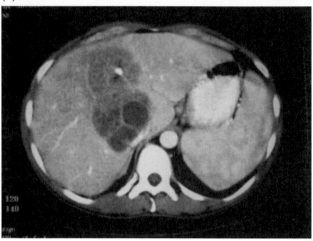

Figure 7.12 Brucellar liver abscess with a characteristic central calcification seen on both ultrasound (a) and CT scan (b). *Source:* Heller et al. (2015), *American Journal of Tropical Medicine and Hygiene.*

smaller abscesses, which often involve the spleen and liver [10]. These 'miliary' lesions may be smaller than 1 cm, show few calcifications, and have been observed in adults and children; the main differential for this pattern is disseminated TB. As the imaging findings are not totally specific, they need to be combined with positive serology before treatment (doxycycline plus rifampicin, both for six weeks) is started. Nevertheless, an abscess with a central calcification should always raise suspicion of brucellosis.

Leptospirosis

Leptospirosis is one of the most prevalent zoonotic infections worldwide. It occurs in tropical and temperate regions, but is about 10 times more common in tropical regions.

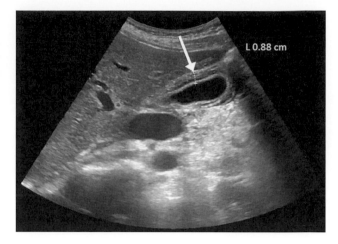

Figure 7.13 Oedematous, thickened gallbladder wall (arrow) in a patient with acute acalculous cholecystitis due to leptospirosis. *Source:* Castelijn, D.A.R., Wattel-Louis, G.H. (2018). An acute acalculous cholecystitis in a returned travel couple. PLoS Negl. Trop. Dis. 12(3): e0006177. Creative Commons Attribution 4.0 International License (http://creativecommons.org/licenses/by/4.0).

Various mammals are natural hosts, but rodents are the most important to human transmission. Transmission occurs through exposure to animal urine, contaminated water, or animal tissues. Portals of entry are skin abrasions or cuts, mucous membranes, and conjunctiva. The clinical picture is variable, ranging from mild, self-limiting disease to multi-organ failure, encompassing hepatitis, myocarditis, acute renal failure, aseptic meningitis, or pulmonary haemorrhage. Acute acalculous cholangitis is an uncommon presentation, but given the high prevalence of leptospirosis in tropical regions, it is important to keep this differential diagnosis in mind. Patients typically present with right upper quadrant pain and a positive Murphy's sign. Ultrasound findings include an oedematous, thickened gallbladder wall, without sludge or stones (Figure 7.13). Additional investigations include serology, PCR, and culture, but these may often be unavailable. The differential diagnosis of acalculous cholecystitis is broad (including dengue fever, which is described later), so it is important to pay close attention to the clinical presentation and local epidemiology. Treatment of leptospirosis is with doxycycline, but abdominal coverage should be considered in severely ill patients as acalculous cholecystitis may be complicated by perforation.

Fungal Infections of the Liver

Fungal liver abscesses are the only notable presentation on ultrasound and may have characteristic ultrasonographic features.

Fungal Liver Abscess

Disseminated fungal infections involving the liver mainly affect immune-compromised hosts, particularly patients with prolonged or recurrent neutropenia. Patients with leukaemia, patients undergoing chemotherapy for lymphoproliferative disorders, and recipients of organ transplants are at high risk. Recognised hepatic fungal pathogens are cryptococcosis, histoplasmosis, mucormycosis, and occasionally aspergillosis, but the most frequent underlying organisms are *Candida* species. These should be suspected in any patient with neutropenia and fever unresponsive to antibacterial treatment. Ultrasound is frequently used as the first-line investigation. When neutropenia is severe, due to the absence of an inflammatory response there may be no focal lesions visible. If focal lesions are present, they are often multiple and small in size. Different sonographic patterns have been described, the most characteristic being the 'wheel-within-a-wheel' appearance, with a hypoechoic or even anechoic central nidus surrounded by an echogenic ring, surrounded again by a hypoechoic halo (Figure 7.14). Histologically this has been shown to represent a central area of necrosis with fungal micelles, surrounded by inflammatory cells and fibrosis. 'Bull's eyes' lesions, believed to be associated with higher neutrophil counts, are another recognised pattern. They measure 1–4cm in size, and have an echogenic centre surrounded by a hypoechoic halo. Also, uniformly hypoechoic nodules and nodules with echogenic foci due to focal calcification are described. Definite diagnosis of systemic fungal infections can be challenging. Targeted aspiration of the focal liver lesions may be falsely negative, but should be attempted if culture of more easily accessible fluids (blood culture, urine culture) remains negative. Treatment with antifungals is guided by culture results.

Viral Infections Affecting the Liver

In this final section, HIV and HIV-associated diseases of the liver are discussed. Dengue is also discussed as it can present with gallbladder wall thickening, while viral hepatitis will be discussed in Chapter 8.

HIV and HIV-Associated Diseases

The liver can be involved in a variety of diseases associated with HIV infection; an increased size of the liver is found most frequently. The changes can be due to viral hepatitis co-infection, opportunistic infections, and cancers associated with immunosuppression, but also metabolic changes like steatosis are frequently seen (partly as a side effect of antiretroviral drugs). Generalised *Pneumocystis jirovecii* infection can present with the so-called 'snowstorm pattern' – multiple diffuse small echogenic foci, often without acoustic shadow in liver and/or spleen. Initially the pattern was thought to be specific for this infection, but it was also found in association with *Candida*, *Aspergillus*, and toxoplasmosis. Hypoechoic lesions are seen with a variety of infections, but also focal infiltration of HIV-associated non-Hodgkin's lymphoma needs to be considered. Owing to the broad differential diagnoses in immune-compromised patients (Table 7.1), ultrasound-guided biopsy is often required to reveal the underlying cause of findings [11].

HIV Kaposi's Sarcoma

Kaposi's sarcoma (KS) is a low-grade mesenchymal tumour involving blood and lymphatic vessels. It primarily affects the skin, but can cause disseminated disease in

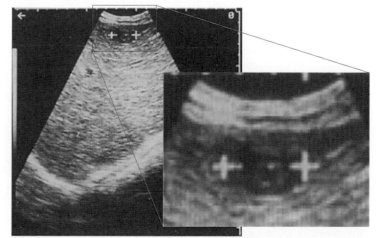

Figure 7.14 Small fungal liver abscess in an HIV-positive patient showing a 'wheel-within-a-wheel' pattern. *Source:* Courtesy of Prof Enrico Brunetti.

Table 7.1 Ultrasound appearance of HIV-associated liver disease.

Diffuse enlargement of the liver	Hyperechoic focal lesion	Hypoechoic focal lesion
Hepatitis B and C	*Pneumocystis jiroveci* ('snowstorm pattern')	Infiltration due to lymphoma
Cytomegalovirus		TB abscesses
Atypical mycobacteria – *Mycobacterium avium* complex (MAC), *M. kansasii*	Calcified toxoplasmosis or TB	Bacterial and fungal abscess
	Kaposi's sarcoma	Syphilitic gummata
Granulomatous hepatitis – tuberculosis (TB)	Hepatocellular carcinoma	Bacillary angiomatosis (peliosis)
Diffuse infiltration in malignant lymphoma		Toxoplasmosis
Fatty infiltration		

(<100/mm^3). Although the aetiology often remains unclear, it is found in association with opportunistic infections, such as cytomegalovirus, *Cryptosporidium*, and possibly *Giardia*, *Microsporidium*, and herpesvirus. The symptoms of biliary disease may often be relatively mild; liver function tests may reveal elevated excretion enzymes like alkaline phosphatase (ALP) and gamma-glutamyl transferase (GGT). Ultrasound is the most cost-effective initial imaging test. The ultrasound findings resemble features of sclerosing cholangitis, such as diffuse thickening of the proximal bile ducts, sometimes associated to bright echogenic thickening surrounding the whole portal triads (Figure 7.16). Thickening of the gallbladder wall can also be present, while involvement of the distal bile ducts is more rarely described. The mainstay of treatment lies not in treating the

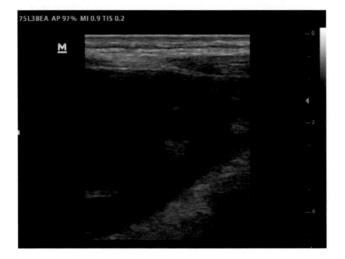

Figure 7.15 Echogenic focal lesions in an HIV-positive patient with disseminated Kaposi's sarcoma involving the liver.

a variety of organs, including the liver and spleen. Human herpes virus type 8 (also called KS-associated herpesvirus) has been identified as a causal link to KS in patients with HIV. Although the development of KS is associated with immunosuppression, it is also seen in patients with normal or only moderately suppressed CD4 cells. Ultrasound may show hepatomegaly with multifocal hyperechoic nodules (5–15 mm in diameter) resembling haemangiomas (Figure 7.15). Similar findings have been described in the spleen.

AIDS Cholangiopathy

The biliary system of HIV patients can be affected in 'acquired immunodeficiency syndrome (AIDS) cholangiopathy'. This refers to an acalculous, secondary cholangiopathy typically affecting patients with very low CD4 counts

(a)

(b)

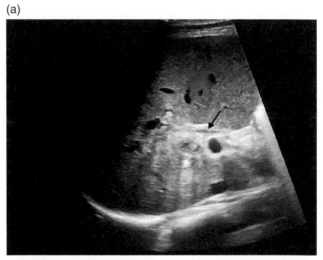

Figure 7.16 HIV cholangiopathy with (a) thickened wall of the common bile duct (arrow) and (b) mild dilatation and bright fibrotic changes in a portal triad towards the left liver lobe (arrows).

specific infection, but in initiating antiretroviral therapy to restore the immune system.

Dengue Fever

Dengue virus, a member of the genus Flavivirus, transmitted by mosquito *Aedes aegypti*, is a common cause of fever in the tropics. The countries with the highest incidence are found in South East Asia, but cases are seen throughout the (sub-)tropics worldwide. Clinically dengue manifests with sudden onset of high fever and intense headache, as well as muscle, joint, and back pain. Elevated transaminases are frequently seen, triggering ultrasonography. Haemorrhagic diathesis, thrombocytopenia, and concurrent haemoconcentration due to capillary leakage are constant findings, especially in more severe cases. As a result of this leakage extravascular fluid accumulation can be found by ultrasound. Besides non-specific hepatosplenomegaly, ultrasound may reveal gallbladder wall thickening (due to wall oedema; Figure 7.17), ascites, and

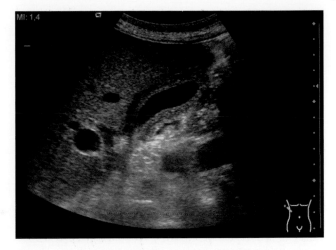

Figure 7.17 Thickened wall of the gallbladder in a patient with dengue fever (small bilateral pleural effusions were additionally noted [not shown], platelet count was 32000/mm^3).

pleural effusions. Whether these findings can be useful as predictors of a more severe clinical course is still debated. Treatment is purely supportive.

References

1 Bélard, S., Tamarozzi, F., Bustinduy, A.L. et al. (2016). Point-of-care ultrasound assessment of tropical infectious diseases – a review of applications and perspectives. *Am. J. Trop. Med. Hyg.* 94: 8–21.

2 Brunetti, E., Kern, P., Vuitton, D.A., and Writing panel for the WHO-IWGE. (2010). Expert consensus for the diagnosis and treatment of cystic and alveolar echinococcosis in humans. *Acta Trop.* 114 (1): 1–16. https://doi.org/10.1016/j.actatropica.2009.11.001.

3 Kratzer, W., Gruener, B., Kaltenbach, T.E. et al. (2015). Proposal of an ultrasonographic classification for hepatic alveolar echinococcosis: echinococcosis multilocularis Ulm classification-ultrasound. *World J. Gastroenterol.* 21 (43): 12392–12402.

4 Niamey Working Group, Richter, J., Hatz, C. et al. (2000). *Ultrasound in Schistosomiasis: A Practical Guide to The Standardized Use of Ultrasonography for The Assessment of Schistosomiasis-Related Morbidity*. Geneva: World Health Organization.

5 Kabaalioglu, A., Ceken, K., Alimoglu, E. et al. (2007). Hepatobiliary fascioliasis: sonographic and CT findings in 87 patients during the initial phase and long-term follow-up. *Am. J. Roentgenol.* 189 (4): 824–828.

6 Lim, J.H. (2008). Toxocariasis of the liver: visceral larva migrans. *Abdom. Imaging* 33 (2): 151–156.

7 Lynser, D., Handique, A., Daniala, C. et al. (2015). Sonographic images of hepato-pancreatico-biliary and intestinal ascariasis: a pictorial review. *Insights Imaging* 6 (6): 641–646.

8 Heller, T., Goblirsch, S., Wallrauch, C. et al. (2010). Abdominal tuberculosis: sonographic diagnosis and treatment response in HIV-positive adults in rural South Africa. *Int. J. Infect. Dis.* 14 (Suppl 3): e108–e112.

9 Maude, R.R., et al. (2012). Prospective observational study of the frequency and features of intra-abdominal abscesses in patients with melioidosis in northeast Thailand. *Trans. R. Soc. Trop. Med. Hyg.* 106: 629–631.

10 Heller, T., Bélard, S., Wallrauch, C. et al. (2015). Patterns of hepato-splenic *Brucella* abscesses on cross-sectional imaging - a review of clinical and imaging features. *Am. J. Trop. Med. Hyg.* 93: 761–766. https://doi.org/10.4269/ajtmh.15-0225.

11 Brunetti, E., Brigada, R., Poletti, F. et al. (2006). The current role of abdominal ultrasound in the clinical management of patients with AIDS. *Ultraschall Med.* 27 (01): 20–33.

8

Ultrasound in Chronic Liver Disease

Matteo Rosselli[1,2], Davide Roccarina[2,3], and Ivica Grgurevic[4]

[1] *Department of Internal Medicine, San Giuseppe Hospital, USL Toscana Centro, Empoli, Italy*
[2] *Division of Medicine, Institute for Liver and Digestive Health, University College London, Royal Free Hospital, London, UK*
[3] *Department of Internal Medicine and Hepatology, Azienda Ospedaliero-Universitaria di Careggi, Florence, Italy*
[4] *Department of Gastroenterology, Hepatology and Clinical Nutrition, University Hospital Dubrava, University of Zagreb School of Medicine and Faculty of Pharmacy and Biochemistry, Zagreb, Croatia*

Chronic liver disease (CLD) is the consequence of persistent inflammation leading to fibrosis, cirrhosis, portal hypertension (PH), and eventually liver failure. The natural history varies according to aetiology, the site of inflammation, fibrosis progression rate and onset, and the severity of PH, which is in general considered the most important clinical endpoint. Ultrasound is the first imaging modality used to diagnose CLD as well as for hepatocellular carcinoma (HCC) screening, and is therefore one of the most important medical tools in clinical hepatology. This chapter aims to describe the sonographic hallmarks of cirrhosis and clinically significant portal hypertension (CSPH), as well as the differences that might be found among various aetiologies and examples of pathological conditions that mimic cirrhosis on ultrasound imaging.

When evaluating patients with CLD, ultrasound assessment should include liver echotexture, echogenicity, capsule and margins, the relationship between the right and caudate lobes, and eventually the description of hypertrophy/hypotrophy of the right and left liver lobes. The presence or absence of focal lesions should be highlighted. The gallbladder and biliary ducts should also be evaluated. The portal venous system should be assessed, highlighting features compatible with PH including the description of porto-systemic vascular collaterals and splenomegaly. The inferior vena cava (IVC) calibre and hepatic vein patency and flow are also important to exclude features compatible with cardiogenic cirrhosis or Budd–Chiari syndrome. Usually the hepatic artery is not described unless specific findings are seen, such as ectasia, aneurisms, pseudoaneurysms, and arterio-venous communications. Finally, the presence of ascites, its aspect, and its amount should be reported.

General Ultrasonic Features of Chronic Liver Disease

Size, Shape, Echotexture, and Contour

The measurement of liver diameters does not seem to be a significant parameter to specify and its use has been abandoned in general practice, as suggested by international guidelines (see also Chapter 3) [1]. It is preferable to give a general description of hepatic enlargement, and hypertrophy or hypotrophy/atrophy of segments/lobe that might influence the shape and general appearance of the liver. In general, although there might be some variability among different aetiologies, morphological signs of cirrhosis include hypotrophy/atrophy of the right liver lobe, and compensatory hypertrophy of the caudate and left lobe. At first glance the morphological appearance is sufficient usually to suggest cirrhosis, although a caudate to right liver lobe width ratio >0.65 using the main bifurcation of the portal vein (PV) as a landmark between the two lobes is more precise and has high accuracy in diagnosing an advanced fibrotic process (Figure 8.1) [2]. Other morphological signs are related to retraction and hypertrophy of different areas of the liver and include enlargement of the gallbladder fossa secondary to atrophy of the right liver lobe, medial segment of the left lobe, and hypertrophy of the caudate lobe; enlargement of the periportal space secondary to atrophy of the left lobe's medial segments [3]; focal capsular retraction, which might be more pronounced in certain areas as it is observed eventually along the posterior margin of the liver adjacent to the right kidney and is known as 'notch sign' [4]; and areas of confluent fibrosis corresponding to wedge-shaped areas with capsular retraction that might be seen in advanced cirrhosis.

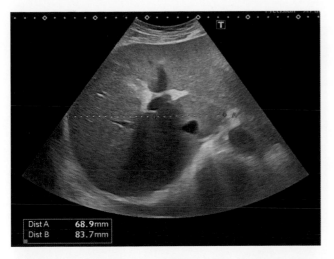

Figure 8.1 At a glance the morphological appearance of the liver shows hypertrophy of the caudate lobe and hypotrophy of the right lobe. The caudate to right liver lobe ratio is 0.82, which more specifically suggests chronic liver disease changes in keeping with cirrhosis.

One of the most common findings in CLD is the heterogeneity of liver echotexture as an expression of the backscattering of the ultrasound beam on uneven surface, secondary to inflammatory changes, fibrosis, and nodular regeneration. The heterogenic echotexture can vary from mild to very pronounced ('coarse echopattern'), usually according to the severity of CLD (Figure 8.2). However, it is also of note that the underlying aetiology has an impact on tissue damage, inflammatory response, and distribution of fibrosis, and hence can influence the echotexture heterogeneity, as will be described later in this chapter. In addition, the inappropriate regeneration of the hepatocytes in response to tissue damage is associated with nodularities, which can be very subtle, more obvious, or sometimes so pronounced as to be confounded with a lesion of a different nature, requiring contrast imaging for differential diagnosis.

In normal conditions the margins of the liver are usually sharp, while in CLD and advanced cirrhosis they become rounded and the outline is typically irregular or even nodular

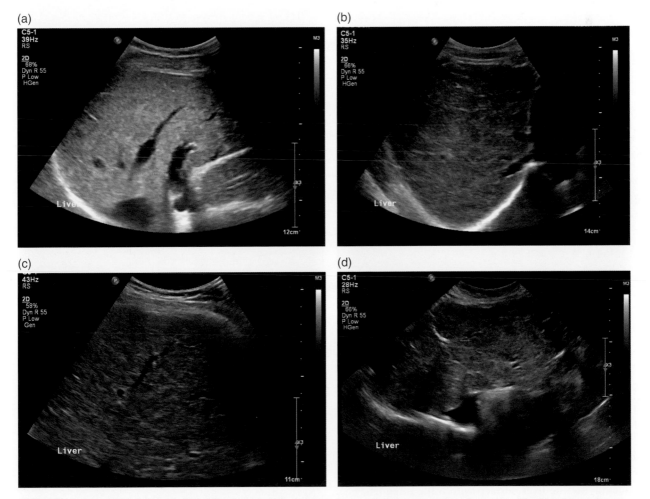

Figure 8.2 Examples of heterogenic echotexture of liver parenchyma of different grades of severity. (a) Mild; (b) moderate–severe; (c) severe; (d) severe with an extremely heterogenic echotexture and a mixed macronodular pattern.

(a) (b)

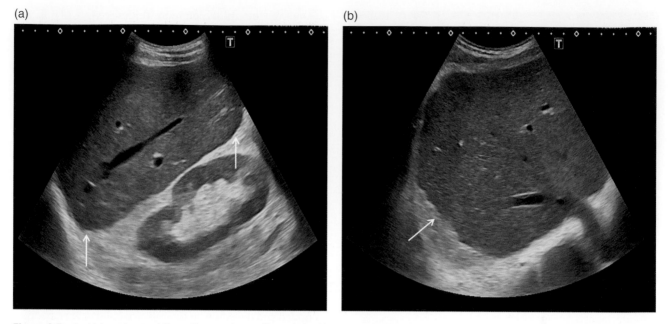

Figure 8.3 (a, b) In advanced liver disease the outline of the liver is irregular and nodular, with less distinct and rounded margins (arrows) owing to parenchymal and capsular retraction.

(a) (b)

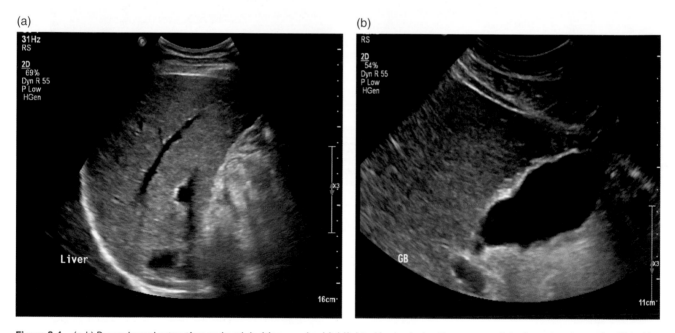

Figure 8.4 (a, b) Parenchymal retraction and nodularities are also highlighted by exploring the contour of the hepatic veins and gallbladder.

(Figure 8.3). The hepatic veins and gallbladder contour irregularities are also very sensitive signs of CLD (Figure 8.4). It is of note that sometimes irregularities of the liver outline and parenchymal changes might be very subtle. The accuracy of ultrasound in detecting early stages and micronodular regeneration can be missed in about 30% of cases [5]. Along these lines, magnifying the liver surface with a high-frequency transducer will highlight structural modifications and help to avoid false-negative results (Figure 8.5) [1].

Echogenicity

The echogenicity of liver parenchyma refers to its brightness, a feature that is most commonly found and used to describe steatosis. Although the most common cause of steatosis is nutrition-related lipid dysmetabolism, steatosis can also be found in different hepatopathies such as alcohol-related liver disease, viral hepatitis [6], hemochromatosis, or be drug induced [7]. According to its ultrasound

(a)

(b)

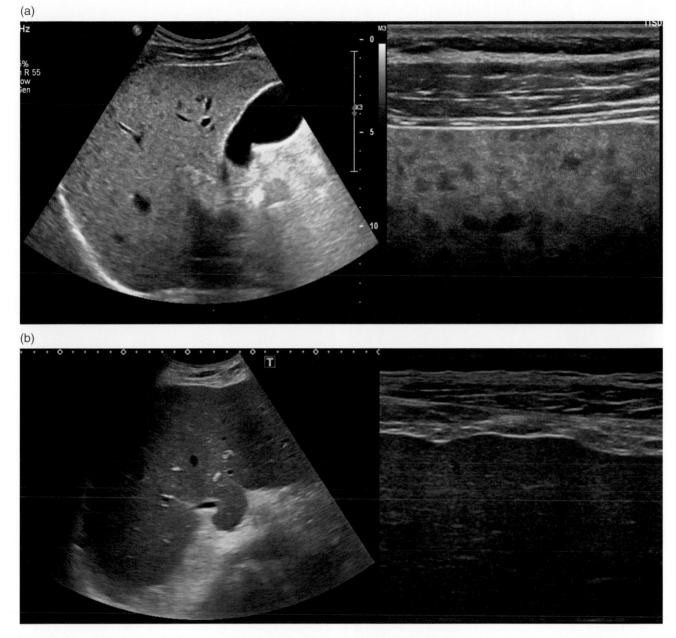

Figure 8.5   (a, b) Parenchymal micronodularities and irregular outline are highlighted by magnifying the liver surface and parenchyma with a high-frequency transducer (typically 8-14 mHz), increasing ultrasound diagnostic accuracy.

appearance, steatosis can be classified as grade I or mild, when liver echogenicity is more pronounced than the renal cortex but there is no or very mild attenuation of the ultrasound beam through the liver parenchyma; grade II or moderate, where fat-induced attenuation reduces the visibility of the posterior segments and the contour of the hepatic veins and portal venous system; or grade III or severe, when posterior attenuation is so severe that the posterior segments of the liver and the outline of the diaphragm cannot be seen or are barely visible (Figure 8.6) [8, 9].

Hepatic steatosis can be diffuse, focal, multifocal, or have a very irregular and ill-defined distribution named the 'geographical' pattern (Figure 8.7). Steatosis in some cases can be well defined as a single area or scattered throughout the liver and mimic neoplastic lesions, sometimes requiring second-level imaging for diagnostic certainty. Nevertheless, a differential criterion between focal steatosis and a focal lesion is that steatosis never deforms the hepatic structures, in particular the liver capsule, bile ducts, and vasculature (Figure 8.8).

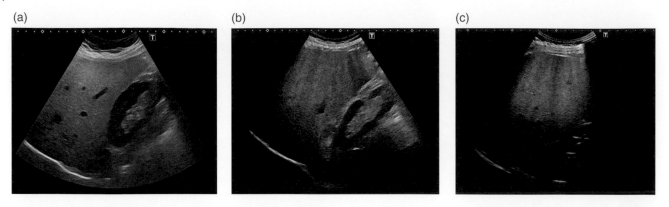

Figure 8.6 Steatosis is graded according to parenchymal brightness and the degree of posterior attenuation. (a) Grade I; (b) grade II; (c) grade III. Note that this grading relies on the description of ultrasound features. More advanced applications are now available and can be used to accurately quantify steatosis (See chapter 15).

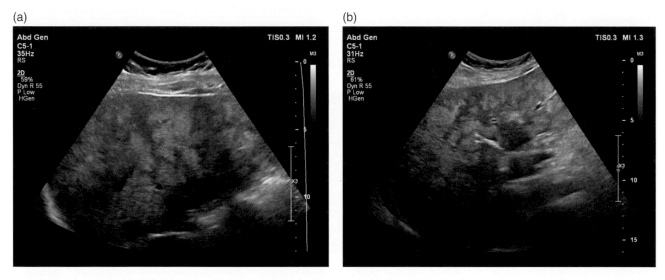

Figure 8.7 (a, b) Diffuse ill-defined hepatic steatosis with a geographical pattern of distribution.

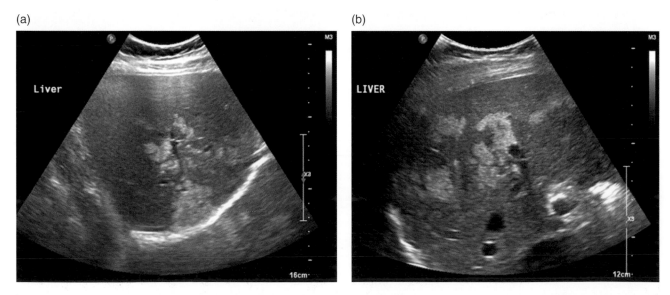

Figure 8.8 (a, b) A more focal but ill-defined distribution of hepatic steatosis with no capsular or vascular distortion.

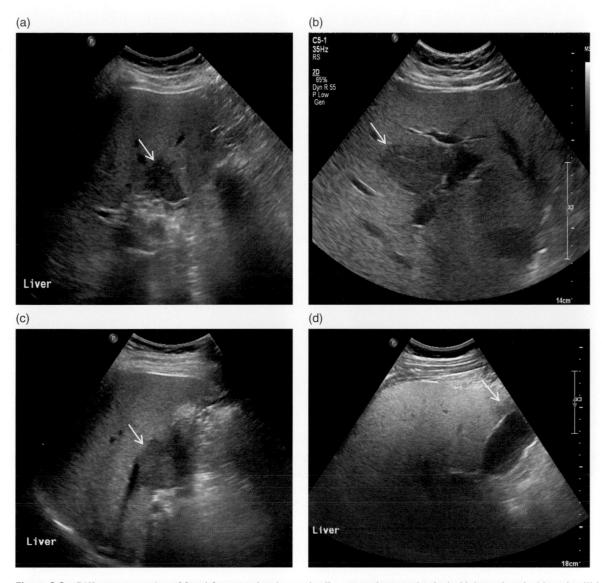

Figure 8.9 Different examples of focal fatty sparing (arrows) adjacent to the portal vein (a, b), hepatic vein (c), and gallbladder (d).

In cases of diffuse steatosis, there might be fat-sparing areas that can be located anywhere in the liver parenchyma, but most typically near the PV bifurcation, subcapsular regions, or around the gallbladder and hepatic veins (Figure 8.9).

It should be borne in mind that increased echogenicity can also be secondary to fibrotic changes, which can be more diffuse or localised according to the underlying liver pathology. As will be further described, periportal and peribiliary fibrosis is typically characterised by peribiliary and perivascular hyperechoic thickening that might extend to the adjacent liver parenchyma.

Ultrasound Features of Portal Hypertension

Increased pressure in the portal venous system accompanies the structural changes of CLD, while haemodynamic factors

subsequently contribute to its further progression. The gold standard for PH assessment in cirrhosis is measurement of the hepatic venous pressure gradient (HVPG) obtained by evaluating the difference between wedged hepatic venous pressure and free hepatic venous pressure by means of hepatic vein catheterisation. An HVPG ≥ 10 mmHg defines the threshold of CSPH, which is associated with the risk of clinical decompensation and onset of the most feared complications such as ascites, variceal bleeding, hepatic encephalopathy, and hepatorenal syndrome [10–12]. However, HVPG is invasive, costly, implies risks, and is not widely available. Although more innovative methods such as elastography have been validated to non-invasively assess CLD in its different stages (see Chapter 9), ultrasound also has an important role in the diagnosis of PH. In fact, not only can ultrasound highlight the presence of signs of CLD, but it can distinguish features that are in keeping with other chronic conditions suggesting an alternative diagnosis, distinguish features that are more specific of certain aetiologies, and evaluate the presence of PV thrombosis, which can be a cause of non-cirrhotic PH as well as a complication of cirrhosis [10].

B-Mode Signs of Portal Hypertension

Abundance of the accumulated fibrous tissue, nodular regeneration, and parenchymal distortion result in resistance to blood flow through the liver with increased pressure in the portal venous system and its tributaries.

The portal venous flow velocity decreases proportionally with the severity of PH, while its calibre often becomes

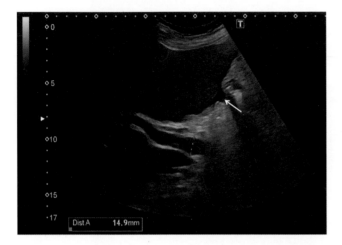

Figure 8.10 Dilated portal vein (calibre 14.9 mm) in a patient with advanced liver disease highlighted by contour irregularities, and ascites (arrow).

wider (>13 mm) (Figure 8.10) [13,14] as well as for the splenic and superior mesenteric veins (>11mm) [10].

It is of note that less commonly a normal or even slightly narrow PV can be found despite the severity of PH in cirrhosis (Figure 8.11). Increased pressure in the portal venous system leads to congestion of splanchnic organs such as stomach, bowel, gallbladder (Figure 8.12) and spleen (Figure 8.13) [15].

Splenomegaly is one of the most common signs of PH and its increase in size over time is described as a marker of PH progression. It is defined by a bipolar cranio-caudal diameter > 13 and an anteroposterior diameter > 4 cm. In some individuals spleen morphology might differ being longer but thinner or shorter but wider. Under these circumstances measuring the area with a cutoff of > 45cm^2 to define splenomegaly might be of help. However, spleen size variability has been described among different CLD aetiologies and in 20–30% of cases it might be normal in size despite the presence of CSPH, especially in alcohol-related liver disease [16, 17]. The presence of hyperechoic foci without acoustic shadowing, of a size of less than a millimetre, scattered throughout the splenic parenchyma can sometimes be seen in patients with both severe cirrhotic or non-cirrhotic PH. These findings are remnants of focal splenic microhaemorrhages, histologically proven to be calcific-fibrosiderotic nodules known as Gamna-Gandy bodies. Magnetic resonance imaging (MRI) has been approved as the most sensitive imaging modality for the detection of these nodules due to their iron content (dropout signal in T1). Nevertheless, sonographic features are also quite typical (Figure 8.14) [18, 19]. Ascites can be one

(a)   (b)

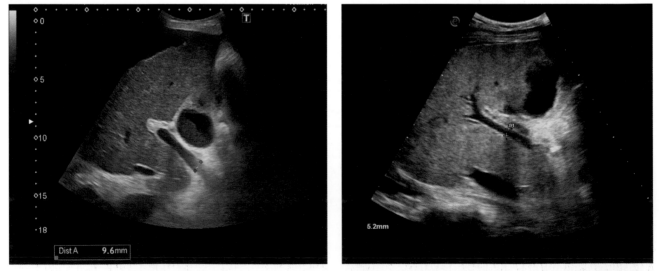

Figure 8.11 Two examples of patients with advanced chronic liver disease highlighted by heterogenic echotexture, irregular outline and ascites, but with a relatively small (a, 9.6 mm) or even narrowed portal vein calibre (b, 5.2 mm), despite the clinical evidence of portal hypertension (both patients have ascites and oesophageal varices on endoscopy).

(a) (b) (c)

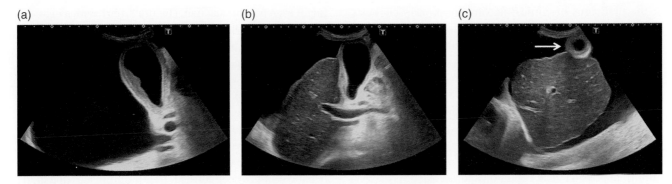

Figure 8.12 (a–c) Gallbladder (GB) thickening secondary to portal hypertension–related congestion. Advanced liver disease is revealed by parenchymal/capsular retraction, irregular outline, ascites, and GB thickening. Different acoustic windows are used to scan the GB on different planes. The arrow points to the GB fundus (transverse section) 'sticking out' from the retracted liver.

(a) (b)

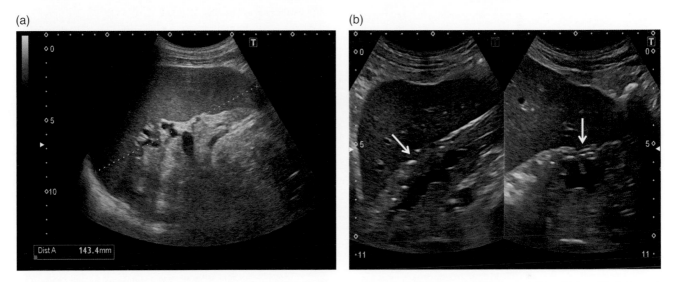

Figure 8.13 (a) An example of homogeneous splenomegaly with a cranio-caudal diameter of 14.4 cm and (b) a thick-walled stomach (arrows) in longitudinal (left) and transverse section (right). Upper endoscopy revealed pronounced portal hypertensive gastropathy.

(a) (b)

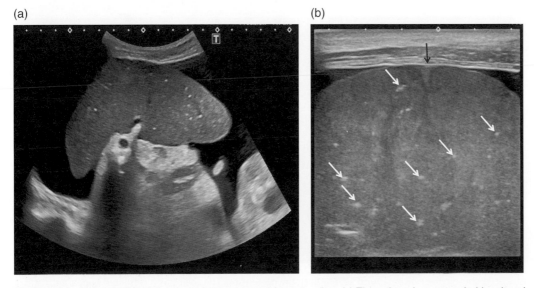

Figure 8.14 Patient with cirrhosis and severe portal hypertension. (a) The spleen is surrounded by abundant ascites and hyperechoic spots are scattered throughout the splenic parenchyma, in keeping with Gamna-Gandy bodies. (b) Magnification helps to improve their definition (arrows), also revealing subtle irregularities of the splenic profile and a fibrous capsular septa (red arrow).

of the first signs of clinical decompensation in cirrhosis with severe PH (Figure 8.15). Nevertheless, in the presence of ascites other signs of advanced cirrhosis and PH should be looked for in patients with CLD, since intraperitoneal fluid might be the consequence of other pathologies such as heart failure, severe hypoalbuminemia, peritoneal carcinomatosis, renal failure, and serositis.

Colour Doppler Signs of Portal Hypertension

In normal physiological conditions portal blood has a constant monophasic or slightly biphasic hepatopetal flow. However, with the worsening of PH, portal vein velocity progressively and proportionally decreases (Figure 8.16a) and it might even become stagnant (Figure 8.16b), with a high risk of thrombosis, or be completely inverted to hepatofugal flow, representing one of the most specific signs of severe PH [13, 20]. Because of the reduced portal venous flow, arterial buffering takes place leading to hepatic parenchymal arterialisation (Figure 8.17). With severe PH, there is an increase in arterial peak systolic velocity and diminished hepatic artery end-diastolic velocity (EDV), resulting in an increased hepatic artery resistive index (RI >0.7) (Figure 8.18a). However, in cases where a shunt between hepatic artery and hepatic vein has been formed, the RI diminishes due to the drop in the peripheral resistance to arterial blood flow, and the resultant waveform in the hepatic artery changes with both high PSV and EDV (Figure 8.18b).

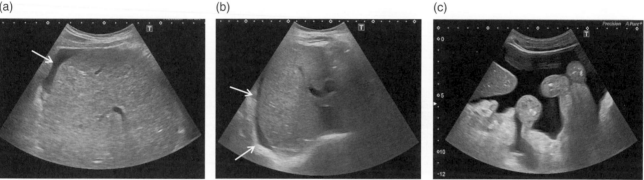

Figure 8.15 Examples of small-volume ascites surrounding the liver (a, b, arrows) and large-volume ascites in which oedematous small bowel loops are seen floating (c).

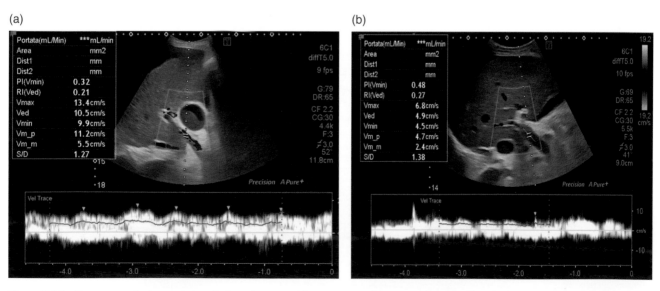

Figure 8.16 Two cases of advanced chronic liver disease with severe portal hypertension. The liver has a retracted appearance and is surrounded by ascites. (a) Colour Doppler reveals a very slow hepatopetal flow (max velocity 13.4 cm/s). (b) There is no detectable colour signal. Doppler analysis depicts an extremely low flow with a max velocity of 6.8 cm/s, which is in keeping with almost stagnant flow and high risk of portal vein thrombosis.

(a)

(b)

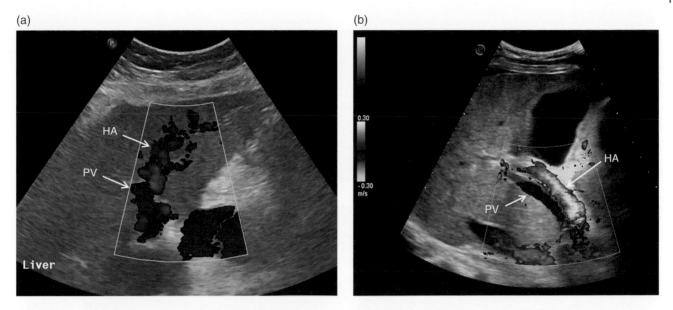

Figure 8.17 (a, b) Two examples of portal blood flow inversion as an expression of severe portal hypertension. There is pronounced hepatic artery (HA) hypertrophy since liver perfusion, in this phase, relies on arterial supply. PV, portal vein.

(a)

(b)

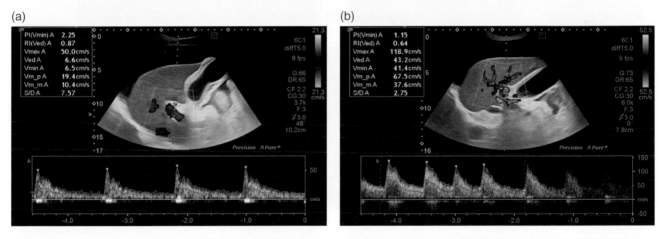

Figure 8.18 (a) Increased hepatic resistive index (RI) in a patient with advanced cirrhosis. (b) High peak systolic velocity and end-diastolic velocity with a low hepatic artery RI in a patient with cirrhosis and intrahepatic arteriovenous shunt.

The hepatic veins are typically narrowed and compressed by collagen deposition and nodular regeneration, therefore the Doppler waveform loses its triphasic appearance and becomes progressively flattened and linear [20]. The flattening of the hepatic vein waveform has been found to correlate with the severity of CLD [21]. Owing to congestion, but also to the hypertrophy and hyperplasia of some tissue elements, resistance to arterial blood flow in the spleen increases together with portal pressure. Therefore, the intrasplenic arterial waveform becomes stretched, with increased PSV and diminished EDV, resulting in a high RI and pulsatility index (PI). The splenic artery PI is easily obtained, automatically calculated by the ultrasound software, and has been demonstrated as a reliable parameter for PH with a cut-off value for significant PH when ≥1

(Figure 8.19) [22]. Owing to splanchnic vasodilation, the RI of the superior mesenteric artery diminishes during fasting. On the other hand, systemic vasodilation results in diminished renal perfusion, leading to intrarenal vasoconstriction and increased intrarenal RI (>0.7). An increase in renal RI in cirrhosis might be one of the first indicators of imminent hepato-renal syndrome [23]. The congestive index is a quite complex Doppler-related measurement obtained by the ratio between the cross-sectional area of the PV and its mean flow velocity (cut-off value of 0.1 cm/s) [24]. Although resistance and pulsatility indexes together with the congestion index are described and have been used in the past, they are considered ancillary findings to be eventually used as integration and not independently for PH diagnosis.

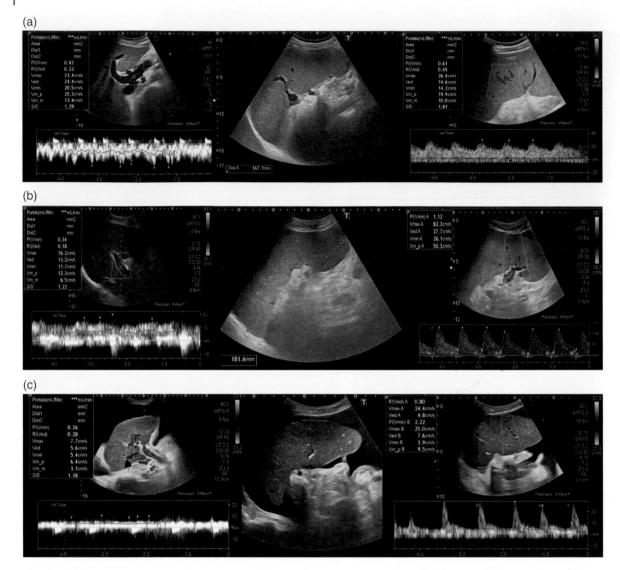

Figure 8.19 (a) Normal portal flow velocity, splenomegaly, and normal splenic pulsatility index (PI) in a patient with parasitic infection and a history of hepatitis C virus, but with no sign of chronic liver disease. Splenomegaly was not secondary to portal hypertension (PH). (b) Cirrhosis with reduced portal flow velocity and splenomegaly with an increased splenic PI. (c) Another case with cirrhosis, ascites, very slow portal venous flow, no sign of splenomegaly, but the PI is very high, suggesting severe PH.

Vascular Modifications as a Sign of Portal Hypertension

With the onset of CSPH the pressure starts forcing the blood flow through low-resistance vascular sites, leading to the formation of gastroesophageal varices and collateral circulation that connects the portal venous system to the inferior and superior vena cava, diverting the obstructed flow into the systemic circulation. The detection of varices and portal systemic shunts is 100% specific for CSPH, but their absence on ultrasound cannot rule out CSPH. Small varices detected on gastroscopy might not be seen on ultrasound as well as

porto-systemic shunts because of their location or suboptimal acoustic window. The most commonly encountered porto-systemic collaterals include recanalisation of the umbilical vein, which usually originates from the left PV branch passing through the round ligament at the visceral edge of the falciform ligament and then beneath the anterior abdominal wall towards the umbilical region (Figure 8.20). The left gastric or coronary vein represents the shortest pathway for portal blood to enter into the para-oesophageal plexus that communicates with the azygos vein [25]. The left gastric vein might be seen as the anechoic tubular structure rising out from the portal trunk along the

(a)

(b)

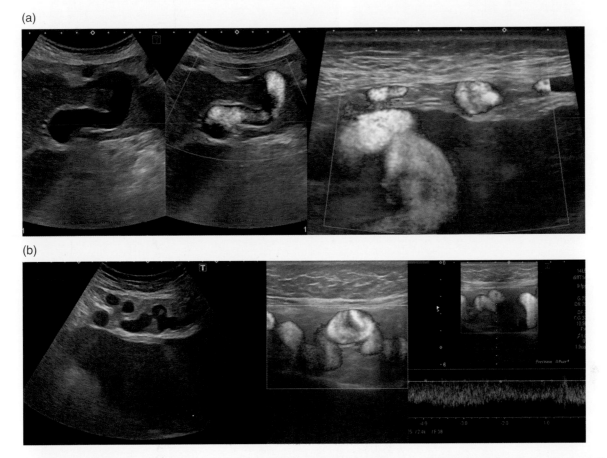

Figure 8.20 Patient with cirrhosis and clinically significant portal hypertension. (a) There is evidence of a large canalised umbilical vein that shunts blood flow from the left branch of the portal vein into smaller subcutaneous collaterals that run beneath the anterior abdominal wall (b).

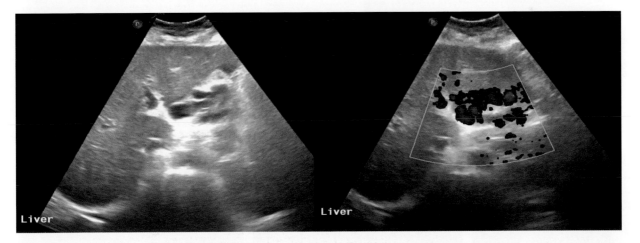

Figure 8.21 Anechoic tubular structures (left side) posterior to the left lobe are in keeping with perigastric varices, as shown on colour Doppler (right side).

minor curvature of the stomach (Figure 8.21). Collaterals in the splenic hilum are seen as tubular anechoic structures, with abundant venous-type flow on Doppler studies. Sometimes these collaterals form a spleno-renal shunt (Figure 8.22), or they connect to para-oesophageal veins and gastric fundal varices, which might be demonstrated by greyscale or Doppler ultrasound. Other collaterals are less frequently seen, including retroperitoneal (Figure 8.23) and pelvic collaterals (between haemorrhoidal and iliac veins). Ectopic varices can be identified in the ileum or colon. Regardless of the presence of porto-systemic collaterals, more rarely an arterio-portal shunt might develop, further contributing to PH (Figure 8.24).

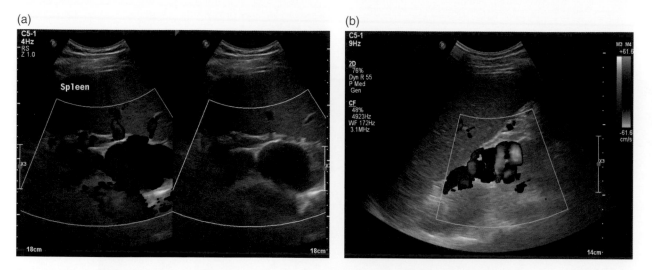

Figure 8.22 (a, b) Two examples of large tubular convoluted vascular collaterals between the spleen and the left kidney in keeping with spleno-renal shunts.

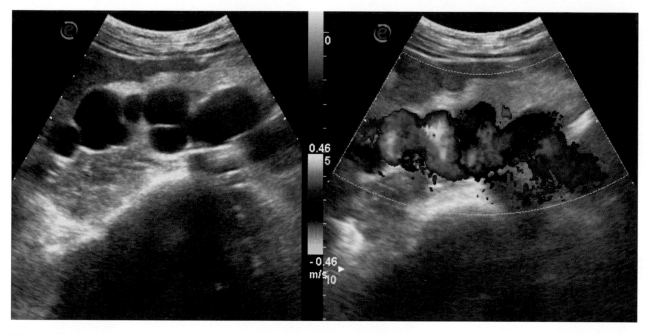

Figure 8.23 Large retroperitoneal shunt in patient with hepatitis C virus/alcohol-related cirrhosis and severe portal hypertension.

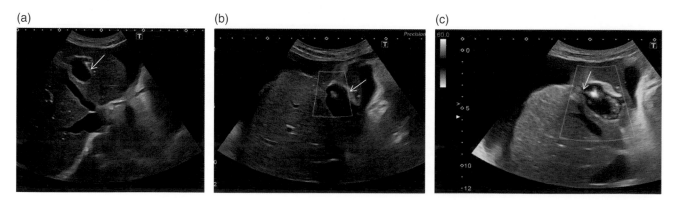

Figure 8.24 Patient with cirrhosis and severe portal hypertension. (a, b) The left portal vein branch (white arrow) is severely dilated with reversed flow. There is evidence of communication between the left branch of the hepatic artery and the left portal vein branch, in keeping with arterioportal fistula, contributing to reversed portal flow (white arrow) and worsening of portal pressure. (c) Directional power Doppler highlights the details of the flow pattern at the site of the arterioportal fistula (white arrow).

Sonographic Differences among Various Liver Disease Aetiologies

The general hallmarks of cirrhosis are usually similar, especially in advanced stages. However, the site, severity, pattern of inflammation and fibrosis are different according to aetiology. This may not only impact the natural history of CLD but also the appearance of the liver.

Viral Hepatitis

Viral hepatitis was one of the most common liver diseases before hepatitis C virus (HCV)-eradicating therapy was available. The course of disease is characterised by subclinical progression, which can last decades until cirrhosis declares itself with ascites, variceal bleeding, or the presence of HCC. If CLD is detected in the early stages, the liver might have a completely normal appearance. Ultrasound findings of overt HCV-related cirrhosis include heterogeneous echotexture, irregular surface, regenerative nodules that are more visible when using a high-frequency transducer, hypertrophy of the caudate lobe, as well as features of CSPH. In some cases, surface irregularities as well as echotexture heterogeneity are more subtle despite quite advanced disease (Figure 8.25) [5]. A certain degree of hepatic steatosis might be found, especially in HCV genotype 3 [6]. The presence of periportal or hepatoduodenal small reactive lymphadenopathies is also a common finding (Figure 8.25). The appearance of hepatitis B virus (HBV)-related cirrhosis in general can be quite similar to HCV, although sometimes the echotexture might be more heterogenic compared to the same stage of HCV and usually, unless there are no other secondary causes,

it is not associated with hepatic steatosis. In HBV CLD, the occurrence of HCC can affect patients even during the non-cirrhotic stage, while that is very unusual for HCV. One distinctive feature in the natural history of HBV is the occurrence of viral-related inflammatory flares that can lead to acute hepatitis or even liver failure. As a consequence of florid inflammation, the hepatic architecture can sometimes undergo dramatic changes over a relatively short time. The co-existence of human immunodeficiency virus (HIV) in both HBV and HCV can accelerate the process to overt cirrhosis, as well as the development of HCC.

Alcohol-Related Liver Disease

Alcohol-related liver disease is a very common cause of CLD in eastern countries. Except in the very advanced stages of cirrhosis where the nodular outline stands out, the echotexture is usually slightly heterogeneous, almost homogeneous in some cases, and the outline might show subtle irregularities more obvious with high-frequency transducers with a possible discrepancy between the liver's appearance and the severity of disease (Figures 8.26–8.28). Hepatic steatosis is usually present as a consequence of alcohol-induced metabolic derangement. Constant alcohol withdrawal leads to rapid reduction and eventually resolution of hepatic steatosis, unless other factors were involved in its development. Despite these frequent findings, in advanced cirrhosis the liver has a shrunken appearance. The PV calibre might be increased, but also normal even in advanced stages, possibly correlating with a normal-sized or small spleen that has been described in alcohol-related liver disease, as previously mentioned.

(a)   (b)   (c)

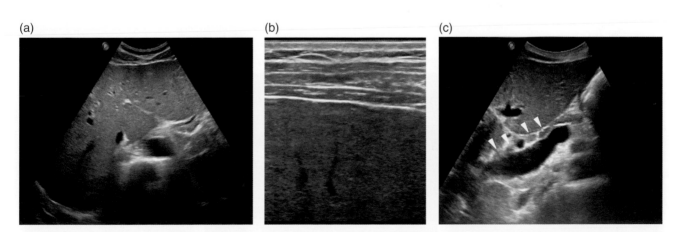

Figure 8.25 An example of hepatitis C virus–related cirrhosis: the liver is quite enlarged and steatotic, with hypertrophy of the caudate lobe (a). The echotexture is relatively homogeneous and the outline is only mildly irregular (b). Multiple small nodes (arrow heads) can be identified anteriorly to the portal vein (c).

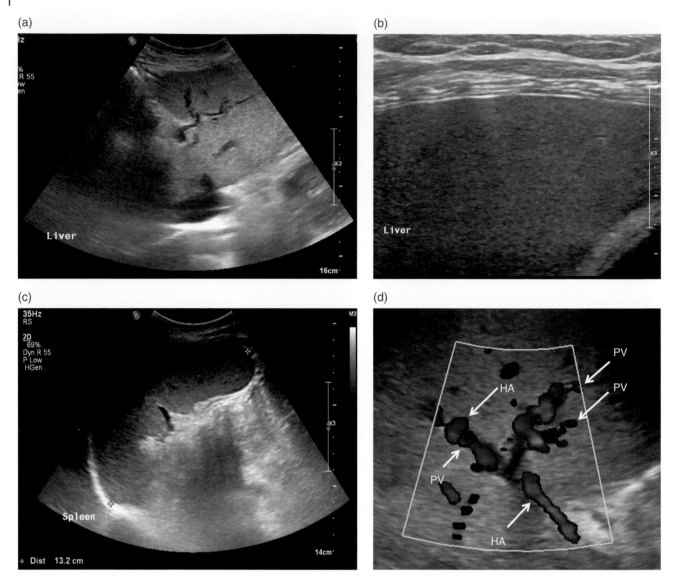

Figure 8.26 Steatotic-looking liver with homogeneous echotexture and almost smooth outline (a, b). Normal-sized spleen (c). However, the portal venous flow is barely visible and inverted, while there is pronounced hypertrophy of the hepatic artery (d). Although the B-mode features were not conclusive, this patient had alcohol-related liver disease cirrhosis with clinically significant portal hypertension.

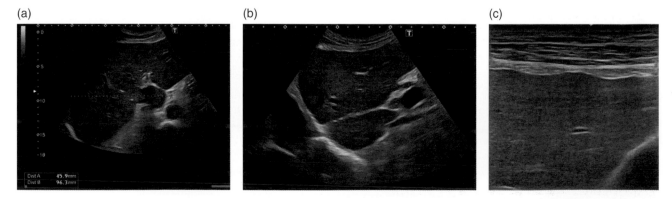

Figure 8.27 There is a clear discrepancy between an almost homogeneous echotexture and caudate lobe hypertrophy (a, b). The liver outline irregularity is highlighted with a high-frequency transducer (c).

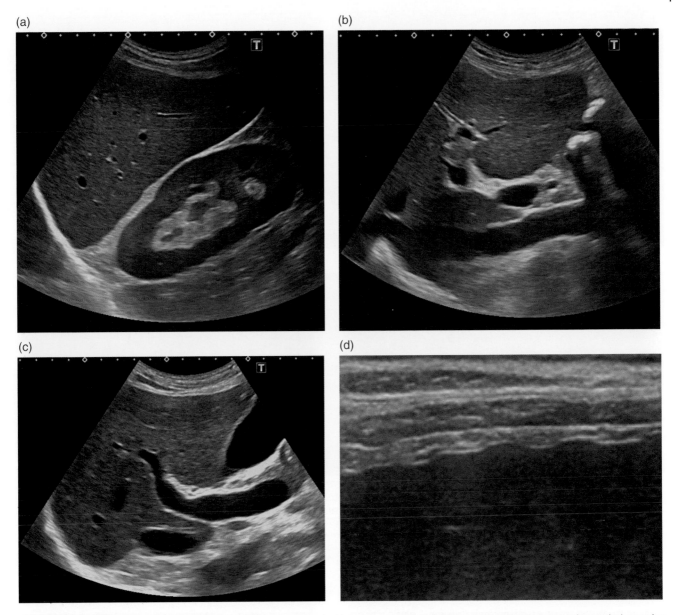

Figure 8.28 Patient with alcohol related liver disease cirrhosis. Note is made of slightly irregular echotexture and rounded margins (a–c), increased calibre of the portal vein (c) and irregular outline at higher magnification with a high frequency transducer (d).

Autoimmune Hepatitis

The sonographic appearance of autoimmune hepatitis is variable, owing to its different clinical presentations and natural history pathways. It might present clinically as fulminant liver failure, severe hepatitis leading to subacute liver failure, have a more indolent progression or a fluctuant course of disease, with flares of severe inflammation leading ultimately to cirrhosis. While a common finding is the presence of reactive hilar, periportal lymphadenopathies [26], morphological changes can range from subtle irregularities of the left liver lobe surface to typical hallmarks of cirrhosis and PH. Alternatively, liver inflammation can be so severe as to cause, in a short period of time, a complete destructuration of the liver parenchyma as a consequence of necroinflammatory changes (Figure 8.29). The resulting coarsened echotexture can be homogeneously or irregularly distributed throughout the liver parenchyma (Figure 8.30). It is of note that sometimes despite a very good biochemical response to immunosuppressive treatment, parenchymal heterogenicity might not be reversible in those cases where severe liver damage has occurred. Parenchymal features might suggest the presence of cirrhosis, although the whole picture could be compatible with 'burn-out inflammation'. Imaging will not be able to distinguish between the two conditions. The history of the patient, biochemistry, and serological testing as well as histology are crucial for diagnosis. Elastography, as it will be further explained in the next chapter, is a very useful tool.

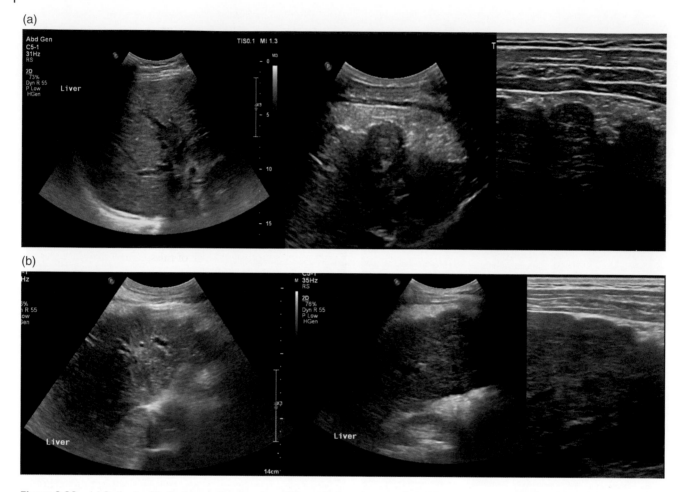

Figure 8.29 (a) Patient with florid autoimmune hepatitis and related severe liver injury showing a heterogeneous echotexture and scattered regenerative nodularities in the subacute phase of disease. (b) The same patient after one year despite good biochemical response to treatment shows diffuse architectural liver distortion with progressive parenchymal retraction, nodular contour and pronounced heterogeneicity of the echotexture.

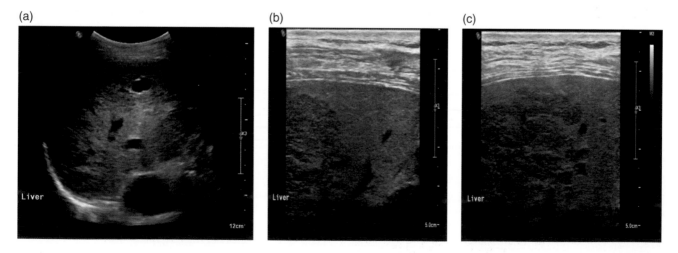

Figure 8.30 (a–c) Severe liver injury with uneven distribution of the necroinflammatory process corresponds to the heterogenic areas of liver parenchyma echotexture.

Non-alcoholic Fatty Liver Disease/Metabolic Dysfunction-Associated Steatotic Liver Disease

The term non alcoholic fatty liver disease (NAFLD) has only recently been changed to metabolic dysfunction-associated steatotic liver disease (MASLD) [27]. This is in order to distinguish a condition characterised by the presence of hepatic steatosis and cardiometabolic risk factors from other non-alcoholic causes of steatosis related hepatopathies, and in general improve stratification of patients with steatotic liver disease. Even the most current literature still refers to NAFLD at time of publishing this chapter, thus we will continue to use this older terminology (See also Chapters 9.2 and 10), bearing in mind that it will be abandoned in the near future for the more appropriate term MASLD.

NAFLD is one of the most common liver disease aetiologies worldwide and is a rising indication for liver transplant once advanced cirrhosis is reached or HCC cannot be managed otherwise [28]. One of the main issues in these patients is the underestimation of the risk of developing steatohepatitis and progressing to advanced CLD. In general, sonographic findings include hepatomegaly, steatosis of different grades, outline irregularities, and parenchymal micronodularities, together with a heterogeneous echotexture (Figure 8.31). However, often the outline is just slightly irregular and there are micronodularities that are difficult to depict as a consequence of adipose infiltration and thickened subcutaneous tissue, with increased skin-to-liver capsule distance. Therefore these sonographic limitations might lead to underdiagnosis in some patients with NAFLD until gross parenchymal irregularities and signs of PH become more obvious or until a first episode of clinical decompensation such as ascites or variceal bleeding declares the severity of CLD. As mentioned, one of the most important limitations in these patients is the difficulty to visualise the whole liver parenchyma. It is very important to acknowledge this limitation, since ultrasound HCC screening might yield suboptimal results due to posterior attenuation, and the inability to visualise appropriately the deeper segments of parenchyma carries a risk of missed pathology.

Primary Biliary Cholangitis

Primary biliary cholangitis is an autoimmune cholestatic chronic liver disease with inflammation and destruction of the small biliary ducts, and histopathological evidence of non-suppurative granulomatous cholangitis [29]. The echotexture of liver parenchyma in the early stages is unremarkable; however, outline irregularities and

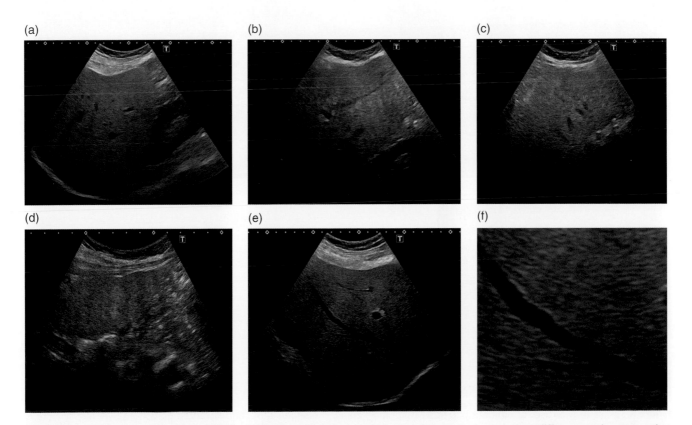

Figure 8.31 Cirrhosis secondary to metabolic dysfunction-associated steatotic liver disease: the images show diffuse posterior attenuation of the ultrasound beam (a–c), nodular regeneration (d), and outline irregularities of the hepatic veins (e, f), in keeping with cirrhosis. Posterior attenuation prevents appropriate visualisation of the deeper segments.

pronounced echotexture heterogeneity are usually present even in the pre-cirrhotic stage, while one distinctive feature is early development of PH due to the pre-sinusoidal increase in intrahepatic resistances. Overt cirrhosis is characterised by obvious parenchymal irregularities and severe PH. Periportal lymphadenopathies are often present (Figure 8.32) and their size and number have been described as correlating with the severity of disease [30].

Primary Sclerosing Cholangitis

Primary sclerosing cholangitis (PSC) is a chronic cholestatic liver disease of unknown aetiology characterised by inflammation and fibrosis of the biliary epithelium extending to liver parenchyma with progression to cirrhosis and its complications [31]. The biliary system can be affected diffusely or more often follow a patchy segmental distribution. Inflammation and fibrosis can involve the extrahepatic

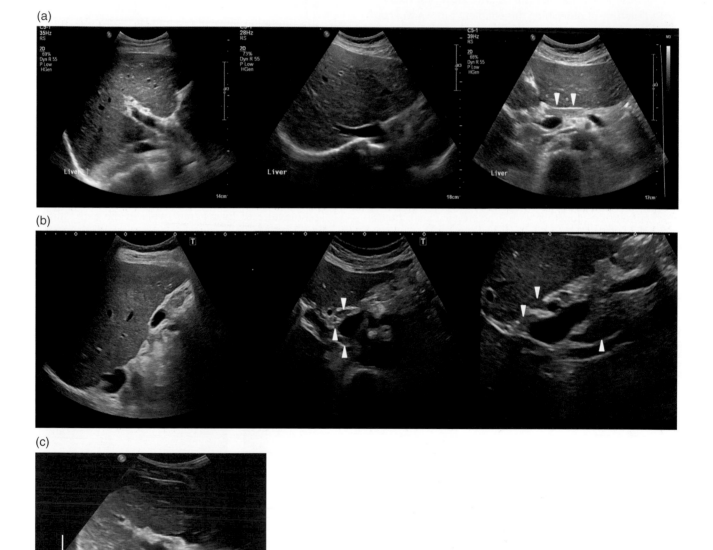

Figure 8.32 (a, b) Two cases of different patients with primary biliary cholangitis (PBC) and advanced fibrosis on liver biopsy. Note is made of the presence of reactive nodes at the hepatic hylum (arrowheads). (c) A case of advanced cirrhosis secondary to PBC complicated by portal hypertension and a hepatic hydrothorax (arrow).

biliary duct or the intrahepatic ducts or both, they can involve the biliary tree of one entire lobe with sparing of the other, or they can have a more homogeneous 'parenchymal' distribution. PSC diagnosis should always rule out other pathological conditions that affect the biliary system, such as choledocolithiasis, immunoglobulin IgG4-related cholangiopathy, acquired immunodeficiency syndrome (AIDS)-related cholangitis, and cholangiocarcinoma. The gold

standard for diagnosis is magnetic resonance cholangiopancreatography (MRCP) and endoscopic retrograde cholangiopancreatography (ERCP), especially when biliary stricturing requires stenting [31]. Ultrasound findings in PSC include thickening, stricturing, and pre-stenotic dilatation of the intrahepatic ducts (Figures 8.33 and 8.34). In the case of distal hepatic duct involvement, ultrasound highlights periportal thickening surrounded by a 'hyperechoic

(a)   (b)

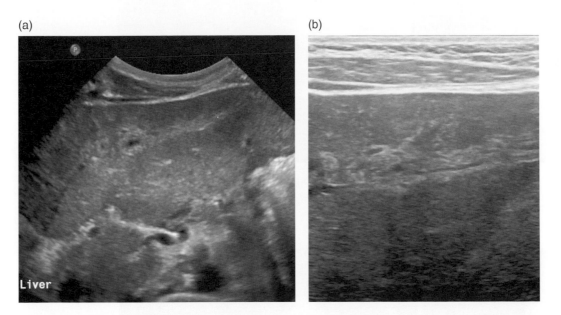

Figure 8.33 (a) Extensive thickening of the left lobe distal biliary ducts in a patient with primay sclerosing cholangitis. (b) Higher magnification with a high frequency transducer shows the details of a left bile duct fibrotic changes.

(a)   (b)

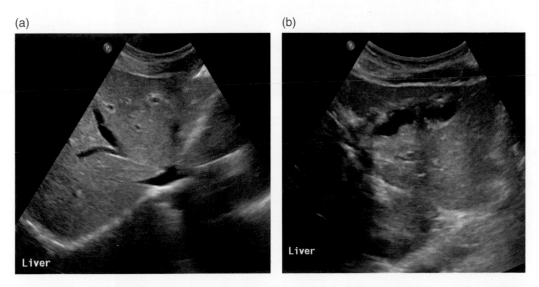

Figure 8.34 Patient with primary sclerosing cholangitis with dissociation of the biliary tree involvement. (a) There is relative sparing of the right liver lobe bile ducts, while there is evidence of extensive involvement of the left liver lobe where a sclerotic and dilated biliary duct is clearly visible (b).

blush' (Figure 8.35). This finding is thought to be secondary to biliary fibrotic changes extended to the adjacent liver parenchyma. Usually the extrahepatic common bile duct is not dilated, but appears thickened with narrowing and threading of its lumen. In PSC two different patterns of parenchymal changes have been described: one characterised by diffuse heterogeneity of liver parenchyma compatible with secondary biliary cirrhosis, and the other characterised by an irregular distribution of patchy echogenic areas (Figures 8.36 and 8.37). Autoptic findings and

(a)   (b)

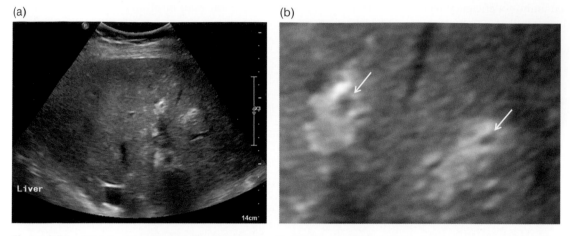

Figure 8.35 Patient with primary sclerosing cholangitis. (a) The distal portal branches are surrounded by a 'hyperechoic blush' that corresponds to peribiliary and periportal fibrosis. (b) The arrows highlight the distal portal branches that stand out against the fibrotic changes as a consequence of biliary sclerosis.

(a)

(b)

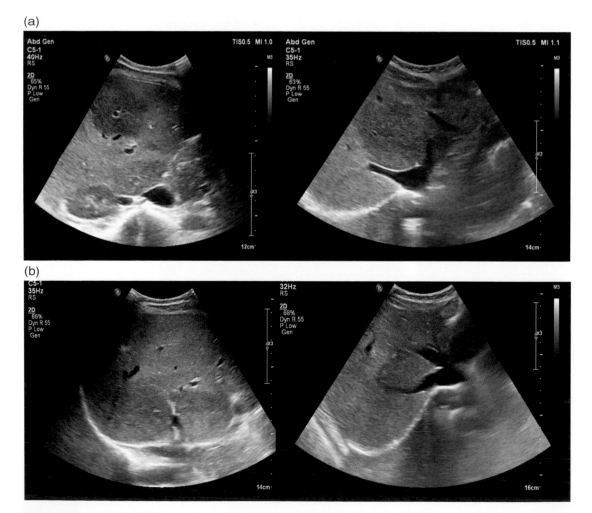

Figure 8.36 (a, b) Two different patients with primary sclerosing cholangitis with a 'parenchymal patchy pattern'. In both cases different areas of echogenicity correspond to different areas of biliary involvement.

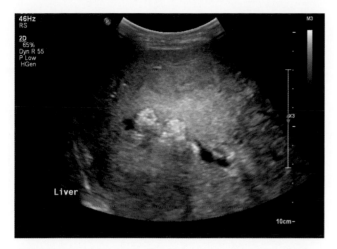

Figure 8.37 Pronounced fibrotic changes extending from the right biliary duct to the adjacent hepatic parenchyma. Note is made of focal large calcifications and debris within the bile ducts.

MRCP investigations showed that the echogenic areas correspond to peribiliary fibrotic areas [32]. In conclusion, sonographic findings in PSC are very variable, ranging from diffuse parenchymal disease, patchy distribution of parenchymal changes, and intra- or extrahepatic biliary stricturing and dilatation. Features of PH are found in advanced disease, and splenomegaly might also be present in patients without significant PH at the time of presentation, especially in patients with coexisting inflammatory bowel disease. It is of note that patients with PSC often have signs of chronic cholecystitis, gallbladder wall thickening, sludge, and cholelithiasis.

Wilson's Disease

Wilson's disease is a rare autosomic recessive disease secondary to a mutation involving the copper transporter, leading to tissue accumulation (liver, brain, pancreas, heart, eye), inflammation, and damage [33]. Wilson's-related liver disease can evolve in a rather indolent manner and be diagnosed when cirrhosis is already developed. In this case the ultrasound appearance shows general features of CLD and multiple well-defined hypoechoic nodularities that have been shown to be compatible with copper deposits on histology (Figure 8.38). Under other unpredictable circumstances, Wilson's-related liver disease can present clinically as fulminant liver failure, with a

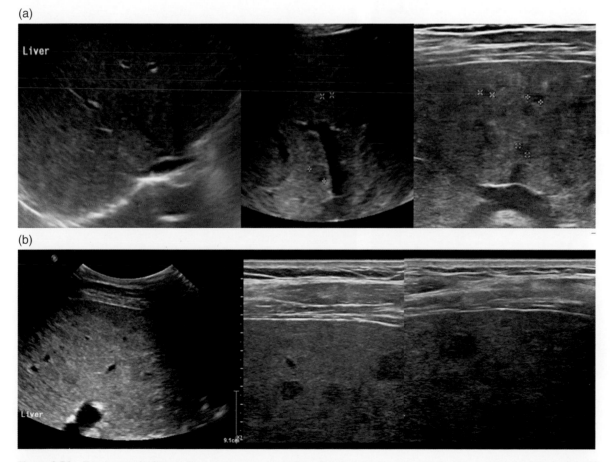

(a)

(b)

Figure 8.38 Two cases of Wilson's disease characterised (a) by slightly heterogeneic echotexture and hypoechoic nodularities compatible with moderated fibrosis and copper deposits on histology; and (b) by pronounced heterogeneic echotexture and well-defined nodularities compatible with cirrhosis and copper deposits.

shrunken ultrasound appearance of the hepatic parenchyma surrounded by ascites.

Cardiogenic Cirrhosis

Chronic venous outflow obstruction secondary to right heart impairment might lead to post-sinusoidal blood congestion, stasis, fibrosis, and cirrhosis. It is secondary to chronic severe pulmonary hypertension, severe tricuspid regurgitation, pericardial constriction, and in general severe heart failure [34, 35].

In cardiogenic cirrhosis usually the echotexture is quite homogeneous, while subtle irregularities of the liver outline and hepatic vein profiles are more indicative of fibrosis and CLD. The liver might be surrounded by a variable amount of ascites, depending on the severity of heart failure, liver congestion/fibrosis, and other comorbidities. One distinctive feature is the distension of the IVC and hepatic veins and demodulation of the triphasic hepatic venous flow together with the pulsatile flow in the PV, as a sign of severe post-sinusoidal increased hydrostatic pressure (Figure 8.39) [15].

Mimics of Cirrhosis

Irregular surface, diffuse parenchymal nodularities, ascites, splenomegaly, and PH are described as hallmarks of cirrhosis. Nevertheless, there are several pathological

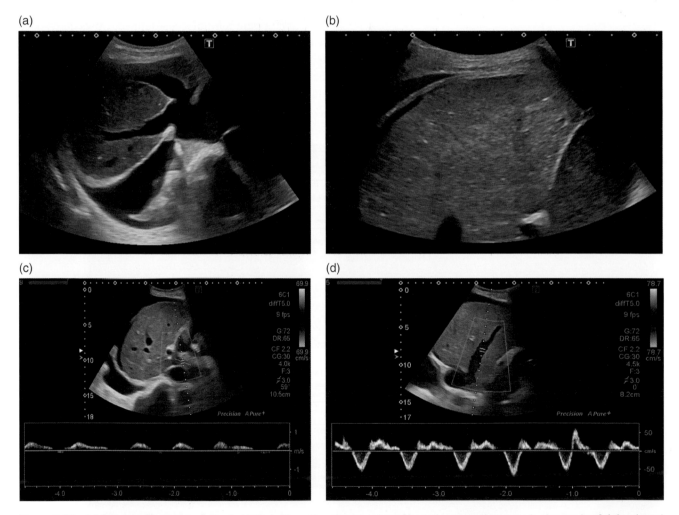

Figure 8.39 (a) Patient with grossly distended IVC and hepatic veins as a sign of hepatic congestion; note is also made of right pleural effusion (arrow). (b) The liver echotexture is heterogeneous and the outline slightly irregular. (c) The liver is surrounded by ascites and there is pulsatile flow in the portal vein as well as hepatic vein flow demodulation due to combined tricuspid regurgitation and right heart failure (d) in a patient with cardiogenic cirrhosis.

conditions with similar findings that resemble cirrhosis on imaging, despite being completely different kinds of diseases, with different aetiologies, natural history, pathogenesis, and outcome. It is crucial to keep in mind these conditions, since misleading diagnosis can lead to incorrect clinical management and influence the outcome.

Sarcoidosis

Sarcoidosis is a non-caseous granulomatous inflammatory systemic disease that might affect the liver and the spleen. Hepato-splenic involvement is usually asymptomatic, leading to subclinical progression and development of PH and variceal bleeding. The most common finding is the presence of hepatomegaly, increased diffuse echogenicity mimicking hepatic steatosis, or a heterogenic echotexture and irregular outline secondary to granulomatous infiltration [36]. Sometimes large, well-defined nodularities can also be seen within the hepatic parenchyma, mimicking neoplastic disease. The spleen can be affected too, with the most common finding being multiple hypoechoic, sometimes confluent nodularities, which can range from a few millimetres to 1–2 cm in diameter (Figure 8.40). Isoechoic lesions can be missed on ultrasound but are easily highlighted by contrast computed tomography (CT), MRI, as well as contrast-enhanced ultrasound (CEUS). The latter has been shown to have a similar accuracy to both CT and MRI with contrast and can be very useful to follow up treatment response.

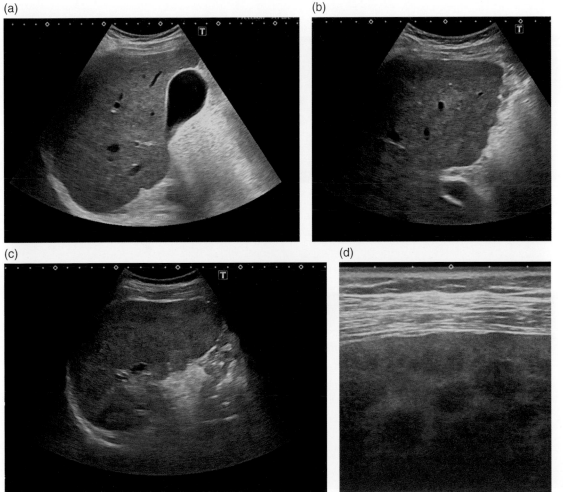

Figure 8.40 Hepatosplenic sarcoidosis: the liver has a slightly heterogeneic echotexture, increased echogenicity, irregular outline, and rounded margins, resembling advanced chronic liver disease (a, b). The spleen has a heterogeneous echotexture and magnification by high-frequency transducer revealed multiple hypoechoic centimetric confluent nodularities (c, d). Liver biopsy confirmed non-caseating granulomas in keeping with hepatic sarcoidosis. A positron emission tomography (PET) scan showed extensive hepatosplenic involvement.

Common Variable Immunodeficiency and Liver Disease

Common variable immunodeficiency (CVID) is a primary B-cell immunodeficiency disorder, characterised by remarkable hypogammaglobulinemia. At least 10% of CVID patients present with liver involvement secondary to autoimmune reactions, granulomatous inflammation, lymphoproliferation, or nodular regenerative hyperplasia (NRH), which can lead to chronic damage, and the development of PH [37]. Imaging is not conclusive, but resembles cirrhosis, especially in advanced stages of liver damage (Figure 8.41). Biopsy can show non-specific inflammation, granulomatous inflammation, or NRH, which is attributed to CVID in the presence of its typical immunodeficiency pattern.

Pseudo-Cirrhosis Secondary to Metastatic/Infiltrative Neoplastic Liver Disease

Micrometastasis and infiltrative neoplastic disease can mimic advanced cirrhosis. Ultrasound features range from irregular outline to heterogenic echotexture, multiple nodularities, and ascites. In some cases PH can develop and variceal bleeding has been observed. This condition can be a consequence of a variety of metastatic tumours, but has more frequently been described in metastatic breast cancer, especially after chemotherapy [38], as well as in the presence of neoplastic infiltration (Figures 8.42 and 8.43).

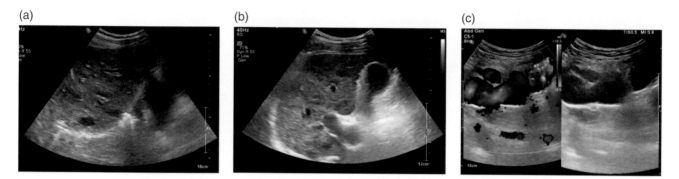

Figure 8.41 Common variable immunodeficiency–related chronic granulomatous liver involvement and severe portal hypertension. The echotexture is very heterogeneous, and there is periportal thickening revealed by increased periportal echogenicity surrounded by hypoechoic areas (a, b). Note is made of a large retroperitoneal porto-systemic shunt (c).

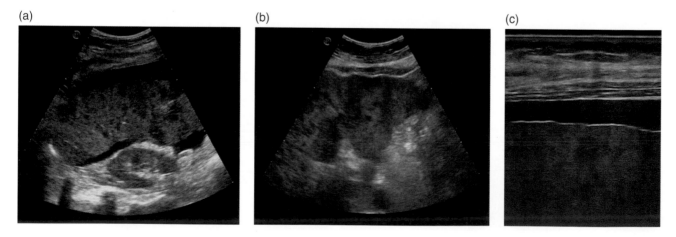

Figure 8.42 Heterogeneic appearance of hepatic parenchyma where multiple ill-defined hypoechoic areas can be identified. The patient was known to have liver metastatic breast cancer, for which she underwent chemotherapy. The appearance of the liver closely resembles cirrhosis for both heterogeneic echotexture (a), nodular contour (b), and ascites (c).

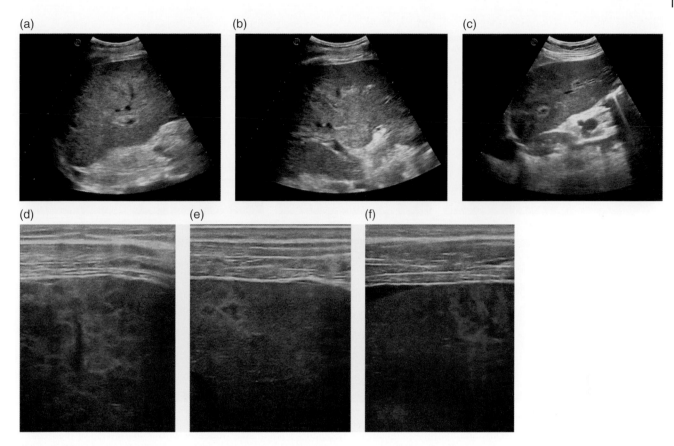

Figure 8.43 Heterogeneic echotexture and irregular outline (a–c) were detected in this patient with no past medical history who was admitted with suspected decompensated chronic liver disease. Magnification with high-frequency transducer revealed diffuse clusters of confluent sub-centimetric nodularities and small-volume ascites (d–f). Liver biopsy revealed Hodgkin's lymphoma related liver involvement.

Sinusoidal Obstruction Syndrome

Sinusoidal obstruction syndrome previously known as hepatic veno-occlusive disease is a rare vascular condition secondary to stem cell transplantation, radiotherapy, or drug toxicity, especially chemotherapeutics [39]. Toxic damage of sinusoidal endothelial cells leads to occlusion of the terminal hepatic vein and congestive dilatation in centrilobular areas, with hepatocyte dysfunction, perisinusoidal fibrosis, and PH. The key diagnostic clinical criteria are occurrence of hepatomegaly, ascites, and jaundice in patients with a compatible medical history and no previous evidence of these abnormalities at baseline. Ultrasound B-mode findings include hepatosplenomegaly, gallbladder wall thickening >6 mm, portal vein diameter >12 mm, narrowing of the hepatic veins (<3 mm), ascites, and eventually visualisation of a collateral circulation. In addition, the most confounding findings that resemble cirrhosis are a heterogeneous liver echotexture, irregular outline and diffuse parenchymal nodularities, that are usually described in the subacute/chronic phases of sinusoidal obstruction syndrome (Figure 8.44).

Colour Doppler findings can provide useful clues for the diagnosis and follow-up in patients who have undergone a bone marrow transplant, especially, to predict and follow up sinusoidal obstruction syndrome. These changes include: (i) threaded hepatic veins with dampened monophasic flow; (ii) slow demodulated PV flow (<10 cm/s) that sometimes might even be reversed (hepatofugal); (iii) hepatic artery RI >0.75 [40].

Liver elastography has also been shown to have a high predictive value for the diagnosis of sinusoidal obstruction syndrome and can be useful for follow up (See Chapters 9.2 and 11).

Essentially, B-mode ultrasound together with Doppler and elastography, can provide highly predictive information for the diagnosis, albeit in the presence of a supportive medical history. Nevertheless, HVPG measurements and liver biopsy remain the gold standard.

(a)   (b)   (c)

(d)   (e)   (f)

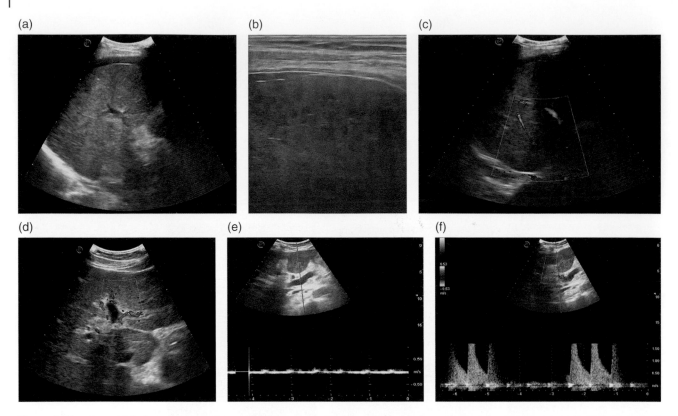

Figure 8.44 sinusoidal obstruction syndrome (SOS) in a patient who underwent chemotherapy for breast cancer. (a, b) Heterogeneic echotexture, irregular outline, ascites and multiple parenchymal nodularities are present together with (c) narrowing of the hepatic veins, (d, e) severely reduced portal venous flow and (f) increased hepatic artery peak systolic velocity (>1.5 m/s). These features suggest the presence of underlying chronic liver disease with clinically significant portal hypertension. However, in light of her medical history and new onset of progressive liver dysfunction she underwent both transjugular liver biopsy and magnetic resonance imaging that confirmed the diagnosis of SOS. Ultrasound findings in patients who do not have a previous history of chronic liver disease and who develop rapidly progressive liver dysfunction after being exposed to specific risk factors are predictive of SOS.

Acute Fulminant Liver Failure and Subacute Liver Failure

Both fulminant and subacute liver failure are secondary to diffuse hepatocellular necrosis due to drug toxicity, autoimmunity, viral infections, and metabolic pathologies such as Wilson's disease, as well as other rarer or unknown conditions. On ultrasound as well as on other imaging modalities, the liver might have a retracted appearance with a heterogenic echotexture and an irregular outline, often surrounded by ascites. The appearance might be indistinguishable from cirrhosis (Figure 8.45), but the differential diagnosis is crucial for management purposes, since acute or subacute liver failure has high transplant priority compared to liver failure in cirrhosis. Diagnosis relies on biopsy when possible (with a transjugular approach, since patients usually are coagulopathic and

have ascites) and on medical history and previous imaging if available.

Congenital Fibrosis

Congenital hepatic fibrosis is an autosomic recessive disorder due to duct plate malformation and abnormal cholangiocyte proliferation, leading to periportal fibrosis and PH [41]. Diagnosis is made by liver biopsy. Sonographic features include hepato-splenomegaly, increased parenchymal echogenicity with hypoechoic periportal areas, and 'periportal cuffing'; regenerative nodules are present in advanced disease. Usually at the time of diagnosis PH is already clinically significant, with evidence of large porto-systemic shunting. The outline is typically quite regular, but the echotexture is heterogeneous, with

(a)

(b)

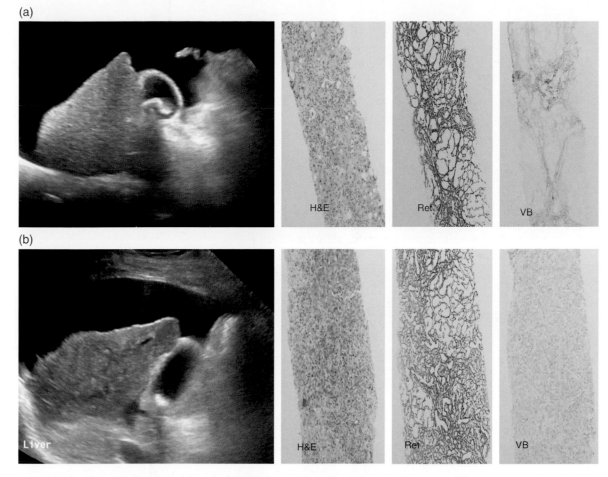

Figure 8.45 The ultrasound appearance of a liver with advanced cirrhosis (a) is compared to (b) the image of a liver that underwent extensive necrosis as a consequence of severe drug-induced liver injury, and who clinically presented with subacute liver failure. In this case the ultrasound appearance of the necrotic liver is not distinguishable from the cirrhotic one. Because of the presence of ascites liver biopsy was carried out using a transjugular approach. The histologic appearance of the cirrhotic liver (a, right side) is similar to the histologic appearance of the necrotic liver (b, right side) on the H&E and reticulin stained sections as the condensation of the extracellular matrix due to confluent hepatocyte loss can mimic a fibrous septum. Cirrhosis can be distinguished from extensive hepatic necrosis using Victoria Blue (VB) staining which stains elastic fibres in blue: the fibrous septa in the cirrhotic liver (a, right side) are clearly blue as they contain mature elastic fibres, while the condensation of the extracellular matrix in the collapsed necrotic areas are negative for elastic fibres (b, right side). *Source:* Courtesy of Dr Tu Vinh Luong.

hypoechoic areas that typically surround and follow the portal venous system, which stands out against a background of a hyperechoic fibrotic-looking parenchyma (Figure 8.46).

Porto-sinusoidal Vascular Disorder

Porto-sinusoidal vascular disorder (PSVD) is a broad term encompassing vascular liver diseases characterised by different histopathological features affecting the sinusoidal and portal vasculature. In its more advanced stages, it presents with variceal bleeding or less frequently, ascites, secondary to PH (See Chapter 11) [42]. On ultrasound, especially in advanced disease, the liver echotexture is heterogeneous and there can be hypertrophy of segments I and IV. At first glance, in light of these morphological changes and signs of PH, PSVD can be labelled erroneously as cirrhosis. However, the presence of pronounced periportal fibrotic thickening, which stands out against a background of a relatively smooth hepatic outline, should raise the possibility of underlying PSVD (Figure 8.47). Liver and spleen elastography may provide important information to

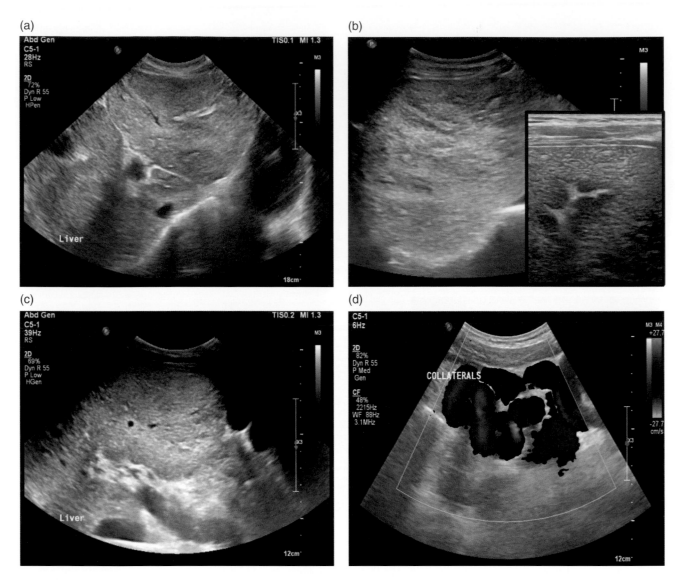

Figure 8.46 (a) Hepatomegaly with heterogeneous echotexture and extensive fibrotic changes. Periportal fibrosis stands out compared to a hypoechoic parenchymal ill-defined halo that follows the entire intrahepatic portal venous system (b, c). Extensive periportal fibrosis leads to severe portal hypertension, which often is present at the time of diagnosis, as shown in (d) where a large retroperitoneal porto-systemic shunt is present.

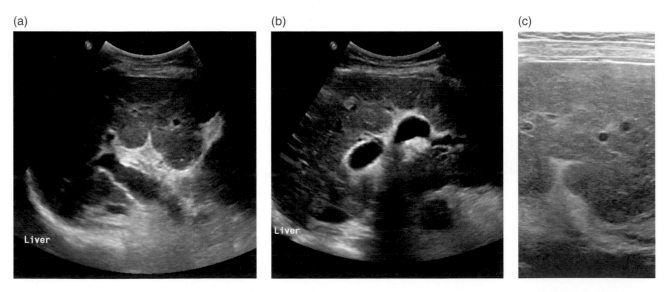

Figure 8.47 A case of porto-sinusoidal vascular disorder diagnosed on liver biopsy. Ultrasound findings show extensive periportal fibrosis and portal vein dilatation (a, b). Fibrotic septa are visualised together with a relatively smooth outline (c).

(a)   (b)

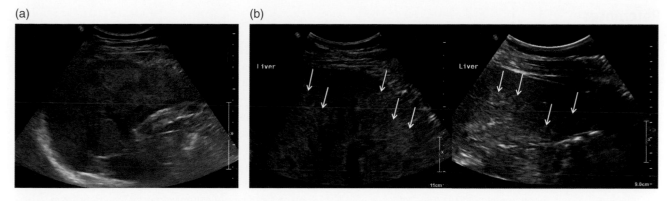

Figure 8.48 Sonographic appearance of biopsy-proven nodular regenerative hyperplasia (NRH). (a) Rounded hyperechoic and confluent nodularities standout against normal liver parenchyma. (b) At higher magnification subtle hyperechoic halos, corresponding to the coral atoll-like sign, are more clearly visible (arrows).

help distinguish the differential diagnosis of cirrhosis (See Chapter 9.2 and 11). Nevertheless, the definitive diagnosis is established via liver biopsy as well as a normal or relatively low HVPG compared to the severity of PH.

Among the histopathological findings associated with PSVD, NRH is characterised by numerous small hyperplastic nodules, sometimes confluent, that are thought to be a response to obliterative vasculopathy, with consequent increase of intrahepatic pressure and development of PH.

On ultrasound, NRH can occasionally appear in the form of multiple isoechoic nodules surrounded by a hyperechoic rim, a finding known as the 'coral atoll-like' sign (Figure 8.48). However, these ultrasonic findings are rarely described and biopsy remains crucial for diagnosis [43].

Pitfalls

When assessing the liver for cirrhosis and PH, the following scenarios need to be kept in mind:

- Not all patients with compensated advanced CLD who have CSPH show overt signs of cirrhosis or PH, yielding potentially false-negative ultrasound results. Therefore, the absence of signs cannot definitely rule out CSPH.

- Many of the ultrasound features are not specific for PH and diagnostic accuracy is increased when correlated with other clinical findings and confirmatory tests.
- The presence of portal venous flow inversion and porto-systemic collateral circulation is pathognomonic of severe PH. However, both collateral circulation and portal venous flow inversion can also be found in non-cirrhotic PH and there are a variety of pathologies that resemble advanced CLD on ultrasound.

Conclusion

Ultrasound provides fundamental information for assessing liver disease. There are classical features that would suggest CLD and PH and these have been highlighted. Some liver disease aetiologies have distinct features, however some of these differences are less obvious when advanced stages of cirrhosis are reached. There is a variety of liver pathologies or systemic conditions with liver involvement that can mimic cirrhosis, and although some ultrasound features can be of help, in the majority of cases careful integration with clinical history, biochemistry and histology are required to provide a definitive diagnosis. Elastography is a fundamental tool to stage liver disease, especially when imaging can underestimate its severity (see Chapter 9).

References

1 Dietrich, C.F., Serra, C., and Jedrzejczyk, M. (2012). Ultrasound of the liver. In: *EFSUMB – European Course Book*, 2e (ed. C.F. Dietrich), 1–30. London: EFSUMB.

2 Harbin, W.P., Robert, N.J., and Ferrucci, J.T. Jr. (1980). Diagnosis of cirrhosis based on regional changes in hepatic morphology: a radiological and pathological analysis. *Radiology* 135 (2): 273–283.

3 Ito, K., Mitchell, D.G., and Gabata, T. (2000). Enlargement of hilar periportal space: a sign of early cirrhosis at MR imaging. *J. Magn. Reson. Imaging* 11 (2): 136–140.

4 Ito, K., Mitchell, D.G., Kim, M.-J. et al. (2003). Right posterior hepatic notch sign: a simple diagnostic MR sign of cirrhosis. *J. Magn. Reson. Imaging* 18 (5): 561–564.

5 Dietrich, C.F., Wehrmann, T., Zeuzem, S. et al. (1999). Analysis of hepatic echo patterns in chronic hepatitis C. *Ultraschall Med.* 20 (1): 9–14.

6 Asselah, T., Rubbia-Brandt, L., Marcellin, P., and Negro, F. (2006). Steatosis in chronic hepatitis C: why does it really matter? *Gut* 55 (1): 123–130.

7 Chalasani, N., Younossi, Z., Lavine, J.E. et al. (2012). The diagnosis and management of non-alcoholic fatty liver disease: practice guideline by the American Gastroenterological Association, American Association for the Study of Liver Diseases, and American College of Gastroenterology. *Gastroenterology* 142 (7): 1592–1609.

8 Hernaez, R., Lazo, M., Bonekamp, S. et al. (2011). Diagnostic accuracy and reliability of ultrasonography for the detection of fatty liver: a meta-analysis. *Hepatology* 54: 1082–1090.

9 Ferraioli, G. and Soares Monteiro, L.B. (2019). Ultrasound-based techniques for the diagnosis of liver steatosis. *World J. Gastroenterol.* 25 (40): 6053–6062.

10 Berzigotti, A. and Piscaglia, F. (2011). Ultrasound in portal hypertension – part 1. *Ultraschall Med.* 32: 548–571.

11 Bosch, J., Abraldes, J.G., Berzigotti, A. et al. (2009). The clinical use of HVPG measurements in chronic liver disease. *Nat. Rev. Gastroenterol. Hepatol.* 6: 573–582.

12 D'Amico, G., Garcia-Tsao, G., and Pagliaro, L. (2006). Natural history and prognostic indicators of survival in cirrhosis: a systematic review of 118 studies. *J. Hepatol.* 44: 217–231.

13 Piscaglia, F., Donati, G., Serra, C. et al. (2001). Value of splanchnic Doppler ultrasound in the diagnosis of portal hypertension. *Ultrasound Med. Biol.* 27 (7): 893–899.

14 Zironi, G., Gaiani, S., Fenyves, D. et al. (1992). Value of measurement of mean portal flow velocity by Doppler flowmetry in the diagnosis of portal hypertension. *J. Hepatol.* 16: 298–303.

15 Allan, R., Thoirs, K., and Phillips, M. (2010). Accuracy of ultrasound to identify chronic liver disease. *World J. Gastroenterol.* 16 (28): 3510–3520.

16 Berzigotti, A., Zappoli, P., Magalotti, D. et al. (2008). Spleen enlargement on follow-up evaluation: a noninvasive predictor of complications of portal hypertension in cirrhosis. *Clin. Gastroenterol. Hepatol.* 6: 1129–1134.

17 Kashani, A., Salehi, B., Anghesom, D. et al. Spleen size in cirrhosis of different etiologies. *J. Ultrasound Med.* 34 (2): 233–238.

18 Sagoh, T., Itoh, K., Togashi, K. et al. (1989). Gamna-Gandy bodies of the spleen: evaluation with MR imaging. *Radiology* 172 (3): 685.

19 Laurent, O., Lubrano, J., de Beauregard, M. et al. (2011). Gamna-Gandy bodies in cirrhosis: a meaningless finding? *J. Radiol.* 92 (10): 909–914.

20 DA, M.N. and Abu-Yousef, M.M. (2011). Doppler US of the liver made simple. *RadioGraphics* 31: 161–188.

21 Kim, M.Y., Baik, S.K., Park, D.H. et al. (2007). Damping index of Doppler hepatic vein waveform to assess the severity of portal hypertension and response to propranolol in liver cirrhosis: a prospective nonrandomized study. *Liver Int.* 27 (8): 1103–1110.

22 Bolognesi, M., Sacerdoti, D., Merkel, C. et al. (1996). Splenic Doppler impedance indices: influence of different portal hemodynamic conditions. *Hepatology* 23 (5): 1035–1040.

23 Kastelan, S., Ljubicic, N., Kastelan, Z. et al. (2004). The role of duplex-doppler ultrasonography in the diagnosis of renal dysfunction and hepatorenal syndrome in patients with liver cirrhosis. *Hepatogastroenterology* 51 (59): 1408–1412.

24 Moriyasu, F., Nishida, O., Ban, N. et al. (1986). Congestion index of the portal vein. *Am. J. Roentgenol.* 146 (4): 735–739.

25 Wachsberg, R.H. and Simmons, M.Z. (1994). Coronary vein diameter and flow direction in patients with portal hypertension: evaluation with duplex sonography and correlation with variceal bleeding. *Am. J. Roentgenol.* 162: 637–641.

26 Dong, Y., Potthoff, A., Klinger, C. et al. (2018). Ultrasound findings in autoimmune hepatitis. *World J. Gastroenterol.* 24 (15): 1583–1590.

27 Rinella, M.E., Lazarus, J.V., Ratziu, V. et al. (2023). A multi-society Delphi consensus statement on new fatty liver disease nomenclature. *J. Hepatol.* doi: https://doi.org/10.1016/j.jhep.2023.06.003.

28 Younossi, Z., Anstee, Q.M., Marietti, M. et al. (2018). Global burden of NAFLD and NASH: trends, predictions, risk factors and prevention. *Nat. Rev. Gastroenterol. Hepatol.* 15: 11–20.

29 Onofrio, F.Q., Hirschfield, G.M., and Gulamhusein, A.F. (2019). A practical review of primary biliary cholangitis for the gastroenterologist. *Gastroenterol. Hepatol.* 15 (3): 145–154.

30 Dietrich, C.F., Leuschner, M.S., Zeuzem, S. et al. (1999). Peri-hepatic lymphadenopathy in primary biliary cirrhosis reflects progression of the disease. *Eur. J. Gastroenterol. Hepatol.* 11 (7): 747–753.

31 Karlsen, T.H., Folseraas, T., Thorburn, D., and Vesterhus, M. (2017). Primary sclerosing cholangitis – a comprehensive review. *J. Hepatol.* 67: 1298–1323.

32 Singcharoen, T., Baddeley, H., Benson, M., and Ward, M. (1986). Primary sclerosing cholangitis: sonographic findings. *Australas. Radiol.* 30: 99–102.

33 European Association for Study of Liver (2012). EASL clinical practice guidelines: Wilson's disease. *J. Hepatol.* 56: 671–685.

34 Witczak, A., Prystupa, A., Ollegasagrem, S., and Dzida, G. (2015). Cardiohepatic interactions – cirrhotic cardiomyopathy and cardiac cirrhosis. *J. Pre-Clin. Clin. Res.* 9 (1): 79–81.

35 Samsky, M.D., Patel, C.B., DeWald, T.A. et al. (2013). Cardiohepatic interactions in heart failure an overview and clinical implications. *J. Am. Coll. Cardiol.* 61 (24): 2397–2405.

36 Tana, C., Dietrich, C.F., and Schiavone, C. (2014). Hepatosplenic sarcoidosis: contrast-enhanced ultrasound findings and implications for clinical practice. *Biomed. Res. Int.* 2014: 926203.

37 Song, J., Lleo, A., Yang, G.X. et al. (2018). Common variable immunodeficiency and liver involvement. *Clin. Rev. Allergy Immunol.* 55 (3): 340–351.

38 Jeong, W.K., Choi, S.-Y., and Kim, J. (2013). Pseudocirrhosis as a complication after chemotherapy for hepatic metastasis from breast cancer. *Clin. Mol. Hepatol.* 19 (2): 190–192.

39 Senzolo, M., Germani, G., Cholangitas, E. et al. (2007). Veno occlusive disease: update on clinica management. *World J. Gastroenterol.* 13 (29): 3918–3924.

40 Zhang, Y., Yan, Y., and Song, B. (2019). Noninvasive imaging diagnosis of sinusoidal obstruction syndrome: a pictorial review. *Insights Imaging* 10: 110.

41 Akhan, O., Karaosmanoglu, A.D., and Ergen, B. (2007). Imaging findings in congenital hepatic fibrosis. *Eur. J. Radiol.* 61: 18–24.

42 De Gottardi, A., Sempoux, C., and Berzigotti, A. (2022). Porto-sinusoidal vascular disorder. *J. Hepatol.* 77 (4): 1124–1135.

43 Caturelli, E., Ghittoni, G., Ranalli, T.V., and Gomes, V.V. (2011). Nodular regenerative hyperplasia of the liver: coral atoll-like lesions on ultrasound are characteristic in predisposed patients. *Br. J. Radiol.* 84 (1003): e129–e134.

9.1

Shear Wave Elastography for Liver Disease: Part 1

Giovanna Ferraioli

Department of Clinical, Surgical, Diagnostic and Pediatric Sciences, University of Pavia, Pavia, Italy

Introduction to Liver Elastography and Different Elastographic Techniques

Liver fibrosis is the common pathway of several chronic liver diseases. Assessment of the severity of liver fibrosis is crucial for determining the prognosis of patients and for evaluating the need for treatment.

Elastography techniques are able to non-invasively evaluate differences in the elastic properties of soft tissues by measuring the tissue behaviour when a mechanical stress is applied. Elasticity is an intrinsic biomechanical property of every tissue, including the liver. Due to fibrosis, the liver becomes stiffer than normal, and there is a close relationship between liver stiffness and fibrosis stage.

Several studies and meta-analysis have shown the important role played by shear wave elastography (SWE) techniques in the staging of liver fibrosis, and such techniques are increasingly replacing liver biopsy in clinical practice. Indeed, guidelines have accepted that, in several clinical scenarios, SWE can be used instead of liver biopsy for assessing the severity of liver fibrosis.

Elastography techniques show the biomechanical properties of the tissue: under a stress, stiffer tissue shows less longitudinal displacement and higher speed of transverse displacement. B-mode ultrasound, in contrast, shows the acoustic properties of tissue. Thus, B-mode ultrasound and elastography give different and complementary information about the status of the liver.

The term SWE includes all the techniques based on the assessment of the shear wave speed (SWS) [1]. The shear wave displacement is generated (i) by an external mechanical stress, as in vibration-controlled transient elastography (VCTE) – which is performed with a dedicated system, the FibroScan® (Echosens, Paris, France) – or in magnetic resonance elastography (MRE); or (ii) by using the push-pulse of a focused ultrasound beam, as in the acoustic radiation force impulse (ARFI)-based techniques integrated into standard ultrasound systems.

The shear waves travel at a speed between 1 and 10 m/s depending on the tissue stiffness: in stiffer tissue they propagate faster [2, 3].

Physical Principles of Shear Wave Elastography

SWE relies on the generation of shear waves determined by the displacement of tissue induced by external pressure (VCTE) or by the force of a focused ultrasound beam (ARFI-based techniques).

Vibration-Controlled Transient Elastography

VCTE is performed with a dedicated device, the FibroScan. Vibrations of mild amplitude and low frequency (50 Hz) are transmitted by the tip of the transducer through the liver, inducing an elastic shear wave that propagates through the underlying tissue. The FibroScan is not a real-time ultrasound device; however, A-mode and time-motion mode are used to locate the area of liver parenchyma to perform the measurement and to monitor the SWS propagation (Figure 9.1.1). Pulse-echo ultrasound acquisitions are used to follow the propagation of the shear wave and to measure its velocity [4].

Software for the quantification of liver steatosis, the controlled attenuation parameter (CAP), has been developed and is available in the new generation of FibroScan devices. The CAP is based on the properties of ultrasound signals acquired by FibroScan using the hypothesis that fat affects

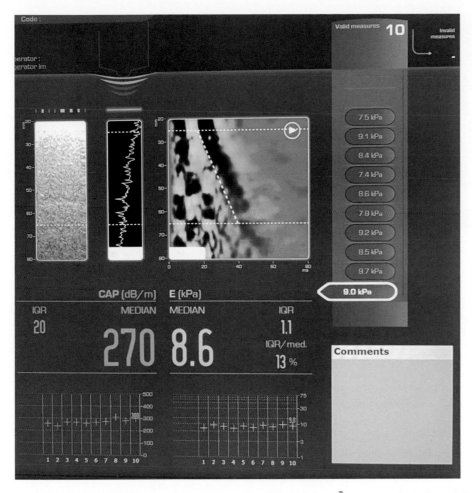

Figure 9.1.1 Transient elastography readings (FibroScan 502 Touch®, Echosens, Paris, France). On the monitor, all the measurements are displayed. The system automatically filters out invalid measurements and their number, if any, is shown on the top right. The median value of the measurements (in kPa) is reported together with the interquartile/median (IQR/M) ratio. The system also quantifies the attenuation of the ultrasound beam, in dB/m, using a proprietary algorithm (controlled attenuation parameter, CAP). The median CAP value, together with the IQR, is shown. Above the readings and from left to right: TM-mode, A-mode, and shear wave propagation speed reported in a distance-time graph.

ultrasound propagation. The CAP is evaluated using the same radio-frequency (RF) data and region of interest (ROI) that are used for liver stiffness measurement (LSM).

Acoustic Radiation Force Impulse–Based Shear Wave Elastography

In ARFI-based techniques, a dynamic stress is applied with short-duration acoustic forces (pushing pulses). It causes localised displacements deep within tissue; the shear waves that are generated are tracked and their speed, thus the elasticity of the tissue, is estimated. The ultrasound beams designed to create a measurable displacement with acoustic radiation force have longer pulses (50–1000 μs) able to generate micron-level tissue displacements [2, 3]. The shear waves are transverse waves, with a motion perpendicular to the direction of the force that has generated them; that is, perpendicular to the direction of the ultrasound beam. In soft tissue, shear waves propagate at a speed 1000 times slower than the speed of sound and they attenuate very fast.

The speed of the shear wave can be measured in a small ROI, as in point shear wave elastography (pSWE). B-mode ultrasound is used to select the area of liver parenchyma to perform the measurement (Figures 9.1.2–9.1.6). With 2D-SWE, quantitative images of the SWS (or stiffness) in a large ROI are obtained by placing the ARFI focus (push) at multiple sequential locations and, at each, detecting the shear wave arrival time at multiple lateral locations [2, 3]. An image, which is a colour-coded map of the SWS, is built. A measurement box is then positioned inside the ROI to obtain the values of shear wave speed/stiffness (Figures 9.1.7–9.1.12).

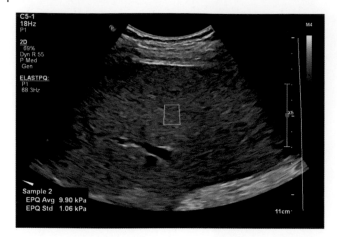

Figure 9.1.2 Point shear wave elastography (ElastPQ®, EPIQ Elite ultrasound system, Philips Healthcare, Eindhoven, Netherlands). The region of interest (the yellow rectangle) has a fixed size. The mean value of the push-track sequences is given together with the standard deviation (SD). An SD ⩽ 30% of the mean value indicates an acquisition of good quality. When the signal-to-noise ratio of an acquisition is very low, the mean value is not shown.

SuperSonic Imagine (Hologic, USA) has a proprietary radiation force technique termed supersonic shear imaging. Ultrasound plane-waves, which enable an ultrafast frame rate (typically faster than 1000 frames per second), are transmitted. The tissue displacement is generated at all positions along the acoustic axis almost simultaneously. This produces a shear wave in the shape of a cone, known as a Mach cone, which decays less rapidly with distance than that from a single push-pulse [5].

ARFI-based techniques are all implemented in ultrasound systems, either pSWE or 2D-SWE. The manufacturers usually have registered names for their elastography products.

Units of Measure

SWS is displayed in metres/second (m/s). Assuming that the tissue has a very simple behaviour (i.e. it is linear, isotropic, and homogeneous) and is incompressible, the velocity of shear wave propagation can be converted to tissue stiffness through the Young's modulus, $E = 3 \ (\rho \times vS^2)$, where E is the Young's modulus, ρ is the density of tissue, and vS is the SWS [2, 3].

The Young's modulus is a measure of stiffness, and it indicates how difficult it is to deform a material by stretching or compression (E = uniaxial stress/uniaxial strain). The unit of measurement is the kilopascal (kPa); that is, the unit of pressure.

It should be underlined that speed may also be converted to the shear modulus G, which measures the ability of a material to resist transverse deformations: shear stress/shear strain. The shear modulus has the same unit of measure as

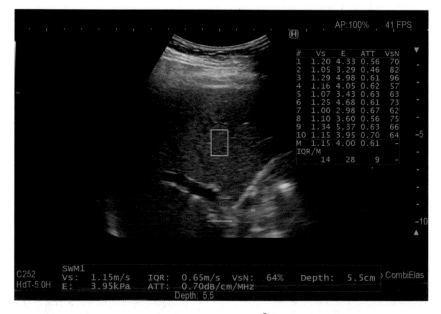

Figure 9.1.3 Point shear wave elastography (SWM®, Arietta 850 ultrasound system, Hitachi, Tokyo, Japan). The region of interest (the yellow rectangle) has a fixed size. All measurements and the final report with median value and interquartile/median (IQR/M) ratio of the parameters are shown directly on the image (or in a separate report). 'VsN' is a reliability index that indicates the percentage of effective push-track sequences. When the signal-to-noise ratio of an acquisition is very low, the mean value is not shown. The system simultaneously quantifies the attenuation of the ultrasound beam in dB/cm/MHz with a proprietary algorithm (attenuation coefficient, ATT).

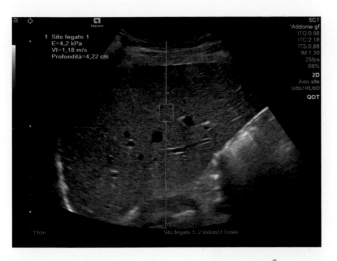

Figure 9.1.4 Point shear wave elastography (VTQ®, Sequoia ultrasound system, Siemens Healthineers, Erlangen, Germany). The region of interest (the white rectangle) has a fixed size. The system automatically filters out the measurements that are not good. In these cases, the numerical value of the shear wave speed is replaced by an 'XXX' sequence.

the Young's modulus, kPa, but it is three times smaller: $G = \rho \times vS^2$. The shear modulus G is used in MRE.

The choice of whether to display speed or modulus is usually under user control. It is preferable to report results in m/s rather than kPa. In fact, the ultrasound system measures the SWS. The conversion to kPa using a simple equation is based on many assumptions that may not be correct [3]. Nonetheless, the measure of stiffness using the Young's modulus in kPa has become quite

common in clinical practice since the availability of the FibroScan.

Finally, we assume a linearly elastic, homogeneous, isotropic, infinite, continuous medium, but biological tissues are viscoelastic. The assessment of viscoelastic properties is still a research field. Some studies are focused on the evaluation of shear wave dispersion as a marker of necroinflammation.

Confounding Factors and Current Limitations

Liver stiffness is related to liver fibrosis; however, there are other physiological or pathological conditions that can determine an increase of stiffness not due to liver fibrosis. As recommended by the European Federation for Ultrasound in Medicine and Biology (EFSUMB) and World Federation for Ultrasound in Medicine and Biology (WFUMB) guidelines and Society of Radiologists in Ultrasound (SRU) consensus, these confounding factors should be excluded before performing LSM with SWE, in order to avoid overestimation of liver fibrosis, and/or should be considered when interpreting the SWE results [6–10].

An increase in liver stiffness not related to liver fibrosis is observed in the following conditions: exacerbations of acute hepatitis associated with transaminase flares, therefore the effect of necroinflammation should be taken into account, and the results should always be evaluated in clinical settings; infiltrative liver diseases such as amyloidosis, lymphomas, and extramedullary hemopoiesis; congestive heart

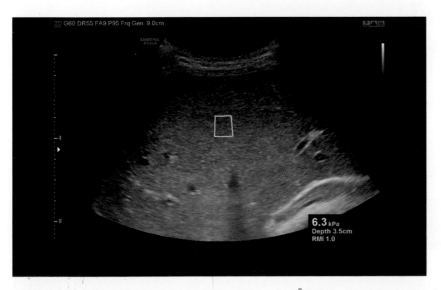

Figure 9.1.5 Point shear wave elastography (S-Shearwave®, RS80A ultrasound system, Samsung Medison, Gangwon, South Korea). The region of interest (the yellow rectangle) has a fixed size. The quality of each measurement is assessed with the performance index, the 'Reliability Measurement Index' (RMI), which is calculated by the weighted sum of the residual of the wave equation and the magnitude of the shear wave. *Source:* Courtesy of Prof Vito Cantisani.

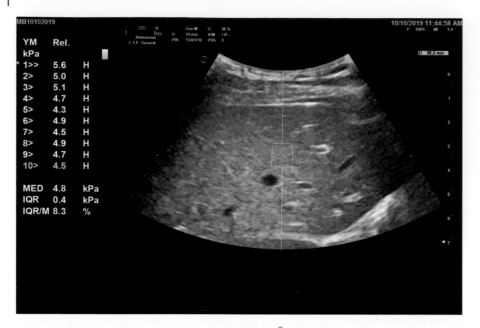

Figure 9.1.6 Point shear wave elastography (QElaXto®, MyLab™9 ultrasound system, Esaote, Genoa, Italy). The region of interest (the white rectangle) has a fixed size. The quality of each acquisition is assessed with the reliability index, which is shown together with each value of stiffness by the alphabetical letter H, M, or L, indicating high quality, medium quality, or low quality of the acquisition.

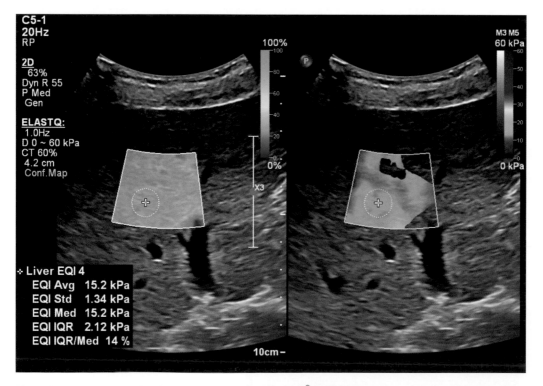

Figure 9.1.7 Two-dimensional shear wave elastography (EQI®, EPIQ Elite ultrasound system, Philips Healthcare, Eindhoven, Netherlands). Colour-coded image of liver stiffness (right side) and confidence map (left side) in a large and modifiable region of interest. The colour-coded confidence map is an evaluation of the quality of the acquired signals. The confidence threshold (CT) is set at 60%: areas of poor quality (red and yellow) are filtered out and left blank on the colour-coded image of liver stiffness assessment (right side); the yellow colour on the confidence map is a warning, indicating that the acquisition in that area is not the most effective and can be filtered out, as in this image.

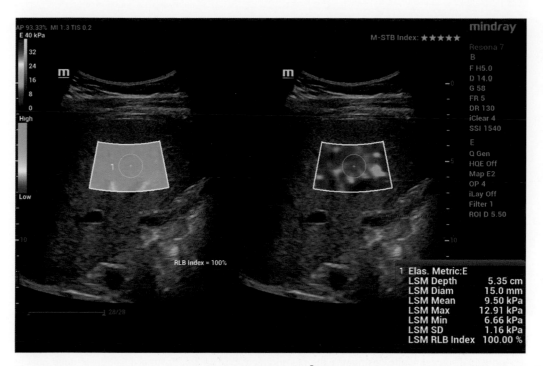

Figure 9.1.8 Two-dimensional shear wave elastography (STE®, Resona 7 ultrasound system, Mindray Medical Systems, Shenzhen, China). Two quality criteria are provided. The Motion Stability (M-STB) index (right upper part of the image) is indicated by stars: the highest stability of the acquired elasticity image is indicated by five green stars, whereas red stars indicate motion. The Reliability (RLB) map (left side) goes from purple, which indicates poor reliability, to green, which indicates the highest reliability. The M-STB is guidance for choosing the most stable image in a cineloop, whereas the RLB is guidance for placement of the measurement box (circle).

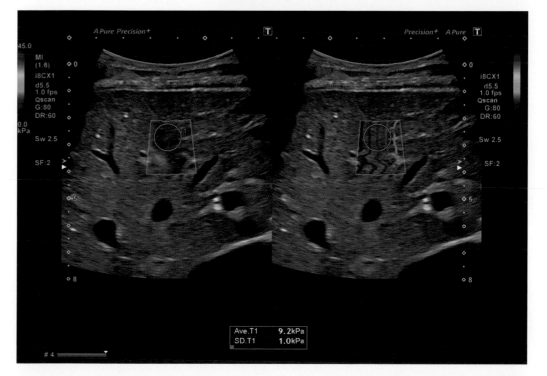

Figure 9.1.9 Two-dimensional shear wave elastography (Aplio i800 series ultrasound system, Canon Medical Systems, Tochigi, Japan). The system filters out values with a low signal-to-noise ratio and these areas are left blank. The system has a proprietary quality parameter: the propagation map (right side). The colour map and the propagation map are shown side by side on the screen. A proper propagation map is displayed by parallel lines, with the intervals between the lines constant. When these criteria are not fulfilled, the reliability of the data obtained is low. The propagation map is guidance for placing the measurement box (circle).

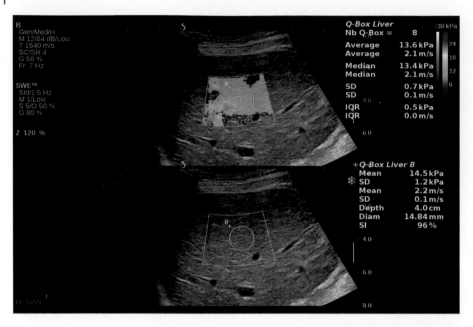

Figure 9.1.10 Two-dimensional shear wave elastography (SSI, Aixplorer® ultrasound system, Supersonic Imagine, Aix-en-Provence, France). The system filters out values with a low signal-to-noise ratio and these areas are left blank. The stability index (SI) is an indicator of temporal stability, and it is displayed while positioning the measurement box (Q-Box™). An acquisition of good quality should have an SI >90%.

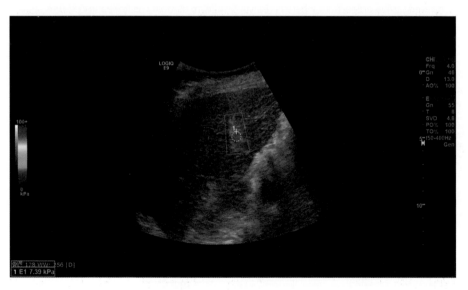

Figure 9.1.11 Two-dimensional shear wave elastography (LOGIQ® E9 ultrasound system, General Electric, St Paul, MN, USA). A quality threshold prevents areas with low-quality measurements from being displayed. *Source:* Courtesy of Prof Ioan Sporea.

failure; and extrahepatic cholestasis. Due to the increase in portal blood flow, food ingestion also increases the stiffness, as does deep inspiration, so that transiently stopping breathing in a neutral position is optimal for measurement. The increase in liver stiffness observed in patients with alcoholic hepatitis usually decreases following 1–4 weeks of abstinence.

As for the influence of steatosis, it is still a matter of debate with conflicting data in the literature: some studies suggest that steatosis determines an increase in liver stiffness, whereas others do not.

Cut-Off Values for Staging Liver Fibrosis and Sources of Variability

There is significant intersystem variability in LSM. In the viscoelastic phantoms developed by the Radiological Society of North America (RSNA) Quantitative Imaging Biomarker Alliance (QIBA) ultrasound Shear Wave Speed (SWS) committee, the greatest outlier system in each phantom/focal depth combination ranged from 12.7% to 17.6% [11].

Figure 9.1.12 Two-dimensional shear wave elastography (Acuson Sequoia™ ultrasound system, Siemens Healthineers, Erlangen, Germany). The system filters out values with a low signal-to-noise ratio and these areas are left blank. The blue relates to softer tissue.

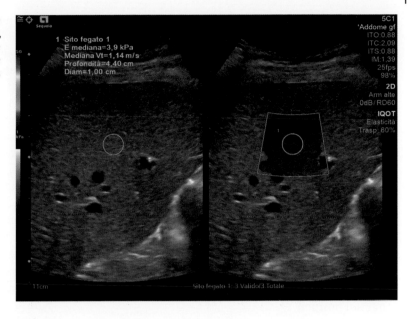

In a study that has evaluated the intersystem variability in LSM, agreement between measurements performed with different systems was good to excellent, and the overall interobserver agreement was above 0.90 in expert hands. However, a high concordance merely indicates that the values follow the same direction, not that the absolute values are the same [12].

Therefore, cut-off values for staging liver fibrosis with SWE techniques are system specific and cannot interchangeably be applied across different ultrasound systems.

The best cut-off values depend also on the aetiology of the underlying liver disease, and on the prevalence of the disease in the target population.

As recommended by EFSUMB and WFUMB guidelines and SRU consensus, elastography values should always be interpreted by a liver specialist aware of the clinical aspects of the liver disease and of the peculiarities of elastography in general and each elastography technique in particular.

There are several sources of variability [3, 6–10]:

- *Measurement depth*: the results with the lowest variability are obtained at a depth of 4–5 cm with a convex transducer. On the other hand, the ARFI pulse is attenuated as it traverses the tissue, therefore measurements taken at a greater depth have less signal-to-noise ratio.
- *Frequency of the transducer*: the linear transducer gives higher values.
- *Position of the transducer*: the highest intra- and interobserver agreement was obtained for measurements performed through the intercostal space. It should be emphasised that cardiac motion affects results from the left lobe of the liver, whereas compression of the liver with the transducer is likely to occur when the measurement is performed subcostally.

- *Position of the patient*: the supine position has been used in most published studies.
- *Respiration phase*: deep inspiration affects measurement; it has been suggested to perform measurement in a breath hold for a few seconds during quiet breathing.
- *Food ingestion*: this increases stiffness because there is a post-prandial increase in portal blood flow.
- *Fibrosis stage*: using VCTE, it has been reported that reproducibility decreases in the lower stage of liver fibrosis.
- *Liver steatosis and liver fibrosis*: due to the attenuation of the ultrasound beam, examination is more difficult in a case of severe steatosis or severe fibrosis.
- *Operator experience*: this also plays an important role. Guidelines have emphasised that experience in B-mode ultrasound is mandatory, and the operator must acquire appropriate knowledge and training in ultrasound elastography.
- *Operator training*: for pSWE, several studies have shown that the operator requires only a short period of training to perform reliable LSM. For 2D-SWE the learning curve is longer.

Moreover, there are several factors affecting data quality and producing speed errors or loss of signal, including strength of push; variations in attenuation, absorption, and reflection of the pushing beam; ultrasound scatterer density; very high or very low shear wave speed; shear wave scattering; and reflection or refraction of the shear waves. The user should be aware of these artefacts. Some of them may be avoided following correct protocol for acquisitions.

An estimation of the quality of SWS assessment is generally provided by the manufacturers (Figures 9.1.1–9.1.12).

Practical Advice

Protocol for Acquisitions [3, 6–10]

The following protocol is recommended for acquisitions:

- Patients should be fasting for at least two hours.
- Examination should be performed in the supine or slight left lateral position (not more than 30°), with the right arm raised above the head to increase the intercostal space.
- Measurements should be obtained with an intercostal approach and the best acoustic window, without shadowing due to the ribs or the lung, should be chosen.
- Measurements should be taken 1.5–2.0 cm below the liver capsule to avoid reverberation artefact.
- The patient should breathe normally while looking for the best acoustic window; the measurement is performed while the patient holds their breath in a neutral position.
- The optimal location for maximum strength of the push-pulse is 4.0–5.0 cm from the transducer.

- The transducer should be positioned at 90° with respect to the liver capsule.
- Placement of the ROI should avoid large blood vessels, bile ducts, and masses.
- The ROI should be positioned in the middle of the image.
- For VCTE the appropriate transducer should be selected based on the skin-to-liver capsule distance (this assessment is automatically made by the VCTE software).
- Ten measurements should be obtained from ten independent images, in the same location, with the median value used for transient elastography and pSWE techniques.
- Five measurements may be appropriate for 2D-SWE when the manufacturer's quality assessment parameter is used.
- The interquartile/median (IQR/M) ratio, which assesses the variability in a set of acquisitions, should be used as a measure of quality. For measurements in kPa the IQR/M should be ≤30% and for measurements in m/s it should be ≤15%. This is the most important quality criterion for reliable measurement.

References

1 Ferraioli, G. (2019). Ultrasound techniques for the assessment of liver stiffness: a correct terminology. *Hepatology* 69 (1): 461.

2 Bamber, J., Cosgrove, D., Dietrich, C.F. et al. (2013). EFSUMB guidelines and recommendations on the clinical use of ultrasound elastography. Part 1: basic principles and technology. *Ultraschall Med.* 34 (2): 169–184.

3 Dietrich, C.F., Bamber, J., Berzigotti, A. et al. (2017). EFSUMB guidelines and recommendations on the clinical use of liver ultrasound elastography, update 2017 (long version). *Ultraschall Med.* 38 (4): e16–e47.

4 Sandrin, L., Oudry, J., Bastard, C. et al. Non-invasive assessment of liver fibrosis by vibration-controlled transient elastography (Fibroscan®). In: *Liver Biopsy* (ed. H. Takahashi), n.p. London: IntechOpen www.intechopen.com/chapters/18782.

5 Bercoff, J., Tanter, M., and Fink, M. (2004). Supersonic shear imaging: a new technique for soft tissue elasticity mapping. *IEEE Trans. Ultrason. Ferroelectr. Freq. Control* 51 (4): 396–409.

6 Dietrich, C.F., Bamber, J., Berzigotti, A. et al. (2017). EFSUMB guidelines and recommendations on the clinical use of liver ultrasound elastography, update 2017 (short version). *Ultraschall Med.* 38 (4): 377–394.

7 Ferraioli, G., Filice, C., Castera, L. et al. (2015). WFUMB guidelines and recommendations on the clinical use of ultrasound elastography, Part 3: liver. *Ultrasound Med. Biol.* 41 (5): 1161–1179.

8 Ferraioli, G., Wong, V.W., Castera, L. et al. (2018). Liver ultrasound Elastography: an update to the world federation for ultrasound in medicine and biology guidelines and recommendations. *Ultrasound Med. Biol.* 44 (12): 2419–2440.

9 Barr, R.G., Ferraioli, G., Palmeri, M.L. et al. (2015). Elastography assessment of liver fibrosis: society of radiologists in ultrasound consensus conference statement. *Radiology* 276 (3): 845–861.

10 Barr, R.G., Wilson, S.R., Rubens, D. et al. (2020). Update to the society of radiologists in ultrasound liver elastography consensus statement. *Radiology* 296 (2): 263–274.

11 Palmeri, M., Nightingale, K., Fielding, S. et al. RSNA QIBA ultrasound shear wave speed Phase II phantom study in viscoelastic media. In: *Proceedings of the 2015 IEEE Ultrasonics Symposium*, 397–400. New York: Institute of Electrical and Electronics Engineers.

12 Ferraioli, G., De Silvestri, A., Lissandrin, R. et al. (2019). Evaluation of inter-system variability in liver stiffness measurements. *Ultraschall Med.* 40 (1): 64–75.

9.2

Shear Wave Elastography for Liver Disease: Part 2

Matteo Rosselli[1,2], Ioan Sporea[3], and Giovanna Ferraioli[4]

[1] Department of Internal Medicine, San Giuseppe Hospital, USL Toscana Centro, Empoli, Italy
[2] Division of Medicine, Institute for Liver and Digestive Health, University College London, Royal Free Hospital, London, UK
[3] Department of Gastroenterology and Hepatology, Victor Babes University of Medicine and Pharmacy, Timisoara, Romania
[4] Department of Clinical, Surgical, Diagnostic and Pediatric Sciences, University of Pavia, Pavia, Italy

Clinical Use and Interpretation of Shear Wave Elastography in Liver Disease

Elastography has marked a milestone in the management of liver disease, by dramatically reducing the number of biopsies for staging purposes [1], predicting the severity of portal hypertension (PH) [2], and providing information on the risk of clinical decompensation in cirrhosis [3]. It has also proven to be a useful tool in the follow-up of liver transplant patients [4], as well as in the paediatric population with chronic liver disease (CLD) [5]. Furthermore, the liver can be a target in systemic diseases and elastography can reveal its possible involvement. This chapter aims to provide an overview on the applications of elastography, highlighting its indications, benefits, and limitations, in line with the most recent guidelines and practical experience in various clinical scenarios.

Elastography Assessment of Liver Fibrosis

Elastography was validated by comparing liver stiffness (LS) results to the amount of fibrosis found on biopsy. According to histological staging, four different ranges of LS were defined as surrogate markers of fibrosis (F0/F1 no or low-grade fibrosis, F2 moderate fibrosis, F3 severe fibrosis, and F4 cirrhosis). However, the diagnostic accuracy of elastography is higher in identifying no or minimal fibrosis (F0/F1), severe fibrosis or cirrhosis (F3–F4), and in general in 'ruling in' and 'ruling out' cirrhosis. The intermediate ranges of LS correlate with a continuum of moderate to severe fibrosis, in which there could be a certain degree of overlap, especially if one considers that the fibrosis scoring system traditionally follows a scale of descriptive 'semi-quantitative' measurements, while LS is a quantitative method (Figure 9.2.1). Hence, when stiffness values fall in

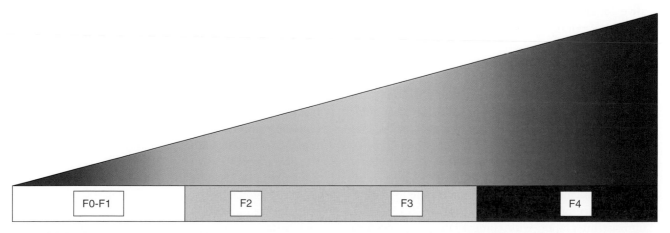

| F0-F1 | F2 | F3 | F4 |

Figure 9.2.1 Elastography is considered accurate in detecting minimal or absent fibrosis and advanced fibrosis/cirrhosis. Intermediate stages of fibrosis (F2–F3) may fall in a grey zone of low diagnostic accuracy where an overlap of values can potentially be found.

this 'grey zone' particular caution is recommended, suggesting additional tests and eventually even liver biopsy in case of ongoing diagnostic uncertainty [6].

The interpretation of LS results needs to take several elements into account:

- *Equipment-related variability*: there are several available elastographic techniques and manufacturers, for which LS measurements and fibrosis cut-off values are different and therefore they must not be considered interchangeable [7]. For example, the stiffness values that correlate with moderate or severe fibrosis measured by a specific software could instead relate to minimal and moderate fibrosis, respectively, obtained with another software. Therefore the report should always specify which technique and equipment were used. However, while a difference in stiffness ranges of fibrosis is found among different kinds of software, all elastographic techniques agree that a stiffness value <5 kPa will surely exclude fibrosis, if the reliability criteria are satisfied. With regard to cirrhosis, all systems are highly accurate in distinguishing no fibrosis from severe fibrosis/cirrhosis, although variability of cut-off values is not only related to the elastographic software, but also to aetiology and confounding factors [7].
- *Liver disease aetiology*: it is extremely important to acknowledge differences in aetiology-related liver disease. In fact, although the endpoint of CLD is cirrhosis, the timing and natural history might be different, depending on the kind of inflammatory process, distribution of fibrosis, and development of PH, as well as the malignant potential. One of the issues in using different systems is that not all of them have been validated against biopsy or in all liver disease aetiologies, advising caution, integration, and careful interpretation of the results.
- *Confounding factors*: as previously mentioned, LS is relative to the biomechanical properties of liver parenchyma, therefore a higher measurement should not be considered an absolute value attributable solely to fibrosis. This is a very important point when interpreting elastography results, since hepatic congestion, cholestasis, inflammation, and parenchymal infiltration can all increase stiffness, regardless of fibrosis through different mechanisms [1]. Under these circumstances, elastography can yield false-positive results when fibrosis is not even present or overestimate the severity of underlying liver disease (Figure 9.2.2). Along these lines, it can be very difficult and sometimes impossible to evaluate the presence or severity of liver disease in relation to fibrosis. Integration with clinical/laboratory investigations, background history, and ultrasound findings provides the necessary information to evaluate the presence or absence of superimposed elements. The clinical

response to dynamic changes and delta stiffness value during a specific treatment (antiviral treatment, diuretics, immune suppression, biliary obstruction resolution, alcohol withdrawal) might be of help, although caution and strict follow-up are highly recommended (Figures 9.2.3–9.2.5) (Videos 9.2.1 and 9.2.2).

Elastography Assessment of Portal Hypertension

PH is a crucial clinical landmark in the natural history of liver disease, representing the physiopathological base of cirrhosis-related complications [8]. Therefore once CLD is diagnosed, it is extremely important to know if the patient has cirrhosis and if the threshold of clinically significant portal hypertension (CSPH) is reached. However, it is also important to bear in mind that the timeframe between these two endpoints is difficult to define, that imaging is usually unable to assess the degree of PH, and that liver disease might clinically declare itself with a decompensating event (variceal bleeding, ascites, hepatic encephalopathy) if its severity is not predicted accurately. It is within this physiopathological landscape that elastography fills a gap of diagnostic uncertainty, in which imaging might underestimate the severity of liver disease, and in which the diagnostic gold standard would be highly invasive (hepatic venous pressure gradient [HVPG] measurement) and endoscopic screening could be carried out unnecessarily, in the absence of high-risk varices. Robust data shows that liver elastography is able to predict the presence of both CSPH and high-risk varices in cirrhosis with considerably high accuracy, reducing the number of unnecessary endoscopies [9, 10]. Nevertheless, a few considerations need to be kept in mind.

Physiopathological Background of Cirrhotic Portal Hypertension and Non-invasive Assessment

The development of PH can be roughly distinguished in a first phase characterised by liver fibrosis and nodular regeneration, which increase intrahepatic resistances, and in a second phase related to more advanced cirrhosis, in which extrahepatic factors, mainly vasoactive molecules, influence splanchnic flow, further increasing PH.

LS has a good linear correlation with HVPG until the threshold of CSPH is reached (HVPG ≥10 mmHg). Since varices develop in the presence of severe PH, with a relative increase of bleeding risk for HVPG >12 mmHg, the diagnostic accuracy of LS per se, in detecting high-risk varices, is lower than expected [11]. The accuracy of non-invasive assessment of PH was improved by combining LS and platelet count, as recommended by the Baveno VI

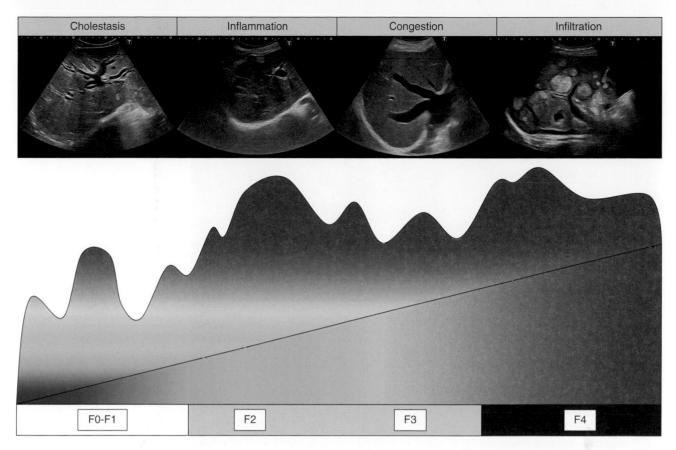

Figure 9.2.2 The presence of confounding factors such as cholestasis, inflammation, congestion, and hepatic infiltration increases liver stiffness (LS), leading to false-positive results. There is no specific cut-off level that allows discrimination of the exact impact of confounding factors on the elastography results related to possible fibrosis. Eventually, if the confounding factor can be reduced/removed, the delta stiffness value will provide information on the magnitude of the interference and the true baseline value of LS, which may or may not reveal underlying fibrosis. The figures of the ultrasound scans above the diagram represent examples of confounding factors that can lead to increased stiffness regardless of the severity of fibrosis. The undulated line represents an example of the potential stiffness variability induced by the impact of confounding factors.

(a)

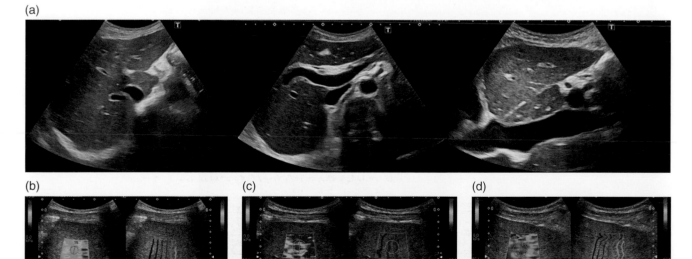

Figure 9.2.3 (a) B-mode ultrasound shows features in keeping with chronic liver disease (CLD) in a 58-year-old woman with a suspected diagnosis of autoimmune hepatitis. Elastography shows dynamic changes of liver stiffness (LS) according to the severity/worsening and improvement of hepatic inflammation over a period of three weeks. (b) At time 0 the patient was assessed showing high LS results in keeping with cirrhosis (20 kPa). However, transaminase levels were significantly high (>500 U/L), suggesting possible interference. (c) At one week biochemistry showed further worsening of liver function tests and transaminase, with a simultaneous increase of LS (37 kPa). Liver biopsy was carried out and the patient was commenced on high-dose steroids, with a dramatic improvement of LS (13 kPa) after just three days of immunosuppressive treatment (d). Findings in keeping with CLD secondary to autoimmune hepatitis with severe inflammatory flare and significant treatment response.

(a)

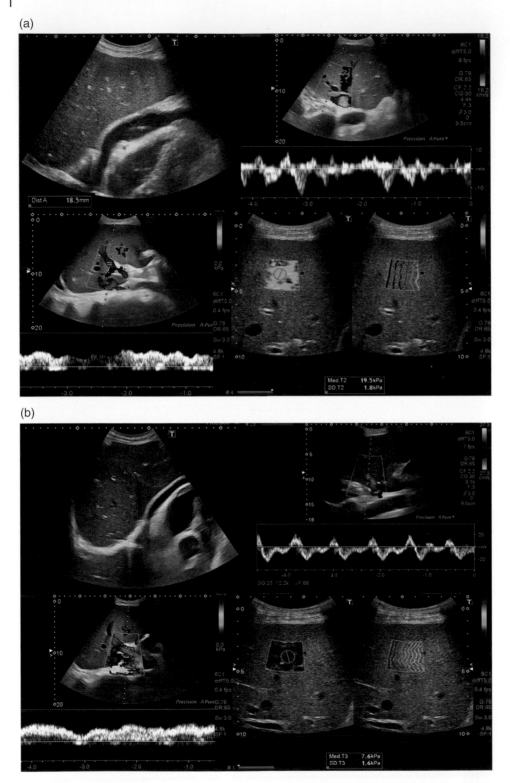

(b)

Figure 9.2.4 Patient with polyserositis complicated by pericardial effusion and severe hypotension. (a) At presentation the patient was severely hypotensive with an arterial pressure of 70/40 mmHg, clinically dehydrated, in atrial fibrillation, and with an almost 2 cm pericardial effusion, which caused hepatic congestion secondary to dynamic cardiac outflow obstruction (Video 9.2.1). There was pulsatile portal venous flow and deranged spectral waveform of the hepatic veins. Liver stiffness (LS) was significantly increased (19.5 kPa) and there was no clear sign of chronic liver disease on B-mode ultrasound. (b) After large-volume fluid infusion and anti-inflammatory treatment, there was significant reduction of the pericardial effusion, with consequent improvement of heart rate and venous return recruitment (Video 9.2.2). Haemodynamic improvement was accompanied by an almost complete normalisation of LS, as shown by 2D shear wave elastography (7.6 kPa).

(a)

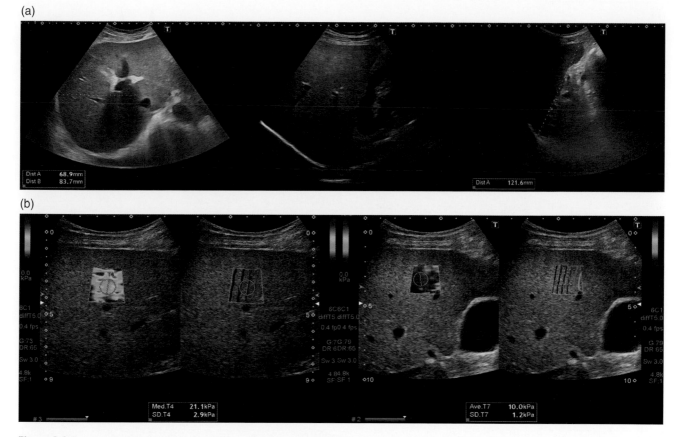

(b)

Figure 9.2.5 A patient admitted to hospital with clinical and biochemical features of alcohol hepatitis and no known history of liver disease. (a) Ultrasound showed caudate lobe/right lobe ratio (CL/RL) >0.65 and initial margin retraction in keeping with chronic liver disease (CLD), but a smooth liver contour and no splenomegaly. (b) Elastography on admission revealed a liver stiffness value of 21.1 kPa (left side) and subsequent significant reduction of almost 10 kPa at one week after detoxification (right side). Features in keeping with alcohol-induced hepatitis against the background of CLD and no signs of clinically significant portal hypertension.

Consensus Conference (and confirmed in Baveno VII), which initially proposed a vibration-controlled transient elastography (VCTE) LS cut-off ≤20 kPa and a platelet count ≥150 000/mm^3 to rule out patients without high-risk varices, hence who could safely avoid an endoscopic screening. These recommendations have been validated extensively with VCTE in hepatitis B (HBV) and hepatitis C (HCV)-related cirrhosis, as well as in alcohol-related cirrhosis, with the prerequisite of the absence of superimposed alcoholic hepatitis [9, 10]. However, even better results were obtained by measuring spleen stiffness (SS), which proved to be independently correlated to CSPH, accurately predicting the presence of high-risk varices as well as the risk of clinical decompensation in cirrhosis [12, 13]. In other terms, when the threshold of CSPH is reached significant variability can be found among LS values, although the integration with platelet count increases the diagnostic accuracy of diagnosing CSPH. Nevertheless, SS has a stronger, progressive, and independent correlation with the severity of PH (Figure 9.2.6). The rationale behind the higher accuracy of SS compared to LS in predicting severe PH is thought to be secondary to the following reasons:

- While PH develops, the resistance to blood flow is transmitted through the splenic vein to the splenic parenchyma, which becomes highly congested, with a consequent increase in intrasplenic pressure and therefore SS.
- The more advanced cirrhosis is, the more nodular, fibrotic, and irregular hepatic parenchyma will be. Such irregularities can influence LS values, yielding high results or relatively low ones, regardless of the severity of CLD, since measurements might be taken on large regenerative nodularities or areas of scarring (Figure 9.2.7) [7]. SS instead seems to have a more homogeneous distribution of stiffness throughout splenic parenchyma (Figure 9.2.8), likely because the increase of SS in PH is mainly secondary to congestion, as shown by its significant reduction after transjugular portal-systemic shunt placement and even more after liver transplantation [14].
- The severity of PH in advanced stages of cirrhosis is less dependent on hepatic structure and more on extrahepatic factors [13, 15]. In addition, SS has proven to be an independent marker of PH, regardless of the underlying cause [2]. This is clinically very relevant, because it permits the distinction of non-cirrhotic PH in which LS, even in the presence of severe PH, is usually relatively

(a)

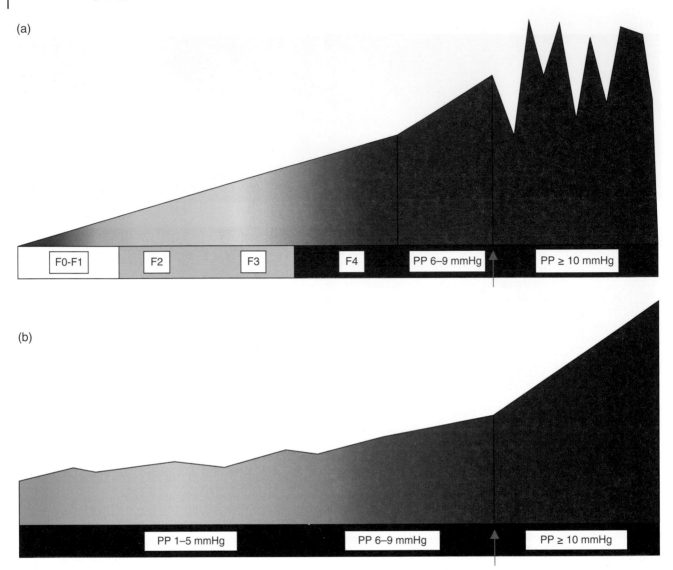

| F0–F1 | F2 | F3 | F4 | PP 6–9 mmHg | PP ≥ 10 mmHg |

(b)

| PP 1–5 mmHg | PP 6–9 mmHg | PP ≥ 10 mmHg |

Figure 9.2.6 Two schematic diagrams that summarise the trend of (a) liver stiffness (LS) and (b) spleen stiffness (SS) in relation to different degrees of fibrosis and clinically significant portal hypertension (CSPH) in cirrhosis. (a) LS increases progressively together with the severity of fibrosis with a good correlation until the threshold of CSPH is reached (arrow). Beyond this point (≥10mmHg) the correlation is lower owing to increased variability with relatively low values of LS, or very high ones likely secondary to liver parenchymal irregularities. (b) SS is higher than LS in basal conditions and remains stable or slightly higher when severe fibrosis/cirrhosis is reached. However, it is only in the presence of CSPH (arrow) that SS increases significantly, showing a very good correlation with the severity of portal hypertension. In b the values of portal pressure 1-5 mmHg are related to fibrosis in the abscence of portal hypertension; the values 6-9 mmHg instead refer to cirrhosis without CSPH, while values ≥10 mmHg refer to CSPH. PP = portal pressure.

lower compared to cirrhosis (Figure 9.2.9) [16]. In addition, SS would be very useful in evaluating the presence of CSPH in different liver disease aetiologies, where a presinusoidal component might be present, such as in primary biliary cholangitis (PBC) and primary sclerosing cholangitis (PSC), and in which PH could develop prior to advanced cirrhosis. Finally, SS could provide key information in those cases in which confounding factors influence LS reliability, making it an important discriminant for 'ruling in' or 'ruling out' the presence of CSPH.

Non-invasive Liver Disease Assessment and the Importance of Integrating Elastography with Ultrasound Imaging

Ultrasound can detect parenchymal changes of CLD expressed as echotexture heterogeneity and irregular outline. In general, its specificity is high for advanced stages of CLD, where clear modification of liver morphology, signs of PH, and clinical decompensation are more obvious, but its sensitivity is low, especially in the pre-cirrhotic and early stages of cirrhosis.

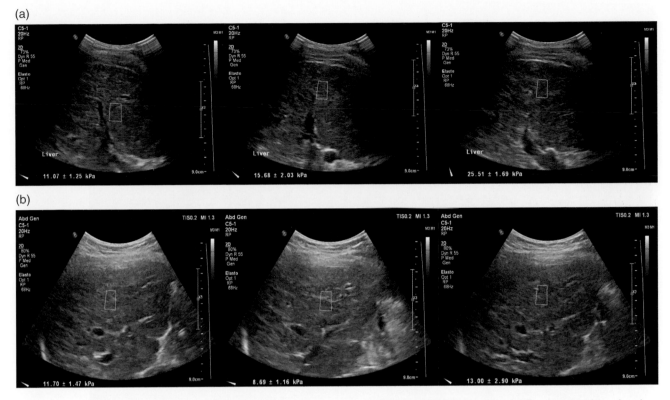

Figure 9.2.7 Two cases of primary biliary cholangitis–related chronic liver disease. (a) Liver stiffness (LS) measured by point shear wave elastography reveals high stiffness results, which however are very variable secondary to the uneven surface of the liver parenchyma. (b) Nodularities and heterogeneity of the liver parenchyma are even more pronounced in the second case, which is an example of advanced cirrhosis in which LS results are lower than expected.

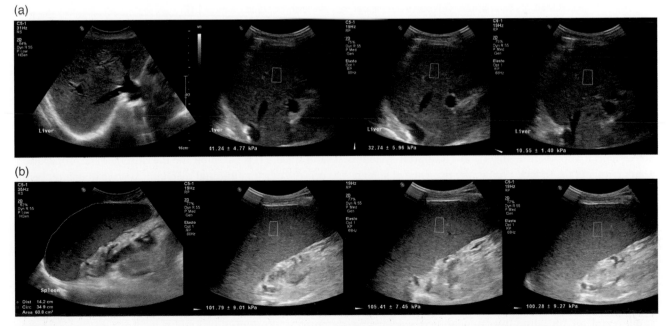

Figure 9.2.8 Patient with primary biliary cholangitis with a heterogeneous liver echostructure and high liver stiffness (LS) variability (a). There is evidence of homogeneous splenomegaly (bipolar diameter of 14.2 cm; area 60.8 cm^2), with very high but low-variability stiffness values (b). An example of the higher accuracy of spleen stiffness in predicting clinically significant portal hypertension compared to LS.

(a)

(b)

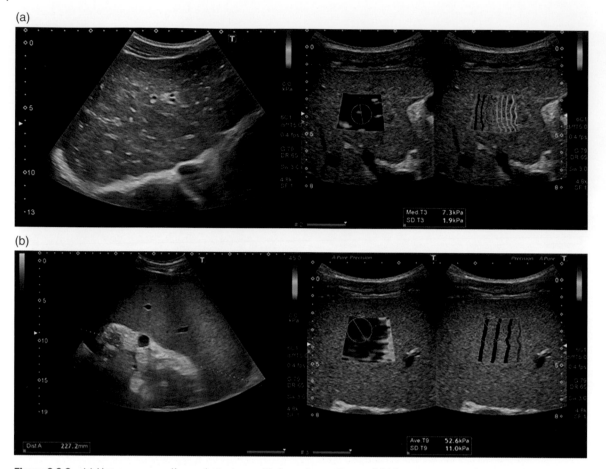

Figure 9.2.9 (a) Heterogeneous liver echotexture with irregular outline and (b) homogeneous splenomegaly. Features highly suspicious for CLD complicated by clinically significant portal hypertension. Elastography shows almost normal liver stiffness results despite obvious parenchymal irregularities (a, right side) and increased spleen stiffness (b, right side) in keeping with non-cirrhotic portal hypertension. Liver biopsy revealed features compatible with porto-sinusoidal vascular disorder (See Chapter 11).

However, it is of note that despite the severity of liver disease, underlying aetiology might influence liver appearance, sometimes showing pronounced parenchymal heterogeneity in pre-cirrhosis, or a relatively smooth outline and homogeneous echotexture when cirrhosis is already established. Similarly, ultrasound cannot establish the degree of PH unless clear signs of its presence can be seen, such as portal venous flow inversion and portal-systemic vascular collaterals. In fact, even in the presence of splenomegaly, dilated portal vein, and morphological changes, which suggest advanced cirrhosis, the chance of significant PH is high, but the accuracy of staging it is insufficient. On the other hand, ultrasound is extremely useful for revealing features that suggest the diagnosis of non-cirrhotic PH, such as portal vein thrombosis, periportal fibrosis, or rarer causes associated to haematological malignancies or parasitic infections. Therefore, while ultrasound is fundamental for revealing liver appearance, spleen size, and splanchnic circulation, elastography is able to overcome imaging limitations by objectively estimating both fibrosis and PH. The most accurate results of non-invasive assessment therefore require the integration of both ultrasound and elastography (Figures 9.2.10–9.2.16).

The use of different elastographic techniques carries benefits and limitations that need to be acknowledged. Although VCTE is the most validated method and is less operator dependent, the majority of the different available versions do not provide an image. Only recently a new system equipped with an ultrasound transducer has been released and is of help in locating and targeting the liver and spleen. It is based on the measurement of propagation velocity of a longitudinal mechanical wave that, after being deployed from its source, passes through the subcutaneous tissue and liver parenchyma. Along this route there could be several elements that interfere with elastography measurements: a small amount of ascites surrounding the right liver lobe, focal lesions, or other mentioned confounding factors such as hepatic congestion and biliary obstruction, which are known to increase intrahepatic pressure and hence stiffness. Therefore it is advisable to employ ultrasound evaluation before transient elastography for the measurement of LS. Point shear wave elastography (pSWE) and 2D-SWE are built into the ultrasound machine and carry the advantage of being able to evaluate the liver and place a region of interest in a selected area. The use of pSWE and 2D-SWE requires more advanced

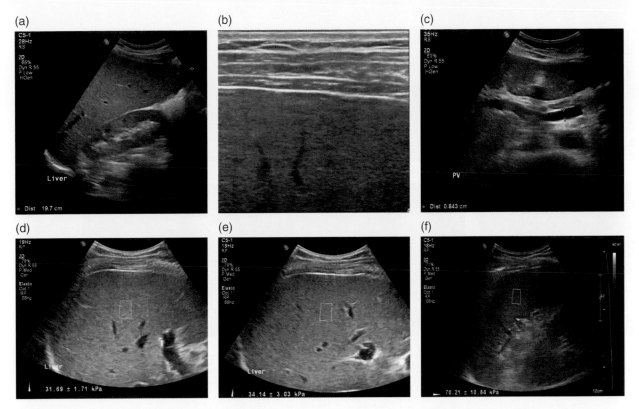

Figure 9.2.10 Patient with chronic liver disease (CLD) secondary to hepatitis C virus. (a) The liver seems to have an almost homogeneous echotexture. However a futher look with a high frequency transducer (b) highlights parenchymal heterogeneicity. (c) The portal vein is not dilated. Nontheless liver stiffness (d, e) is significantly increased at >30 kPa and the spleen (f), that is not enlarged, has a stiffness of 70 kPa in keeping with clinically significant portal hypertension. This is a case in which there are some ultrasound features of CLD but the appearance clearly underestimates its severity which instead is revealed by elastography.

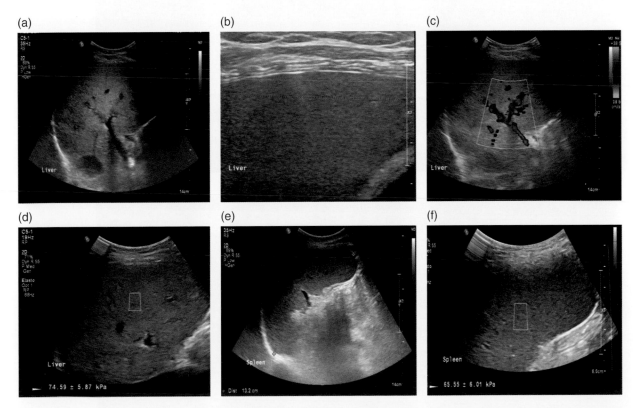

Figure 9.2.11 48 year-old women with alcohol-related chronic liver disease (CLD). (a) B-mode US shows a steatotic looking liver with (b) a homogeneous echotexture and a smooth outline. (c) Colour Doppler showed arterialisation of liver parenchyma as a result of arterial buffering against portal venous flow inversion (subtle blu signals on colour Doppler adjacent to the red arterial ones). (d) Liver stiffness is very high at 74 kPa. (e) The spleen is almost normal in size (bipolar diameter 13.2 cm), however (f) its stiffness is signinficantly increased at 65 kPa. In this csase B-mode features clearly underestimated the severity of liver disease, colour Doppler suggested significant portal hypertension, elastography suppports the definitive diagnosis of advanced CLD complicated by clinically significant portal hypertension (elastography assessment of a case presented in Chapter 8, Figure 8.26).

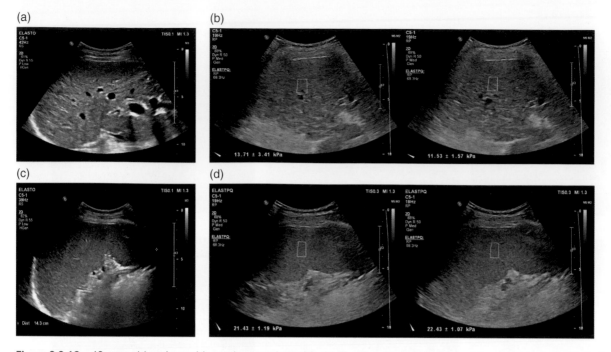

Figure 9.2.12 40 year-old patient with autoimmune hepatitis. (a) The liver has a heterogeneous echotexture although the outline is quite smooth. (b) liver stiffness is increased compatibly with F3-F4 fibrosis. (c) Note is made of moderate splenomegaly. (d) Spleen stiffness is relatively low. Features are compatible with chronic liver disease with no signs of clinically significant portal hypertension.

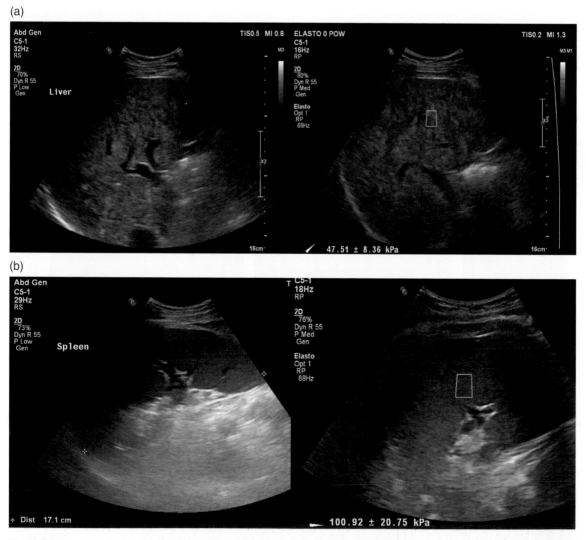

Figure 9.2.13 Non-alcoholic steatohepatitis-related chronic liver disease. (a) The liver has a grossly heterogeneous echotexture and it is significantly increased in stiffness (a, right side). (b) There is homogeneous splenomegaly that has high stiffness values (b, right side). B-mode appearance is compatible with advanced cirrhosis and portal hypertension that is confirmed by the elastography results.

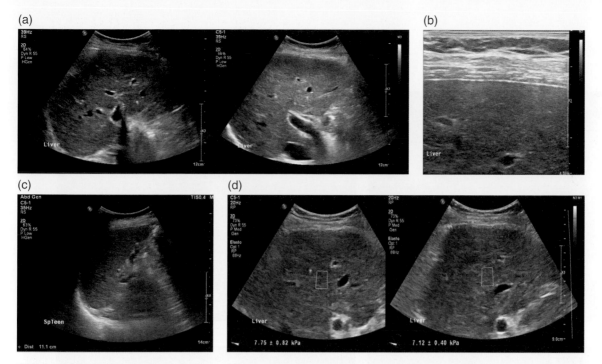

Figure 9.2.14 A 60 year-old woman with primary biliary cholangitis (PBC). (a) The liver has a pronounced heterogeneous echotexture; (b) the outline is smooth; (c) the spleen is normal in size. (d) Liver stiffness is just slightly increased showing a clear discrepancy between the appearance of the liver and the elastography results. PBC can be characterised by an 'early' heterogeneicity of liver parenchyma.

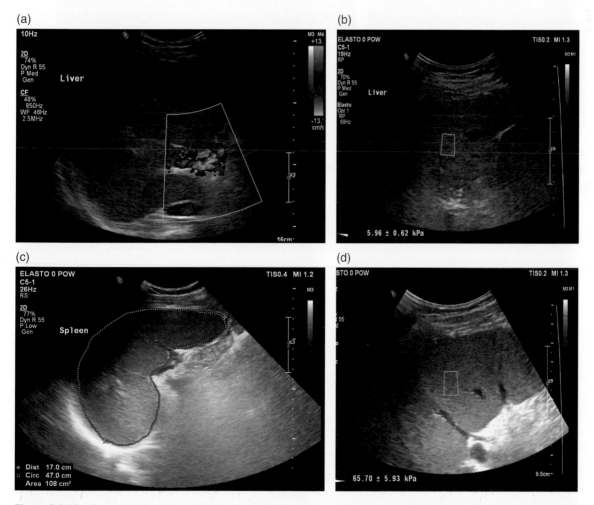

Figure 9.2.15 Presence of portal vein thrombosis (PVT) with cavernous transformation. Although increased liver stiffness (LS) has been described in some cases of PVT, more often, when there is no sign of primary chronic liver disease, LS is within normal range or just slightly increased. However, the resistance to portal flow due to PVT leads to pre-hepatic portal hypertension with a backflow significant increase of spleen stiffness. This is an example where ultrasound shows (a) features of PVT, (b) LS excludes cirrhosis, and there is (c, d) stiff splenomegaly in keeping with severe pre-hepatic portal hypertension.

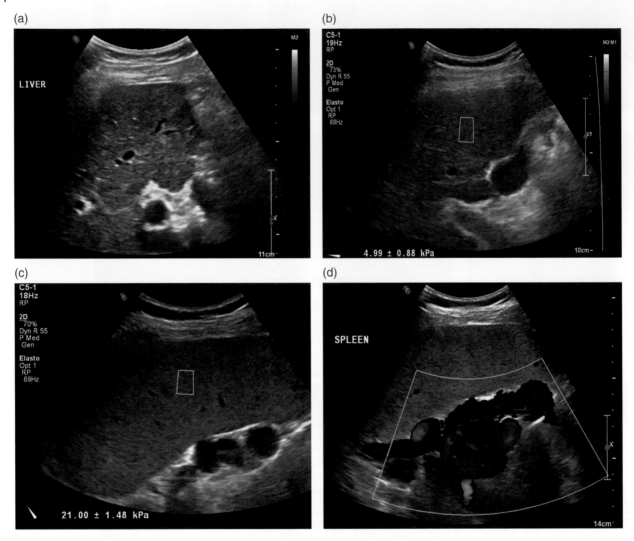

Figure 9.2.16 Patient with (a) pronounced hepatic parenchymal heterogeneicity and splenomegaly (not shown). (b) Liver stiffness is within normal range excluding cirrhosis. (c) Spleen stiffness is relatively low. (d) On color Doppler there is evidence of a large splenorenal portal-systemic shunt as a sign of severe portal hypertension. This is a case of portal-sinusoidal vascular disorder (proved on biopsy) characterized by severe non-cirrhotic portal hypertension causing a large portal-systemic shunt that decongests the spleen reducing its stiffness. In this case the integration of B-mode ultrasound, color Doppler and elastography is important to support the interpretation of the results of non-invasive diagnostic assessment.

training in ultrasound imaging; they are more operator dependent than VCTE, but have the undoubted benefit of imaging the liver while performing elastography (Figures 9.2.17–9.2.19) [1]. With regard to both fibrosis and PH, VCTE is the more validated method. However, the same principles are applicable to other techniques such as pSWE or 2D-SWE, which show promising results in the non-invasive diagnosis of PH by measuring both LS and SS [17, 18].

Elastography in Different Liver Disease Aetiologies

Viral Hepatitis–Related Chronic Liver Disease

CLD secondary to viral hepatitis can be reliably assessed by elastography and although VCTE is the most validated

method, pSWE and 2D-SWE are also considered accurate to assess CLD in this setting, as recommended by international guidelines [18]. With regard to HBV-related CLD, caution is advised since parenchymal necroinflammation is one of the most important confounding factors that can interfere with stiffness measurements, potentially overestimating fibrosis [19, 20]. Therefore liver function tests and especially transaminase values should always be taken into account in this particular aetiology. Elastography has been shown to correlate with the prediction of liver disease–related malignant potential. Nevertheless, since it is also used as a follow-up tool in treatment response, revealing significant reduction of stiffness values in both HBV and HCV CLD, it should not be used to influence decisions on CLD surveillance strategies. In fact, there is insufficient scientific evidence to prove that reducing stiffness

(a)

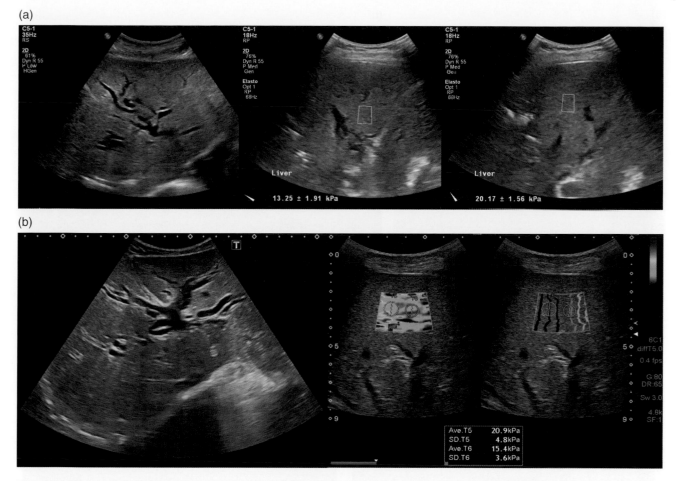

(b)

Figure 9.2.17 Increased liver siffness values are not reliable because of intrahepatic biliary duct dilatation that is a known confounding factor and is revealed by sonographic imaging. (a) point shear wave elastography; (b) 2D shear wave elastography.

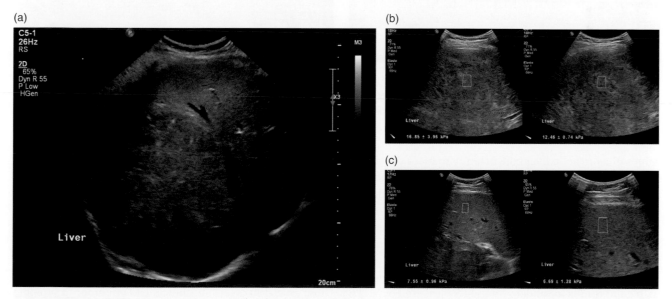

Figure 9.2.18 (a) A large right liver lobe lesion surely interferes with elastography results that are always measured in the right liver lobe. However, imaging allows to distinguish the neoplastic tissue from the healthy parenchyma, and a specific area to be targeted to acquire stiffness measurements of the background liver. (b) Increased stiffness of the neoplastic tissue. (c) Normal/slightly increased liver stiffness values of the background liver.

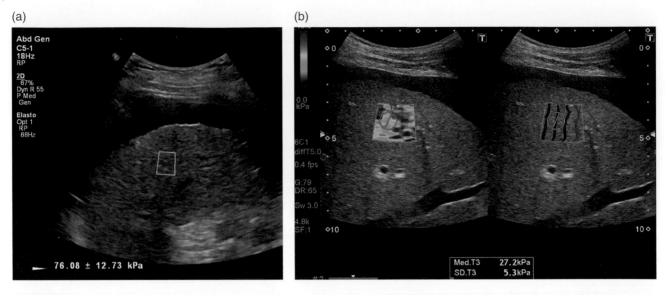

Figure 9.2.19 Two different elastography techniques are used in different patients with different aetiologies. (a) Point shear wave elastography in hepatitis C–related cirrhosis and (b) 2D-shear wave elastography in alcohol-related cirrhosis. In both cases there is a considerable amount of ascites surrounding the liver that can rapidly be assessed with ultrasound and by-passed by the elastographic technique.

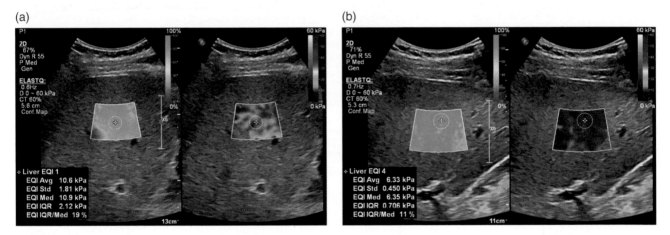

Figure 9.2.20 A 66-year-old patient with chronic hepatitis C and slightly elevated transaminases (alanine aminotransferase [ALT] 64 IU/L; aspartate aminotransferase [AST] 48 IU/L). (a) Liver stiffness (LS) measured a week before starting treatment with direct-acting antivirals reveals severe fibrosis. (b) Elastography follow-up at four months after the end of treatment shows a dramatic decrease of LS, likely due to the resolution of necroinflammation.

values of a cirrhotic liver concurrently reduces the risk of developing hepatocellular carcinoma [18]. This condition is observed particularly in HCV cirrhosis, where a drastic decrease of LS is seen after treatment with direct-acting antivirals (DAAs; Figure 9.2.20), but ongoing ultrasound screening for hepatocellular carcinoma is still highly recommended.

Both HBV and HCV CLD have been used in large trials with good results to validate LS and SS measured by VCTE as non-invasive surrogate markers of PH, against both HVPG and endoscopic evidence of varices. pSWE and 2D-SWE were also recently compared to HVPG and presence of varices, showing a good correlation [18].

Alcohol-Related Liver Disease

Alcoholism is a very common cause of CLD. However, patients are often unaware of their underlying condition, which can progress indolently until a first sign of clinical decompensation such as jaundice, ascites, or variceal bleeding presents, declaring severe liver disease. The presence of fibrosis or cirrhosis in compensated patients is the most important predictor of long-term survival [21]. It is therefore crucial to detect subclinical CLD in order to promote abstinence and improve prognosis [22]. Alcohol-related liver disease (ALD) is a challenging aetiology to accurately diagnose non-invasively and to follow up. Its natural history is characterised by alcohol abuse and LS encompasses fibrosis, but also necroinflammation and hepatocyte ballooning, as a consequence of the toxic effects of alcohol [22]. In addition, the spectrum of disease presentation in ALD ranges from acute alcohol steatohepatitis to acute-on-chronic liver failure and 'stable' fibrosis/cirrhosis. Despite this complex scenario of varying clinical presentation in which even acute alcoholic hepatitis might have an onset of jaundice and ascites, stiffness values provide an important follow-up of biomechanical inflammation. In fact, LS has been shown to improve shortly after alcohol withdrawal in more than 80% of patients (Figure 9.2.5) [22, 23]. Along these lines, correct information on alcohol intake and biochemistry is crucial for differentiating the severity of underlying fibrosis with superimposed steatohepatitis. The aspartate aminotransferase (AST) value seems to be a reliable biochemical marker of superimposed alcoholic steatohepatitis and a useful discriminant to accurately assess liver fibrosis with elastography. More specifically, after abstinence an AST <50 U/L yields high accuracy for diagnosing F3/F4 fibrosis with VCTE, an AST <100 U/L allows a high diagnostic accuracy for F4 fibrosis, while an AST >100 U/L would instead be sufficient to interfere with LS reliability in detecting fibrosis [23]. In conclusion, in ALD an ultrasound evaluation should always be carried out to exclude the presence of advanced cirrhosis, ascites, signs of CSPH, and especially biliary dilatation, since patients often present with jaundice in the acute phase of decompensation. Abstinence should be proven, since it is a cornerstone of clinical management and assessment of these patients. If the patient is actively drinking and undergoing detoxification, liver elastography is useful anyway, focusing on the delta LS values and a target AST of at least <100 U/L, to confirm that a reasonable accuracy of non-invasive assessment of liver fibrosis is achieved.

Non-alcoholic Fatty Liver Disease/Metabolic Dysfunction-Associated Steatotic Liver Disease

Non-alcoholic fatty liver disease (NAFLD) is at present the most prevalent liver disease worldwide and an increasing indication for liver transplantation [24, 25]. Despite this epidemiological burden, its importance is still disregarded among the general population, probably because of the incorrect perception that 'simple' steatosis is a relatively benign and harmless condition. In general two pitfalls can be identified in the management of patients who are at high risk of developing advanced stages of NAFLD. The first is that usually only patients who have increased transaminase eventually undergo an ultrasound scan, meaning that if a patient has CLD and normal liver function tests the diagnosis can be completely missed. In some circumstances, even well-compensated cirrhotic patients could have normal transaminase levels and hence might not undergo routine

assessment, despite being at an advanced stage and even at risk of developing hepatocellular carcinoma. Second, NAFLD CLD ultrasound features might not be detected, unless liver morphological changes are unequivocal for advanced cirrhosis. Once again, elastography provides crucial information in revealing fibrosis non-invasively and hence the presence of CLD (Figure 9.2.21).

Nevertheless, in consideration of the epidemic burden of NAFLD, a selective screening strategy is needed, using scoring systems predictive of fibrosis in primary care. The most accurate scoring system in this context is the NAFLD fibrosis score [26], which discriminates three groups according to low, intermediate, and high risk. While low-risk patients are recommended to have a yearly follow-up with a repeat NAFLD fibrosis score, intermediate- and high-risk patients should undergo specific referral for ultrasound and elastography [24]. Although elastography shows good diagnostic accuracy for staging NAFLD [18], it must be stressed that NAFLD is a technically difficult aetiology to assess, because of the increased skin-to-capsule distance that is usually found in patients with high body mass index (BMI). Patients with a skin-to-capsule distance up to 2.5 cm can be assessed with a VCTE M probe, while for distances >2.5 cm and ≤4 cm, an XL probe is necessary. For a skin-to-capsule distance ≥4 cm VCTE will not always be able to measure LS accurately and other techniques such as pSWE and 2D-SWE are recommended, with good results [24]. Nevertheless, LS measurements using these forms of software must be taken at least 1.5–2 cm below the liver capsule. The presence of severe subcutaneous thickening, and therefore increased skin-to-capsule distance, would imply raising considerably the overall depth of the region of interest (ROI), with consequent difficult acquisitions for low signal-to-noise ratios. Moreover, liver steatosis cannot only lead to posterior attenuation and reverberation artefacts, but also influence stiffness values [18]. Although dedicated software has been developed in order to quantify steatosis objectively, it is difficult to evaluate its exact impact on stiffness values and therefore on the non-invasive assessment of liver fibrosis in this context. Some studies have addressed this issue evaluating LS and controlled attenuation parameter (CAP) and comparing the results to the amount of fibrosis and steatosis found on biopsy [27]. However, it was recently reported that differences in CAP steatosis cut-off values were found according to different study populations. In addition, the cut-off values seem to be influenced by the use of different probes (M and XL) [28, 29]. Considering that LS could be influenced by the severity of steatosis, and that there are still uncertainties regarding the cut-off values of CAP, caution is recommended in interpretation of the results, especially in NAFLD. The non-invasive gold standard to quantify steatosis remains magnetic resonance

(a)

(b)

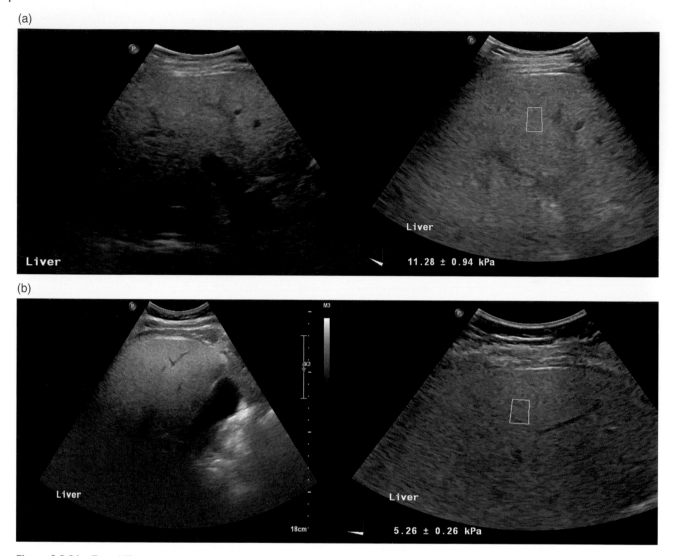

Figure 9.2.21 Two different cases of patients with severe steatosis. Elastography allows the presence of underlying fibrosis to be distinguished. (a) Severe fibrosis; (b) no fibrosis.

imaging (MRI)-derived proton density fat fraction (PDFF), although promising results are being achieved with other ultrasound-related software [30–32]. In patients with NAFLD another issue is the difficulty in obtaining reliable measurements for predicting the severity of PH, especially in obese patients [33]. SS could yield important results in this context, by bypassing the confounding effect of steatosis on LS values. However, technical difficulties could be met both owing to the anatomical position and size of the spleen, and because measurements of SS are also affected by the increased skin-to-capsule distance.

Autoimmune Hepatitis

Autoimmune hepatitis (AIH) has a broad spectrum of presentations that range from severe acute hepatitis to life-threatening liver failure. In other cases liver disease has a

more indolent progression, which might be affected or not by sudden inflammatory flares, which can resolve or accelerate the progression to cirrhosis and liver failure.

Approximately one-third of patients already have severe fibrosis (Figure 9.2.12) or established cirrhosis at diagnosis (Figure 9.2.22) [34]. However, appropriate and timely treatment can lead to resolution of inflammation and regression of fibrosis and even cirrhosis within certain limits (Figure 9.2.23) [35]. Non-invasive assessment in AIH has been shown to be very useful, although it needs to take into account that, similar to other conditions, LS is influenced by superimposed inflammation. Biochemical response together with elastography assessment have been shown to be excellent tools for disease monitoring and their integration is strongly advised (Figure 9.2.3) [36]. It is of note that AIH might have a variable appearance at presentation, with regard to not only the severity of inflammation, but also the

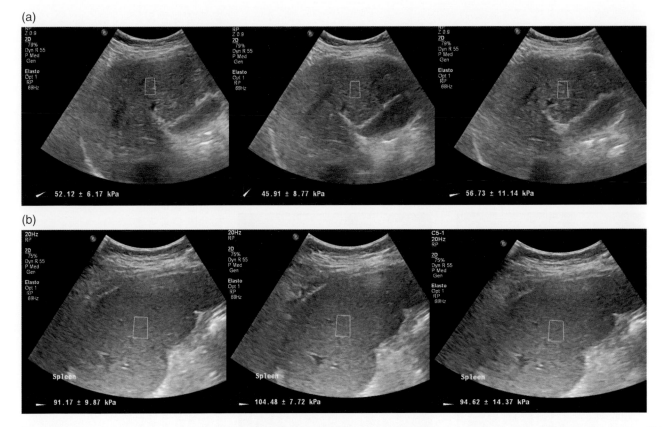

Figure 9.2.22 Autoimmune hepatitis–related cirrhosis. Both liver (a) and spleen (b) elastography confirm stiffness values compatible with clinically significant portal hypertension.

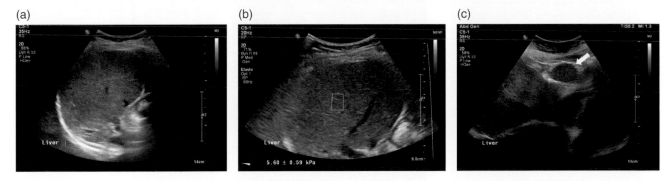

Figure 9.2.23 A 48-year-old woman with a history of acute severe onset of autoimmune hepatitis and liver failure, who showed a very good biochemical and clinical response to immunosuppression. Despite complete biochemical remission and clinical stability, (a) the appearance on ultrasound of the right liver lobe is slightly reduced in size with rounded margins and (b) normal liver stiffness values. (c) The left liver lobe is completely atrophied (white arrow).

distribution of inflammation and fibrosis across the hepatic parenchyma. Although more often inflammation is diffuse, there are other situations in which some areas appear to be more affected than others. There might be areas of confluent fibrosis and areas of parenchymal sparing; some areas subject to severe necroinflammation and others that compensate, reacting with nodular regeneration (Figure 9.2.24). Therefore, elastography results could be influenced not only by the severity of inflammation, but also by its uneven distribution. In addition, the appearance of the liver might confound the operator, especially in those patients in whom significant regression of inflammation and fibrosis was obtained, but in whom the architecture of the liver was modified, showing obvious morphological changes and a heterogeneous echotexture. This can mimic cirrhosis, while instead the picture is rather compatible with burn-out AIH. The clinical history and biochemistry are fundamental in the interpretation of LS results and in cases of uncertainty liver biopsy is indicated to clarify the underlying diagnosis, in terms of fibrosis staging and inflammatory activity.

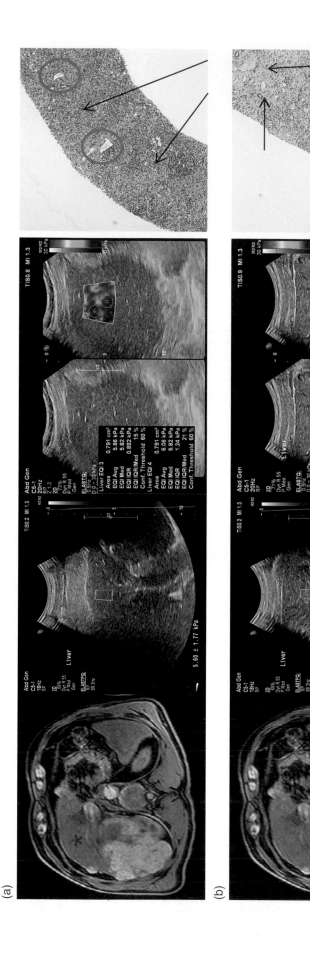
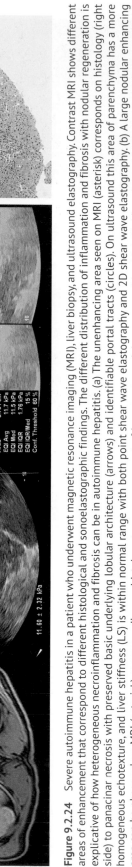

Figure 9.2.24 Severe autoimmune hepatitis in a patient who underwent magnetic resonance imaging (MRI), liver biopsy, and ultrasound elastography. Contrast MRI shows different areas of enhancement that correspond to different histological and sonoelastographic findings. The different distribution of inflammation and fibrosis with nodular regeneration is explicative of how heterogeneous necroinflammation and fibrosis can be in autoimmune hepatitis. (a) The unenhancing area seen on MRI (asterisk) corresponds on histology (right side) to panacinar necrosis with preserved basic underlying lobular architecture (arrows) and identifiable portal tracts (circles). On ultrasound this area of parenchyma has a more homogeneous echotexture, and liver stiffness (LS) is within normal range with both point shear wave elastography and 2D shear wave elastography. (b) A large nodular enhancing area can be observed on MRI (asterisk) corresponding on histclogy to an arrangement of hepatocyte nodules separated by thick fibrous septa with marked ductular proliferation (arrows) and a mild, mainly lymphoplasmacytic inflammatory infiltrate. *Source:* Courtesy of Dr Tu Vinh Luong. On ultrasound the liver has a very heterogeneous echotexture. Elastography reveals significant increase in LS values in keeping with severe fibrosis/cirrhosis.

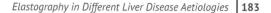

Cholestatic Liver Disease

PBC is a chronic cholestatic liver disease of autoimmune cause, characterised by granulomatous necrotic inflammation of the small bile ducts. Although the evidence is scarce compared to other aetiologies, VCTE has shown good results in predicting different grades of fibrosis and cirrhosis compared to liver biopsy [37–40]. In addition, elastography also seems able to provide useful prognostic information for VCTE stiffness values >9 kPa at the time of diagnosis, and a yearly delta stiffness value >2.1 kPa [35]. With regard to PH, PBC is a disease characterised by the development of presinusoidal PH and therefore, although in a minority of patients, there is an increased risk of varices development and gastroesophageal bleeding in the pre-cirrhotic stage [41]. To date, the evidence of the accuracy of liver elastography in predicting the severity of PH and therefore varices is limited. Consequently caution is advised [42]. Although at present limited data is available, SS could potentially increase the diagnostic accuracy of elastography in predicting the severity of PH and high-risk varices in PBC. Of note that one of the reported findings in PBC, is its patchy distribution of fibrosis, and the heteorgeneicity of liver's echotexture in the early stages of disease which might be confusing at the eyes of the operator. This should always encourage to add elastography during the ultrasound assessment (Figures 9.2.7 and 9.2.14).

PSC is an inflammatory cholestatic disease of unknown cause, characterised by inflammation of the biliary epithelium, with consequent biliary fibrosis and eventually cirrhosis and PH. The distribution of inflammatory and fibrotic changes are random and can affect the right and/or left biliary tree, as well as the extrahepatic common bile duct or the small distal ducts ('small duct PSC'). As in PBC, the data on elastography in PSC is related to a few studies, mainly with VCTE [18, 43, 44]. It is important to stress that although the data available showed a good correlation with liver fibrosis and overall prognosis, according to baseline elastography results and a yearly increase in delta stiffness, in PSC fibro-inflammation might have a variable distribution throughout the liver parenchyma (Figures 9.2.25 and 9.2.26) (see Chapter 8). Therefore, when measuring LS it is crucial to integrate biochemistry, exclude the presence of a dominant biliary stricture and cholangitis, and carefully evaluate the known distribution of disease prior to stiffness acquisition, since sparing of the right lobe can yield false-negative results in patients who might have significant left lobe involvement (Figure 9.2.27). Similarly to PBC, there is a paucity of data regarding the use of elastography in predicting the presence of high-risk varices in PSC [42, 45] and SS could potentially yield interesting and clinically important results, bearing in mind how liver parenchyma is subjected to many interferences in cholestatic liver disease and especially in PSC.

(a)

(b)

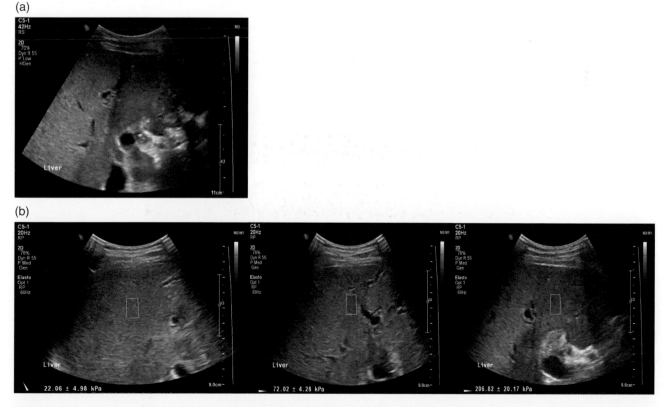

Figure 9.2.25 Primary sclerosing cholangitis might be characterised by biliary dissociation as in this case in which (a) there is a clear difference in liver echogenicity defining the boundary between the two areas. (b) Elastography reveals a progressive increase in liver stiffness according to the area in which biliary obstruction is more pronounced.

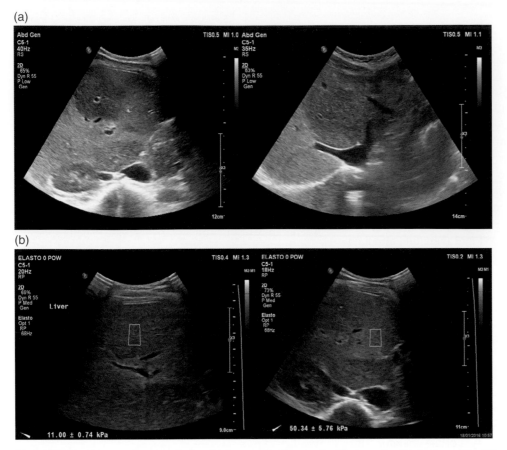

Figure 9.2.26 Primary sclerosing cholangitis is typically characterised by irregular distribution of the biliary tree involvement. As a result, on ultrasound (a) the liver might appear with a well defined pattern of different areas of echogenicity corresponding to the segmental distribution of reduced biliary drainage and/or related fibrosis. (b) Elastography clearly shows there is a difference in stiffness of the involved areas.

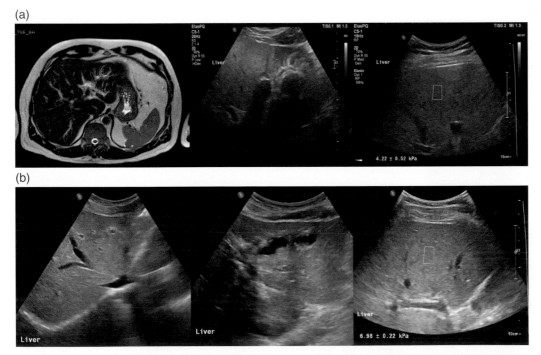

Figure 9.2.27 Two cases of primary sclerosing cholangitis (PSC) show pronounced involvement of the left liver lobe and relative sparing of the right one. Since elastography is perfomed in the right liver lobe, in these cases it cannot provide information on the severity of disease. Integrating ultrasound with elastography in cases like these is crucial. (a) Magnetic resonance cholangiopancreatography shows left side biliary tree involvement corresponding to what is also seen on ultrasound. Liver stiffness (LS) performed with point shear wave elastography (pSWE) on the right liver lobe is unremarkable (right side image). (b) Another patient with PSC who has pronounced involvement of the anterior left bile duct that appears sclerotic and grossly dilated (middle image). LS measured with pSWE in the right liver lobe (right side image) has relatively low values and does not reflect the severity of disease.

Elastography in Liver Transplant

Liver transplant patients need to undergo thorough clinical, laboratory, and imaging follow-up, in order to measure possible signs of rejection, disease recurrence, and fibrosis. Liver biopsy is usually carried out when one of these scenarios is suspected and is routinely performed at 12 months post transplant, although there might be some variability according to the referring centre or the underlying liver disease aetiology [46]. Even if there is no specific guideline or recommendation to use elastography routinely in liver transplant, in a small series of studies it was shown that graft LS provides useful information in the prediction of moderate/severe rejection [47], and there is sufficient evidence to consider it a useful tool for non-invasively diagnosing the recurrence and severity of post-transplant fibrosis at 6–12 months follow-up [48–50]. Nevertheless, it needs to be emphasised that the importance of LS in the management of transplant patients might rely more on the fact that elastography not only provides a measurement of fibrosis recurrence, but rather an evaluation of biomechanical abnormalities occurring within the liver graft (Figure 9.2.28). Along these lines, elastography in liver transplant can be seen as a dynamic repeatable surveillance procedure that accompanies the diagnostic process, rather than 'only' a surrogate marker of fibrosis [51].

Elastography in the Paediatric Population

Paediatric liver disease encompasses a variety of different aetiologies ranging from AIH to PSC, viral hepatitis, and especially NAFLD, owing to the increasing burden of obesity in the paediatric population [52]. Nevertheless, other rarer aetiologies are described, such as biliary atresia, cystic fibrosis–related liver disease, Alagille syndrome, glycogen storage diseases, and cardiac causes, especially as a consequence of Fontan procedure–related liver disease [5]. However, although the cut-off values might be different owing to constitution and different liver disease aetiologies, for which there is scarce evidence in terms of histopathological correlation, the biomechanical principles of elastography are equally applicable in the paediatric population. Therefore, besides viral and NAFLD liver disease in which cut-off values seem to be more defined and used as a 'traditional' fibrosis screening tool [5], elastography has been shown to be a very useful method for monitoring disease progression and treatment response in all those conditions in which confounding factors and liver fibrosis are indistinguishable non-invasively. In this context, the delta LS variability has proven to be a reliable and useful clinical tool for following up patients after liver transplant [53] and other surgical interventions such as Fontan and Kasai procedure [54–56].

Elastography as a Tool to Diagnose Liver Involvement in Systemic Diseases

A variety of pathologies can affect hepatic structure, physiology, and function, leading to secondary liver disease. These conditions range from congestive heart failure to infiltrative diseases, such as amyloidosis or malignancies, as well as vascular haematological disorders, as seen in sinusoidal obstruction syndrome and graft-versus-host disease. When using elastography to quantify fibrosis, all these pathological conditions are considered confounding factors, because they interfere by increasing stiffness values regardless of collagen deposition. Nevertheless, in the presence of a suspected or known underlying disease, the use of elastography becomes a method for detecting liver involvement rather than fibrosis, and for evaluating disease progression or regression in response to treatment. This is particularly helpful in amyloidosis, which is usually undetectable on ultrasound. Only in advanced stages of disease might the liver show morphological changes or even signs of severe PH. Diagnosis of hepatic involvement is confirmed usually by biopsy or non-invasively by serum amyloid protein scintigraphy. In this context an increase in LS, after excluding cardiac involvement and congestive hepatopathy, correlates with the presence of hepatic amyloidosis [57], whereas a reduction in stiffness correlates with a significant response to treatment [58]. Elastography has also shown promising results in predicting the occurrence of sinusoidal obstruction syndrome by detecting LS increase in patients who underwent bone marrow transplantation, even prior to any biochemical and clinical abnormality [59]. In a disease with a mortality rate of 80% [60], where early diagnosis and treatment are vital, liver elastography could therefore represent an important diagnostic resource. LS measurement has also shown potential application in the same field, detecting liver-related graft-versus-host disease involvement in both diagnosis and follow-up [61]. Although elastography is considered an 'off-label' application in this context, the available data is encouraging. It suggests, in fact, that elastography can be used, albeit with caution, as a predictor of hepatic involvement in haematological conditions such as sinusoidal obstruction syndrome and liver graft-versus-host disease. Furthermore, the available data also suggests that elastography can be a follow-up tool in amyloidosis and congestive hepatopathies, in view of its correlation

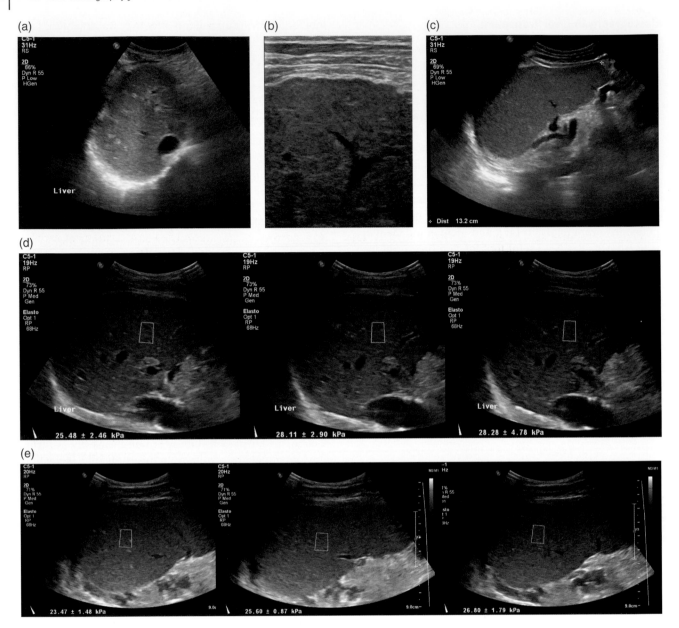

Figure 9.2.28 Patient with acute cellular rejection after two months from liver transplant for autoimmune hepatitis. (a) The liver has a retracted appearance, heterogeneous echotexture, and irregular outline, as it is more obvious after magnification with a high-frequency transducer (b). (c) The spleen is homogeneous and just slightly increased in size. (d) Liver stiffness is significantly increased, compatible with a severe necroinflammatory reaction (as proven on biopsy). (e) Spleen stiffness is relatively low in the absence of portal hypertension.

with central venous pressure and, in general, with venous outflow obstruction syndrome [62].

Elastography in Focal Liver Lesions

Focal lesions present a variety of histological differences that influence their biomechanical properties, therefore elastography can be used for the detection of such differences. Nevertheless, a significant degree of stiffness overlap values among different focal lesions might be found. Hence elastography is not recommended in general, as a single diagnostic tool, in the differential diagnosis between benign and

malignant focal liver lesions [18]. Elastography could instead be used with higher accuracy to evaluate the background liver (Figure 9.2.18), especially when using pSWE and 2D-SWE, to assess the presence of advanced fibrosis or cirrhosis, bearing in mind that CSPH has a considerable impact on postsurgical mortality rate at three and five years and on clinical decompensation at three months [63]. Secondary and/or tertiary centres still use highly invasive techniques such as HVPG, which are considered the gold standard for the assessment of liver cirrhosis and PH. Elastography could add an important tool in this scenario, speeding up presurgical assessment [63, 64]. Nevertheless, caution is advised and more robust data is needed to fully endorse the use of elastography for this purpose [65].

Practical Advice

Liver disease can be assessed non-invasively by shear wave elastography with relatively high accuracy. However, in consideration of the reported variability of LS cut-off values for intermediate fibrosis stages, two approaches are proposed in clinical practice. The first is to look at elastography as a tool to 'rule out' significant fibrosis and 'rule in' cirrhosis, providing an accurate system to discriminate the two extremes of liver disease. The second is to use cut-off values that refer to stages of disease, rather than to stages of fibrosis, and for which a distinction is made between VCTE and acoustic radiation force impulse (ARFI) techniques (pSWE and 2D-SWE). The Baveno VI Consensus Conference in 2015 proposed the term 'compensated advanced chronic liver disease (cACLD)' to describe the spectrum of advanced fibrosis and cirrhosis (F3 and F4) in asymptomatic patients who are at risk of developing CSPH [9].

The World Federation for Ultrasound in Medicine and Biology (WFUMB) 2018 guidelines endorsed the Baveno VI recommendation for ruling in and ruling out cACLD and ruling out varices needing treatment and proposed using five ranges of LS to distinguish five corresponding stages of liver disease with VCTE (Rule of 5) [18]. In practice, in patients with chronic viral hepatitis and NAFLD an LS cutoff < 5kPa rules out fibrosis; an LS between 5-10 kPa identifies varies ranges of fibrosis but rules out cACLD; an LS > 10 and < 15 kPa identifies cACLD that needs further integration with other tests and information for confirmation; an LS > 15 kPa is highly suggestive of cCALD; while an LS > 20 kPa can rule in CSPH [9,18].

In 2021, the Baveno VII Consensus Conference recommendations were to extend the rule of 5 focusing on cACLD: an LS > 20 kPa and ≤ 25 kPa alone or combined with platelet count and spleen size predict the presence of CSPH; an LS > 25kpa is sufficient to predict the presence of CSPH and patients at higher risk of variceal bleeding and clinical decompensation (in patient with viral hepatitis, alcohol-related liver disease and non-obese NASH-related CLD) [66]. With regard to elastography measurements with ARFI techniques, the recent update to the Society of Radiologists in Ultrasound (SRU) Elastography Consensus statement has proposed a vendor-neutral 'Rule of 4' system, based on the probability of cACLD in patients with viral hepatitis or NAFLD: an LS of 5kPa (1.3m/s) or less has high probability of being normal; an LS less than 9kPa (1.7m/s), in the absence of other known clinical signs, rules out cACLD; values between 9kPa (1.7m/s) and 13kPa (2.1m/s) are suggestive of cACLD, but may need further tests for confirmation; and

values greater than 13kPa (2.1m/s) are highly suggestive of cACLD. There is a probability of CSPH with LS values greater than 17kPa (2.4m/s), but additional patient testing may be required. In some patients with NAFLD, the cutoff values for cACLD may be lower and follow-up or additional testing in those with values between 7 and 9kPa is recommended [67].

Despite these important points of reference, when measuring LS, variables such as liver disease aetiology, confounding factors, the equipment used, and reliability criteria need to be considered. Once the elastography results are acquired, it is crucial to know if they are accurate and reliable and therefore can be considered a guide for clinical management. Reliability criteria are based on an accuracy cut-off value related to measurement variability (interquartile range/median [IQR/ Med] < 30% for measurements in kPa, and < 15% for measurements in m/s). The less variable the results, the more accurate the measurement data. Technical and constitutional limitations sometimes make elastographic measurements difficult to acquire, resulting in possible low accuracy. Despite these recommendations, it is also important to pay attention to high LS variability, when these limitations apparently are not present. In fact this situation should be recognised as a measure of possible structural parenchymal abnormalities that could be caused by an extremely uneven surface secondary to focal lesions or other causes, for which the integration of ultrasound and biochemistry is absolutely necessary [68].

In the majority of cases, there is a linear correlation of LS with the progression of liver disease up to the stage of CSPH. Beyond this stage, the strength of the correlation decreases markedly, likely due to the increased relevance of extrahepatic factors on the progression of PH. Because of these reasons, in view of the potential inaccuracy of LS in predicting severe PH and varices needing treatment, attention on the potential role of SS and on its higher accuracy in correlating with the severity of PH has been given. SS is generally higher than LS in healthy subjects and throughout the different stages of liver disease, with a clear diagnostic role once the stage of CSPH is reached (Figure 9.2.6). The Baveno VII consensus suggests that SS measured by VCTE can be used in cACLD due to viral hepatitis (non-treated HCV patients and treated and untreated HBV patients) to rule-out and rule-in CSPH with cutoffs of < 21 kPa and ≥ 50 kPa, respectively.

In patients who are not candidates for NSBBs (contraindication/intolerance) and in whom endoscopy would be required according to the Baveno VI criteria (LSM by TE ≥ 20 kPa or platelet count < 150000/mm3, a SS ≤ 40 kPa can be used to identify those patients with a low probability of high-risk varices, and in whom endoscopy can be avoided [65]. The recent availability of a spleen-dedicated 100 Hz VCTE, specifically designed for SS assessment, will surely lead to a refinement of these cutoffs and the whole range of liver disease aetiologies will likely be explored in future studies.

Due to the variability of SS values among different US systems, no general agreement has yet been reached for the ARFI-based SS cut-offs. Nevertheless, the available studies highlight the importance of SS measurements for stratifying the severity of PH, its improvement (post-transplant, post transjugular intrahepatic portosystemic shunt [TIPS], beta-blockers response) as well as its use in the differential diagnosis between cirrhotic and non-cirrhotic portal hypertension (see Chapter 11).

Note is made of the possible finding of relatively low SS values against a background of advanced cirrhosis or severe

non-cirrhotic PH. In this scenario, low SS values might be a consequence of portal-systemic shunting that decongests the portal venous system (Figure 9.2.16). In theory, portal systemic shunting can be 'protective' against the risk of variceal bleeding. However, at present there is no data on the clinical use of this finding and its interpretation remains speculative.

Videos

Videos for this chapter can be accessed via the companion website: www.wiley.com/go/LiverUltrasound.

References

1 Ferraioli, G., Filice, C., Castera, L. et al. (2015). WFSUMB guidelines and recommendations for the clinical use of ultrasound elastography, Part 3: liver. *Ultrasound Med. Biol.* 41 (5): 1161–1179.

2 Berzigotti, A. (2017). Non-invasive evaluation of portal hypertension using ultrasound elastography. *J. Hepatol.* 67 (2): 399–411.

3 Singh, S., Fujii, L.L., Murad, M.H. et al. (2013). Liver stiffness is associated with risk of decompensation, liver cancer, and death in patients with chronic liver diseases: a systematic review and meta analysis. *Clin. Gastroenterol. Hepatol.* 11: 1573–1584.

4 Rigamonti, C., Donato, M.F., Fraquelli, M. et al. (2008). Transient elastography predicts fibrosis progression in patients with recurrent hepatitis C after liver transplantation. *Gut* 57: 821–827.

5 Ferraioli, G., Barr, R.G., and Dillman, J.R. (2021). Elastography for pediatric chronic liver disease: a review and expert opinion. *J. Ultrasound Med.* 40 (5): 909–928.

6 Ferraioli, G. (2019). Review of liver elastography guidelines. *J. Ultrasound Med.* 38: 9–14.

7 Piscaglia, F., Salvatore, V., Mulazzani, L. et al. (2016). Ultrasound shear wave elastography for liver disease. A critical appraisal of the many actors on the stage. *Ultraschall Med.* 37: 1–5.

8 Berzigotti, A. and Piscaglia, F. (2012). EFSUMB education and professional standards committee. Ultrasound in portal hypertension – part 2 – and EFSUMB recommendations for the performance and reporting of ultrasound examinations in portal hypertension. *Ultraschall Med.* 33 (1): 8–32.

9 De Franchis, R. and on behalf of the Baveno VI Faculty (2015). Expanding consensus in portal hypertension Report of the Baveno VI Consensus Workshop: stratifying risk and individualizing care for portal hypertension. *J. Hepatol.* 63: 743–752.

10 Augustin, S., Pons, M., Maurice, J.B. et al. (2017). Expanding the Baveno VI criteria for the screening of varices in patients with compensated advanced chronic liver disease. *Hepatology* 66 (6): 1980–1988.

11 Choen, E.B. and Afdhal, N.H. (2010). Ultrasound-based hepatic elastography. Origin, limitations and applications. *J. Clin. Gastroenterol.* 44 (9): 637–645.

12 Colecchia, A., Montrone, L., Scaioli, E. et al. (2012). Measurement of spleen stiffness to evaluate portal hypertension and the presence of esophageal varices in patients with HCV-related cirrhosis. *Gastroenterology* 143 (3): 646–654.

13 Colecchia, A., Colli, A., Casazza, G. et al. (2014). Spleen stiffness measurement can predict clinical complications in compensated HCV-related cirrhosis: a prospective study. *J. Hepatol.* 60 (6): 1158–1164.

14 Chin, J.L., Chan, G., Ryan, J.D., and McCormick, P.A. (2015). Spleen stiffness can non-invasively assess resolution of portal hypertension after liver transplantation. *Liver Int.* 35 (2): 518–523.

15 Vizzutti, F., Arena, U., Romanelli, R.G. et al. (2007). Liver stiffness measurement predicts severe portal hypertension in patients with HCV-related cirrhosis. *Hepatology* 45: 1290–1297.

16 Elkrief, L., Lazareth, M., Chevret, S. et al. (2021). Liver stiffness by transient elastography to detect porto-sinusoidal vascular liver disease with portal hypertension. *Hepatology* 74 (1): 364–378.

17 Roccarina, D., Rosselli, M., Genesca, J., and Tsochatzis, E.A. (2018). Elastography methods for the non-invasive assessment of portal hypertension. *Exp. Rev. Gastroenterol. Hepatol.* 12 (2): 155–164.

18 Ferraioli, G., Wong, V.W., Castera, L. et al. (2018). Liver ultrasound elastography: an update to the world federation for ultrasound in medicine and biology guidelines and recommendations. *Ultrasound Med. Biol.* 44 (12): 2019–2040.

19 Arena, U., Vizzutti, F.C., Ambu, G. et al. (2008). Acute viral hepatitis increases liver stiffness values measured by transient elastography. *Hepatology* 47 (2): 380–384.

20 Chan, H.L., Wong, G.L., Choi, P.C. et al. (2009). Alanine aminotransferase-based algo-rythms of liver stiffness measurement by transient elastography (Fibroscan) for liver fibrosis in chronic hepatitis B. *J. Viral. Hepat.* 16: 36–44.

21 Lackner, C., Spindelboeck, W., Haybaeck, J. et al. (2017). Histological parameters and alcohol abstinence determine long-term prognosis in patients with alcoholic liver disease. *J. Hepatol.* 66: 610–618.

22 Moreno, C., Mueller, S., and Szabo, G. (2019). Non-invasive diagnosis and biomarkers in alcohol-related liver disease. *J. Hepatol.* 70: 273–283.

23 Mueller, S., Millonig, G., Sarovska, L. et al. (2010). Increased liver stiffness in alcoholic liver disease: differentiating fibrosis from steatohepatitis. *World J. Gastroenterol.* 16 (8): 966–972.

24 Castera, L., Friedrich-Rust, M., and Loomba, R. (2019). Noninvasive assessment of liver disease in patients with nonalcoholic fatty liver disease. *Gastroenterology* 156: 1264–1281.

25 Pais, R., Barritt, A.S. 4th, Calmus, Y. et al. (2016). NAFLD and liver transplantation: current burden and expected challenges. *J. Hepatol.* 65 (6): 1245–1257.

26 Angulo, P., Hui, J.M., Marchesini, G. et al. (2007). The NAFLD fibrosis score: a noninvasive system that identifies liver fibrosis in patients with NAFLD. *Hepatology* 45 (4): 846–854.

27 Petta, S., Wong, S.W., Camma, C. et al. (2017). Improved noninvasive prediction of liver fibrosis by liver stiffness measurement in patients with nonalcoholic fatty liver disease accounting for controlled attenuation parameter values. *Hepatology* 65 (4): 1145–1155.

28 Petroff, D., Blank, V., Newsome, P.N. et al. (2021). Assessment of hepatic steatosis by controlled attenuation parameter using the M and XL probes: an individual patient data meta-analysis. *Lancet Gastroenterol. Hepatol.* 6: 185–198.

29 Ferraioli, G. (2021). CAP for the detection of hepatic steatosis in clinical practice. *Lancet Gastroenterol. Hepatol.* 6: 151–152.

30 Ferraioli, G., Maiocchi, L., Raciti, M.V. et al. (2019). Detection of liver steatosis with a novel ultrasound-based technique: a pilot study using MRI-derived proton density fat fraction as the gold standard. *Clin. Transl. Gastroenterol.* 10 (10): e00081.

31 Ferraioli, G. and Soares Monteiro, L.B. (2019). Ultrasound-based techniques for the diagnosis of liver steatosis. *World J. Gastroenterol.* 25 (40): 6053–6062.

32 Bende, F., Sporea, I., Victor, S. et al. (2021). Ultrasound-guided attenuation parameter (UGAP) for the quantification of liver steatosis using the controlled attenuation parameter (CAP) as the reference method. *Med. Ultrason.* 23 (1): 7–14.

33 Pons, M., Augustin, S., Scheiner, B. et al. (2020). Noninvasive diagnosis of portal hypertension in patients with compensated advanced chronic liver disease. *Am. J. Gastroenterol.* 00: 1–10.

34 European Association for the Study of the Liver, Asociación Latinoamericana para el Estudio del Hígado (2015). EASL-ALEH clinical practice guidelines: non-invasive tests for evaluation of liver disease severity and prognosis. *J. Hepatol.* 63: 237–264.

35 Dufour, J.F., DeLellis, R., and Kaplan, M.M. (1997). Reversibility of hepatic fibrosis in autoimmune hepatitis. *Ann. Intern. Med.* 127: 981–985.

36 Hartl, J., Ehlken, H., Sebode, M. et al. (2018). Usefulness of biochemical remission and transient elastography in monitoring disease course in autoimmune hepatitis. *J. Hepatol.* 68: 754–763.

37 Corpechot, C., Carrat, F., Poujol-Robert, A. et al. (2002). Noninvasive elastography-based assessment of liver fibrosis progression and prognosis in primary biliary cirrhosis. *Hepatology* 56 (1): 198–207.

38 Poupon, R. and Corpechot, C. (2011). Elastography-based assessment of primary biliary cirrhosis staging. *Dig. Liver Dis.* 43: 839–840.

39 Zhang, D.K., Chen, M., Liu, Y. et al. (2014). Acoustic radiation force impulse elastography for non-invasive assessment of disease stage in patients with primary biliary cirrhosis: a preliminary study. *Clin. Radiol.* 69: 836–840.

40 Yan, Y., Xing, X., Lu, Q. et al. (2020). Assessment of biopsy proven liver fibrosis by two-dimensional shear wave elastography in patients with primary biliary cholangitis. *Dig. Liver Dis.* 52 (5): 555–560.

41 Ali, A.H., Sinakos, E., Silveira, M.G. et al. (2011). Varices in early histological stage primary biliary cirrhosis. *J. Clin. Gastroenterol.* 45 (7): 66–71.

42 Carlos, M.-V., Saffioti, F., Tasayco-Huaman, S. et al. (2019). Non-invasive prediction of high-risk varices in patients with primary biliary cholangitis and primary sclerosing cholangitis. *Am. J. Gastroenterol.* 114 (3): 446–452.

43 Corpechot, C., El Naggar, A., Poujol-Robert, A. et al. (2006). Assessment of biliary fibrosis by transient elastography in patients with PBC and PSC. *Hepatology* 43 (5): 1118–1124.

44 Corpechot, C., Gaouar, F., El Naggar, A. et al. (2014). Baseline values and changes in liver stiffness measured by transient elastography are associated with severity of fibrosis and outcomes of patients with primary sclerosing cholangitis. *Gastroenterology.* 146: 970–979.

45 Roccarina, D., Saffioti, F., Rosselli, M. et al. (2023). Utility of ElastPQ point-shear wave elastography in the work-up of patients with primary sclerosing cholangitis. *JHEP Rep.* doi: https://doi.org/10.1016/j.jhepr.2023.100873.

46 Sebagh, M. and Samuel, D. (2004). Place of the liver biopsy in liver transplantation. *J. Hepatology* 41: 897–901.

47 Crespo, G., Castro-Narro, G., García-Juarez, I. et al. (2016). Usefulness of liver stiffness measurement during acute cellular rejection in liver transplantation. *Liver Transpl.* 22 (3): 298–304.

48 Rigamonti, C., Fraquelli, M., Bastiampillai, A.J. et al. (2012). Transient elastography identifies liver recipients with nonviral graft disease after transplantation: a guide for biopsy. *Liver Transpl.* 18: 566–576.

49 Carrion, J.A., Navasa, M., Bosch, J. et al. (2006). Transient elastography for diagnosis of advanced fibrosis and portal hypertension in patients with hepatitis C recurrence after liver transplantation. *Liver Transpl.* 12 (12): 1791–1798.

50 Della-Guardia, B., Evangelista, A.S., Felga, G.E. et al. (2017 Jan). Diagnostic accuracy of transient elastography for detecting liver fibrosis after liver transplantation: a specific cut-off value is really needed? *Dig. Dis. Sci.* 62 (1): 264–272.

51 Rinaldi, L., Valente, G., and Piai, G. (2016). Serial liver stiffness measurements and monitoring of liver-transplanted patients in a real-life clinical practice. *Hepat. Mon.* 16 (12): e41162.

52 Skinner, A.C. and Skelton, J.A. (2014). Prevalence and trends in obesity and severe obesity among children in the United States, 1999-2012. *JAMA Pediatr.* 168 (5): 561–566.

53 Vinciguerra, T., Brunati, A., David, E. et al. (2018). Transient elastography for non-invasive evaluation of post-transplant liver graft fibrosis in children. *Pediatr. Transplant.* 22 (2): doi:10.1111/petr.13125.

54 Leschied, J.R., Dillman, J.R., Bilhartz, J. et al. (2015). Shear wave elastography helps differentiate biliary atresia from other neonatal/infantile liver diseases. *Pediatr. Radiol.* 45: 366–375.

55 Hahn, S.M., Kim, S., Park, K.L. et al. (2013). Clinical benefit of liver stiffness mesurement at 3 months after Kasai hepatoportoenterostomy to predict the liver related events in biliary atresia. *PLoS One* 18 (8): e80652.

56 Kutty, S.S., Peng, Q., Danford, D.A. et al. (2014). Liver adult-pediatric-congenital-heart-disease dysfunction study (LADS) group. Increased hepatic stiffness as a consequence of high hepatic afterload in the Fontan circulation: a vascular Doppler and elastography study. *Hepatology* 59 (1): 251–260.

57 Loustaud-Ratti, V., Cypierre, A., Rousseau, A. et al. (2011). Non-invasive detection of hepatic amyloidosis: FibroScan, a new tool. *Amyloid* 18 (1): 19–24.

58 Richards, D.B., Cookson, L.M., Alienor, B. et al. (2015). Therapeutic clearance of amyloid by antibodies to serum amyloid P component. *N. Engl. J. Med.* 373 (12): 1106–1114.

59 Colecchia, A., Ravaioli, F., Sessa, M. et al. (2019). Liver stiffness measurement allows early diagnosis of veno-occlusive disease/sinusoidal obstruction syndrome in adult patients who undergo hematopoietic stem cell transplantation: results from a monocentric prospective study. *Biol. Blood Marrow Transplant.* 25: 995–1003.

60 Coppell, J.A., Richardson, P.G., Soiffer, R. et al. (2010). Hepatic veno-occlusive disease following stem cell transplantation: incidence, clinical course, and outcome. *Biol. Blood Marrow Transplant.* 16: 157–168.

61 Zhang, M., Mendiratta-Lala, M., Maturen, K.E. et al. (2019). Quantitative assessment of liver stiffness using ultrasound shear wave elastography in patients with chronic graft-versus-host disease after allogeneic hematopoietic stem cell transplantation: a pilot study. *J. Ultrasound Med.* 38 (2): 455–461.

62 Ferraioli, G. and Barr, R.G. (2020). Ultrasound liver elastography beyond liver fibrosis assessment. *World J. Gastroenterol.* 26 (24): 3413–3420.

63 Berzigotti, A., Reig, M., Abraldes, J.C. et al. (2015). Portal hypertension and the outcome of surgery for hepatocellular carcinoma in compensated cirrhosis: a systematic review and metanalysis. *Hepatology* 61 (2): 526–536.

64 Llop, E., Berzigotti, A., Reig, M. et al. (2012). Assessment of portal hypertension by transient elastography in patients with compensated cirrhosis and potentially resectable liver tumors. *J. Hepatol.* 56 (1): 103–108.

65 Huang, Z., Huang, J., Zhou, T. et al. (2018). Prognostic value of liver stiffness measurement for the liver-related surgical outcomes of patients under hepatic resection: a meta-analysis. *PLoS One* 13 (1): e0190512.

66 De Franchis, R., Bosch, J., Garcia-Tsao, G., Reiberger, T., Ripoll, C., on behalf of the Baveno VII Faculty (2022). Baveno VII – Renewing consensus in portal hypertension. *J. Hepatol.* 76: 959–974.

67 Barr, R.G., Wilson, S.R., Rubens, D. et al. (2020). Update to the society of radiologists in ultrasound liver elastography consensus statement. *Radiology* 296: 263–274.

68 Sporea, I. (2018). Clinical Ultrasonography. *Med. Ultrason.* 20 (3): 263–264.

10

Liver Ultrasound in the Paediatric Population

Andreas Panayiotou[1], Maria E. Sellars[1], and Annamaria Deganello[1,2]

[1] *Department of Radiology, King's College Hospital, London, UK*
[2] *Division of Imaging Sciences, King's College London, London, UK*

Paediatric liver disease is different from liver disease in the adult population, in terms of aetiology (more often genetic or congenital in children versus secondary to environmental exposure in adults) and susceptibility and response to injury; therefore numerous pathologies are unique to this age group. In this chapter, the emphasis will be on hepatobiliary scanning technique in the neonatal and paediatric age group, as well as the ultrasound appearance of the most common diffuse and focal liver pathologies. Ultrasound is the first-line method of imaging of the liver in the paediatric population for obvious reasons: it is relatively inexpensive, does not require sedation, does not involve ionising radiation, and can easily be performed at the patient's bedside (i.e. in the paediatric and neonatal intensive care unit), next to the parents.

To perform ultrasound on children, a high-frequency transducer is used for high-resolution anatomical detail. High-frequency linear probes can be used in neonates to assess the gallbladder and biliary tree, and high-frequency curvilinear probes should be used in older children and to obtain Doppler traces of the hepatic vasculature. A systematic approach is needed with a detailed assessment of the right upper quadrant, including the liver, gallbladder, bile ducts, and portal vein. The ultrasound examination should also include the spleen and the lower abdomen and pelvis, to assess the presence of any associated congenital findings or complications, such as ascites. The liver parenchyma and size need to be assessed as well as the texture of the liver parenchyma. The normal hepatic parenchyma, similarly to adults, is smooth and homogeneous, and the peripheral portal vein branches should be clearly seen, with well-defined, echogenic walls, as opposed to the thin-walled hepatic veins. The gallbladder shape and size should be examined as well as the presence of biliary duct dilatation; the pancreas and pancreatic duct should also be included in the investigation. Calculi, inspissated bile, pericholecystic fluid, and sonographic Murphy's sign should also be assessed. Although normal anatomy is similar to adults, it should be remembered that measurements differ according to paediatric age. The common bile duct is <1 mm in infants to 1 year of age, <4 mm in older children, and <7 mm in adolescents and young adults [1]. The pancreatic duct measures 1–2 mm and the gallbladder length is 1.5–3 cm in infants up to 1 year of age, and 3–7 cm in older children. Normal splenic length ranges from <6 cm in infants up to 3 months of age and <12 cm in older children [2].

Diffuse Liver Disease: Congenital

Biliary Atresia

Biliary atresia is a congenital absence or deficiency of the extrahepatic biliary system which can lead to neonatal cholestasis. If left untreated, it will lead to subsequent biliary cirrhosis, end stage liver disease and death. Therefore early diagnosis is important to achieve a favourable outcome. There are various ultrasound findings that can aid in the diagnosis of biliary atresia. The most sensitive signs include the triangular cord sign (hyperechoic triangular or tubular fibrous tissue along the anterior wall of the portal vein at the porta hepatis) and an abnormal, often small gallbladder with irregular walls (Figure 10.1a). Other findings may include a hypertrophic, hyperdynamic hepatic artery, a cyst at the porta hepatis, asplenia, absent gallbladder, non-visible/absent common bile duct, and sub-capsular flow [3]. Biliary atresia can be associated with other congenital abnormalities such as biliary atresia splenic malformation (BASM) syndrome (Figure 10.1b), for which these signs should be sought: polysplenia, situs inversus, portal vein

(a)　　　　　　　　　　　　　　(b)

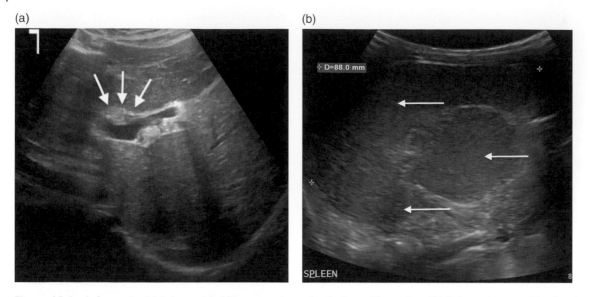

Figure 10.1 A 9-month-old infant with biliary atresia and splenic malformation (BASM) syndrome, with situs inversus. B-mode ultrasound demonstrates a hyperechoic fibrous ductal remnant of the extrahepatic bile duct, 'triangular chord sign' at the bifurcation of the portal vein (a, arrows), and polysplenia (b, arrows).

abnormalities (hypoplastic, pre-duodenal portal vein), interrupted inferior vena cava (IVC) with an azygous continuation, and intestinal malrotation. Patients with biliary atresia should also have a formal cardiac assessment with an echocardiogram to look for cardiac defects [4]. Treatment of biliary atresia entails a surgical procedure to restore bile flow known as 'Kasai portoenterostomy'. Regular ultrasound follow-up of these patients are imperative in order to detect the appearance of any sign of progression to chronic liver disease as a consequence of failure of the procedure. Thus, ultrasound assessment of these patients will aim to highlight signs of portal hypertension such as portal venous flow velocity reduction, increased hepatic artery resistance index and splenomegaly. A thorough liver parenchymal evaluation is also warranted to exclude the presence of focal lesions. Of note, increased liver stiffness, estimated by elastography, has been reported as an early predictor of Kasai procedure related complications and failure (Chapter 9.2).

It is important to highlight that years after the Kasai procedure, the liver architecture may undergo remodelling in the form of central plate hypertrophy (and hence heterogeneity).

Alagille Syndrome

Also known in the past as arteriohepatic dysplasia, Alagille syndrome is a rare genetic multiorgan systemic disorder characterised by a paucity of bile ducts and chronic cholestasis. It is diagnosed by demonstrating a paucity of intrahepatic bile ducts on liver biopsy and other criteria such as abnormal facies, congenital heart defect, ocular

abnormalities, and vertebral anomalies [5]. Alagille syndrome can present with jaundice and hyperbilirubinemia and shares similar findings with biliary atresia and neonatal hepatitis. It is important to differentiate early, because biliary atresia requires early surgical management while Alagille can be managed conservatively. However, 15% of children with Alagille would require liver transplantation due to progression to end-stage liver failure and refractory symptoms. Alagille is principally a clinical diagnosis and ultrasound findings are non-specific and similar to biliary atresia. Both biliary atresia and Alagille syndrome can have evidence of an abnormal gallbladder shape and hypertrophy of the hepatic artery, although in Alagille the triangular cord sign is not present and hypertrophy of the hepatic artery is less commonly seen; in addition, in Alagille signs of portal hypertension are less common [6]. Alagille syndrome can also be differentiated from biliary atresia by the presence of associated congenital abnormalities such as abnormal facies and other visceral anomalies. Ultimately, biopsy and genetic testing are required for diagnosis [5].

Fibropolycystic Liver Disease

Also known as ductal plate malformations, fibropolycystic liver disease is a complex group of congenital liver diseases resulting from abnormal embryonal development of the bile ducts. These disorders include congenital hepatic fibrosis, biliary hamartomas, polycystic liver disease, choledochal cysts, and Caroli disease, and can be associated with autosomal recessive polycystic kidney disease (ARPKD), medullary sponge kidney, and nephronophthisis. They constitute a spectrum of disorders that can co-exist in the same patient and their manifestation and radiological signs will depend on the timing by which they occur during embryogenesis and the size of the bile ducts affected, with hepatic fibrosis being most commonly seen in abnormalities of the small, peripheral bile ducts [7].

Congenital hepatic fibrosis is characterised by periportal fibrosis, which can be seen on ultrasound as increased periportal echogenicity, and often presents in adolescents with signs of portal hypertension, such as splenomegaly and varices. Other ultrasound findings include hypertrophy of the left liver lobe, especially segment IV, with right lobe atrophy, and a hypertrophic hepatic artery with possible development of large intrahepatic regenerative nodules. Renal abnormalities such as polycystic kidney disease and medullary sponge kidney as well as co-existing Caroli disease are often seen in association with this.

Biliary hamartomas, also known as 'von Meyenburg complexes', are small scattered collections of dilated intrahepatic bile ducts that have lost their communication with the biliary tree and are distributed evenly throughout the liver parenchyma, measuring up to 1.5 cm in size. On ultrasound, they can present as multiple small hypoechoic or hyperechoic lesions with comet-tail artefacts (See Chapter 6).

Polycystic liver disease is a group of genetic disorders that can present in isolation, as autosomal dominant polycystic liver disease (ADPLD), or in combination with autosomal dominant or recessive polycystic renal disease (ADPRD or

ARPRD). The disease is characterised by cysts that progressively increase in number and replace the liver parenchyma. Patients with polycystic liver disease show on ultrasound examination an enlarged liver, with bi-lobar thin-walled cysts of various sizes, ranging from a few millimetres to several centimetres in diameter. Possible complications include infection, compression of biliary ducts (even though the cysts do not communicate with the biliary tree), and bleeding or rupture of the cysts.

Caroli disease and *Caroli syndrome* are seen on imaging as multifocal segmental dilatation of the large intrahepatic bile ducts, which still preserve their communication with the biliary tree. In Caroli disease, the arrest of remodelling of the ductal plate affects the larger intrahepatic ducts, whereas in Caroli syndrome, the arrest occurs both early and late during embryogenesis; in the latter, there is almost invariably a concomitant degree of congenital hepatic fibrosis. On ultrasound there is saccular or fusiform dilatation of the intrahepatic bile ducts (Figure 10.2), which may contain inspissated bile or stones. Typical of the disease is the 'central dot sign', better appreciated on magnetic resonance imaging (MRI) but still visible on ultrasound, where a central portal venous radicle and hepatic artery are surrounded by the dilated bile duct. Caroli can be differentiated from primary sclerosing cholangitis by the absence of focal strictures.

Choledochal cysts consist in dilatation of the intra- and/ or extrahepatic bile ducts, and different theories have been proposed to explain their aetiology, including one that sees them as part of ductal plate malformation. A more

(a)　　　　(b)

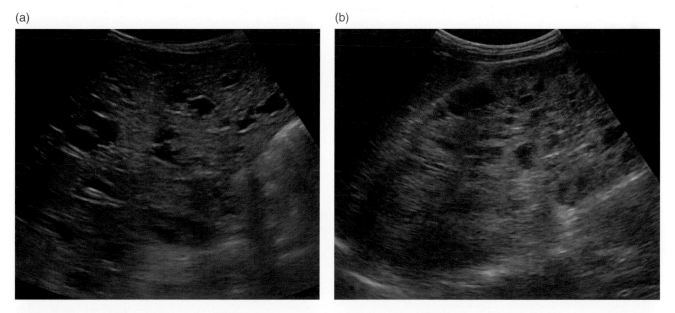

Figure 10.2 A 3-year-old with Caroli syndrome. (a) B-mode image of the liver demonstrates multiple, anechoic saccular dilatations of the intrahepatic bile ducts, with a background of heterogenous liver parenchyma in keeping with congenital hepatic fibrosis. (b) B-mode image of the left kidney demonstrates numerous anechoic cysts and hyperechoic parenchyma in keeping with polycystic kidney disease.

common theory is that they are caused by reflux of pancreatic enzymes and cholangitis due to an abnormal pancreaticobiliary junction with a long common channel, which eventually results in dilatation of the biliary system [8]. To make a diagnosis of a choledochal cyst, there must be a demonstrable communication with the biliary duct system. On ultrasound, choledochal cysts can be seen in different sizes and locations, according to the revised Todani classification (Table 10.1) [9, 10]. The pancreas should be assessed for duct dilatation and pancreatitis. Other complications include abscess, cirrhosis, malignancy, gallbladder, and biliary tract stones, as well as biliary peritonitis from spontaneous rupture of the cyst.

Progressive Familial Intrahepatic Cholestasis

Progressive familial intrahepatic cholestasis (PFIC) is a rare genetic disorder in which the liver fails to adequately secrete bile, resulting in cholestatic jaundice and pruritus. There are three types of PFIC; all patients are at risk of developing portal hypertension, ascites, liver failure, and, especially in PFIC type 2, cirrhosis and liver cancer. Ultrasound is the imaging modality of choice to screen these patients mostly for the early detection of hepatocellular carcinoma (HCC), as well as signs of portal hypertension, gallstones, and complications such as pancreatitis.

Cystic Fibrosis–Associated Liver Disease

Cystic fibrosis–associated liver disease has become a well-recognised complication of cystic fibrosis. Prompt identification and treatment can lead to better outcomes. The aetiology is an abnormal cystic fibrosis transmembrane regulator (CTFR) protein in the biliary epithelium, resulting in the accumulation of viscous bile. This results in injury to the

Table 10.1 Todani classification of bile duct cysts.

Type IA	Dilatation of the entire extrahepatic bile duct
Type IB	Focal, segmental dilatation of the extrahepatic bile duct
Type IC	Smooth, fusiform dilatation of the extrahepatic bile duct
Type II	Diverticuli of the extrahepatic bile duct
Type III	Dilatation of the intraduodenal common bile duct (choledochocele)
Type IVA	Multiple dilatations of the intrahepatic and extrahepatic bile ducts
Type IVB	Multiple dilatations of the extrahepatic bile ducts only
Type V	Dilatation of the intrahepatic bile ducts (Caroli disease)

hepatocytes and biliary epithelium, leading to fibrosis. Hepatic complications in cystic fibrosis are normally seen in older children; such children are usually asymptomatic until they present late with established portal hypertension and liver cirrhosis. Ultrasound may detect focal biliary fibrosis, which manifests as increased periportal echoes of heterogenous liver parenchyma. Additional findings include hepatomegaly, periportal fat deposition, biliary abnormalities including altered gallbladder morphology, and features of liver cirrhosis and portal hypertension (Figure 10.3) [11].

Wilson's Disease

Wilson's disease is an uncommon inherited autosomal recessive disorder of copper metabolism. Excess copper accumulation results in chronic liver disease, although in some cases it can cause acute or even fulminant liver failure. Ultrasound findings include features of hepatic steatosis, acute hepatitis, and cirrhosis. Compared to other causes of chronic liver disease, in Wilson's disease, the caudate lobe is not hypertrophied. A perihepatic fat layer can be observed and the outline of the liver may appear smooth or irregular with parenchymal hypoechoic or hyperechoic nodularities as well as a combination of both (mixed pattern) [12].

Diffuse Liver Disease: Acquired

Acquired diffuse liver disease includes hepatitis of various causes. The most common causes in this age group are non-alcoholic fatty liver disease (NAFLD), viral and autoimmune hepatitis, and sclerosing cholangitis. Diffuse liver disease often has non-specific ultrasound findings ranging from normal to end-stage liver disease. Ultrasound features of end-stage liver disease include nodular liver parenchyma and features of portal hypertension, which are hepatofugal flow in the portal vein, venous collaterals, splenomegaly, and ascites (See Chapter 8). In the acute setting, ultrasound is mainly used as a screening tool to exclude obstructive causes of jaundice in patients who present with cholestasis (See Chapters 6 and 12).

Non-alcoholic Fatty Liver Disease/Metabolic Dysfunction-Associated Steatotic Liver Disease

NAFLD is characterised by excessive build-up of fat in the liver secondary to dysmetabolism or increased caloric intake in the absence of alcohol. There is an increasing prevalence of NAFLD in the paediatric population and it is one of the most common causes of chronic liver disease in children [13]. Steatosis is a hallmark of NAFLD and it is easily diagnosed with ultrasound by comparing the

(a)   (b)

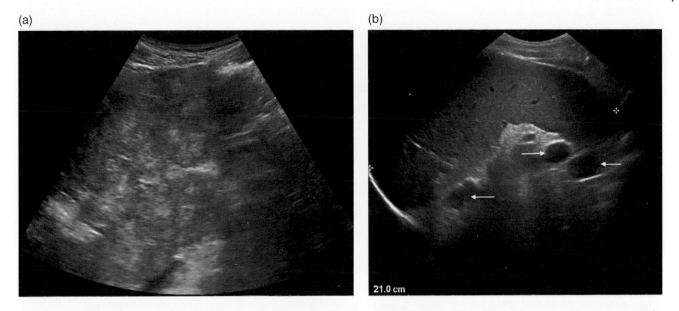

Figure 10.3 Cystic fibrosis–associated liver disease. (a) B-mode image showing liver cirrhosis with heterogeneous macronodular echotexture and atrophy of the left liver lobe. (b) Splenomegaly and peri-splenic varices (arrows).

echogenicity of the right liver lobe to the cortex of the right kidney. In normal conditions the liver parenchyma demonstrates a smooth homogeneous echotexture with similar echogenicity to the renal cortex. Instead, when steatosis is present, the liver's echogenicity appears increased compared to the cortex of the right kidney [14], and it can be graded subjectively according to the severity of posterior attenuation (See Chapter 8). Patients with hepatic steatosis are at risk of developing non alcoholic steatohepatitis (NASH), a condition that if left unchecked can lead to fibrosis and eventually end-stage liver disease.

However, the accuracy of ultrasound in detecting and staging fibrosis is insufficient and elastography is warranted in order to detect any increase in liver stiffness suggesting the presence of, or progression to, chronic liver disease (See Chapters 8 and 9).

Acute Viral Hepatitis

Acute viral hepatitis is a diffuse inflammation of the liver secondary to hepatotropic viruses, most commonly A-E, although epidemiology may vary significantly among different countries. Ultrasound findings in acute hepatitis are normally non-specific, with the only findings usually being diffuse reduced echogenicity of the liver parenchyma and increased reflectivity of the portal triads due to periportal oedema. The liver may be normal in size or enlarged. The biliary ducts and gallbladder are usually unremarkable, but in some cases the gallbladder may be reduced in size due to a decreased volume of bile. Other findings include gallbladder wall thickening, porta hepatis lymph nodes,

and splenomegaly [15–17]. If acute hepatitis is extremely severe (regardless of the underlying cause), it can lead to massive necrosis. On ultrasound, this can lead to changes which include liver parenchymal heterogeneities, ascites and segmental/lobular retraction (although this is usually found in the subacute phase), thus resembling a cirrhotic appearance (See Chapter 8).

Autoimmune Liver Disease

Autoimmune liver disease is an inflammatory disorder secondary to an immune disregulation that affects the liver. It is characterised by a large heterogeneity of clinical, laboratory and histological findings. It may manifest as acute hepatitis, liver failure or cirrhosis. Thus, its sonographic appearance is highly variable and may be normal, with subtle and irregularly distributed parenchymal heterogeneity or have features of advanced liver disease. Regenerative nodules and mild intrahepatic biliary dilatation con also be seen [18]. Periportal lymphadenopathy is a common finding (See Chapter 8).

Sclerosing Cholangitis

Primary sclerosing cholangitis is an inflammatory disease of unknown cause characterised by inflammation and fibrosis of the intra and extrahepatic bile ducts leading to biliary duct stricturing and dilatation. The fibrotic process can extend diffusely to the hepatic parenchyma leading to cirrhosis and portal hypertension. A significant association with inflammatory bowel diseases, especially ulcerative

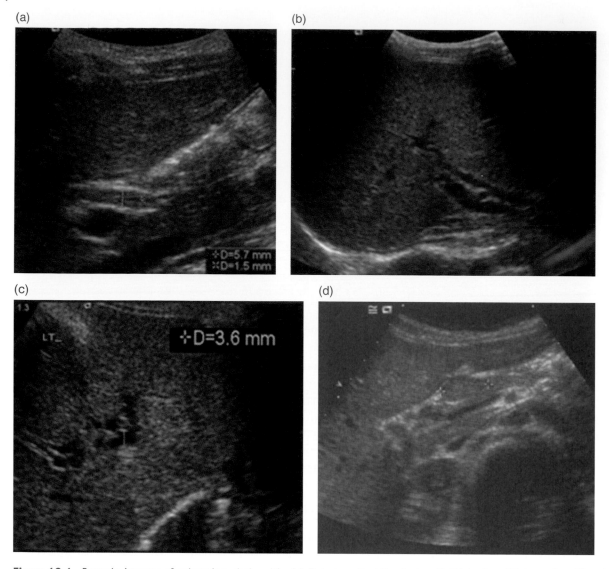

(a)

(b)

(c)

(d)

Figure 10.4 B-mode images of sclerosing cholangitis. (a) Extrahepatic bile duct wall thickening. (b) Irregular, dilated intra- and extrahepatic biliary ducts. (c) Segmental bile duct dilatation. (d) Enlarged peri-portal lymph nodes.

colitis, has been described. The risk of development of cholangiocarcinoma, gallbladder carcinoma and hepatocellular carcinoma is significantly increased in patients with primary sclerosing cholangitis. Note is made of the possibility of overlap syndrome with autoimmune hepatitis. Secondary causes of sclerosing cholangitis in children encompass other disorders such as immunodeficiencies, cystic fibrosis, Langerhan's cell histiocytosis and sickle cell anaemia. Ultrasonically, there may be signs of cholangiopathy in the form of thickened bile duct walls (Figure 10.4a), and intra-or extra-hepatic bile duct dilatation (see Figures 10.4b and c). Parenchymal findings include atrophy of the liver segments secondary to biliary stricturing and fibrotic retraction, as well as compensatory hypertrophy of other

segments. There are often enlarged lymph nodes at the porta hepatis (Figure 10.4d), and there may be signs of portal hypertension (See Chapter 8).

Focal Liver Lesions

In children every effort should be made to reduce ionising radiation, in accordance with the ALARA (As Low As Reasonably Achievable) principle. Ultrasound is a valid and economical screening tool for suspected focal liver masses, although, due to the limitations of conventional ultrasound, further cross-sectional imaging such as computed tomography (CT) and MRI is often required to reach a diagnosis. Contrast-enhanced ultrasound (CEUS) offers a more detailed assessment compared to conventional ultrasound and may obviate the need for the ionising radiation and sedation associated with CT and MRI. Although CEUS is widely used and well established among adults, its use in Europe in the paediatric population is still off-label. Nevertheless, there is mounting evidence of its safety and usefulness in the paediatric setting [19]. In 2016, its use was approved in the USA by the Food and Drug Administration (FDA) for the characterisation of focal liver lesions in both adults and children. CEUS uses an intravascular microbubble contrast agent, which allows better assessment of focal liver lesions through their enhancement characteristics (See Chapters 4 and 5). In addition, CEUS is quick, offers high spatial resolution, and allows real-time and continuous dynamic assessment of the lesion that is not greatly affected by patient movement. Other advantages of CEUS when dealing with a newly detected focal liver lesion include the possibility of immediate reassurance for parents and bedside availability, making it the ideal investigation in children, even in the intensive therapy unit or emergency department.

Age, specific imaging features, and laboratory findings should be taken into consideration when approaching suspected liver masses in paediatrics, as some lesions are unique to children of certain age groups while others are more common in adults. Laboratory findings play a key role, especially α-fetoprotein (AFP), which is a tumour marker elevated in hepatic malignancies; nevertheless, even though elevated levels of AFP virtually rule out a benign lesion (except in neonates, where AFP levels are elevated at birth and then decline during the first weeks of life), not all malignancies produce AFP and therefore the role of imaging is key [20]. Knowledge of the ultrasound appearances of these masses aids in the differential diagnosis and management plan, although ultimately ultrasound- or CT-guided biopsy is required for diagnosis in uncertain cases.

Many focal liver lesions can be reliably assessed with CEUS, with similar accuracy to cross-sectional imaging, including focal nodular hyperplasia (FNH), haemangioma, adenoma, cyst, abscess, regenerative nodule, and focal fatty infiltration or sparing. Occult lesions on conventional ultrasound may also be detected when using CEUS [19]. Many focal liver lesions show enhancement characteristics on CEUS that are similar to CT and MRI; for instance the presence of contrast wash-out in the portal venous phase is strongly suggestive of malignancy [21]. It should be noted that the timing of vascular phases in liver ultrasound differs according to the child's age and to that of adults.

Benign Tumours

Focal Nodular Hyperplasia

FNH is not a neoplasm, but a non-specific reaction to vascular abnormalities [22]. It is more common in adults than in children. FNH is mostly asymptomatic and diagnosed incidentally. On ultrasound, a typical FNH is a homogeneous, well-defined lesion and may be either slightly hypoechoic, isoechoic, or slightly hyperechoic (Figure 10.5a). Internally, a central hypoechoic scar may be seen with increased flow on colour Doppler that radiates outwards in a spoke–wheel pattern (Figure 10.5b). CEUS shows early arterial centrifugal enhancement with a characteristic spoke–wheel pattern (Figure 10.5c), and homogeneous enhancement on the late arterial phase (Figure 10.5d). Persistent enhancement is seen on the portal venous phase with no washout (Figure 10.5e), which is isoenhancing and inconspicuous compared to the adjacent liver parenchyma [21, 23, 24].

Haemangioendothelioma

Haemangioendothelioma is a vascular neoplasm and the most common benign liver tumour in children. Although benign, it could have serious clinical implications such as high-output cardiac failure. The majority of cases are diagnosed in the first six months of life, and 50% of cases are multiple [25]. Haemangioendothelioma has characteristic ultrasound and Doppler findings that can often result in a confident diagnosis without the need for cross-sectional imaging. It can present as unifocal, multifocal, or diffuse, each with corresponding imaging features. Focal masses tend to appear heterogeneous owing to haemorrhage, necrosis, fibrosis, and calcifications (Figure 10.6a), whereas multifocal lesions tend to appear as small, well-defined hypoechoic masses. Diffuse involvement will appear as diffusely nodular, heterogeneous liver parenchyma, and hepatomegaly. The imaging features reflect their vasculature nature, with evidence of high flow on colour Doppler (Figure 10.6b) and enlarged feeding arteries and draining veins. There is typically tapering of the abdominal aorta inferior to the coeliac axis and the hepatic artery is hypertrophic, with high peak systolic velocity on Doppler trace. CEUS may show peripheral rim or nodular enhancement (Figure 10.7a [greyscale], b [CEUS]), with full or partial centripetal filling on portal venous and late phases (Figure 10.7c) [26, 27]. A central unenhanced, hypoechoic region is seen in the late phase, owing to central haemorrhage or necrosis (Figure 10.7d). Unlike haemangioendotheliomas, multifocal haemangiomas and FNH demonstrate early hyperenhancement and isoenhancement to hyperenhancement on the portal and late phases [28].

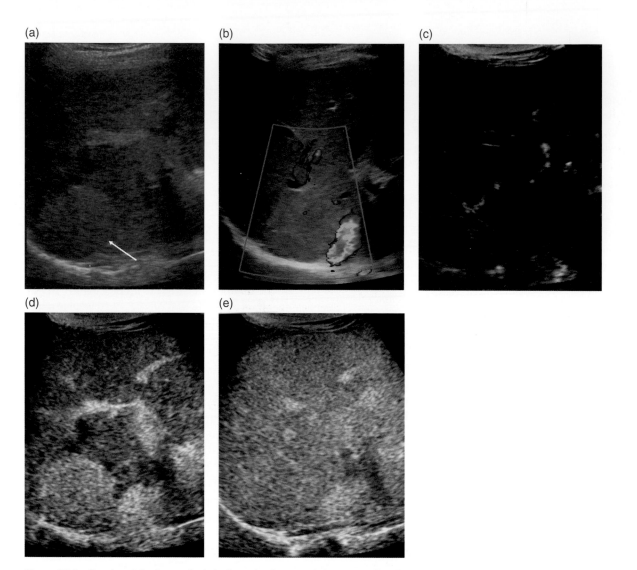

Figure 10.5 Focal nodular hyperplasia in B-mode ultrasound shows a well-defined hyperechoic nodule (a, arrow), with minimal internal vascularity on colour Doppler (b). Contrast-enhanced ultrasound at 14 seconds showing a characteristic 'spoke–wheel pattern' (c). There is a centrifugal homogeneous enhancement in the late arterial phase at 26 seconds (d), isoenhancing to the adjacent liver parenchyma on the venous phase, with no evidence of washout (e).

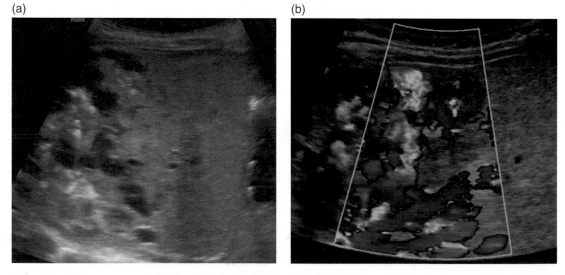

Figure 10.6 Haemangioendothelioma. Conventional ultrasound showing a mixed echogenic mass with solid and cystic components on B-mode ultrasound (a), and prominent vascular channels on colour Doppler ultrasound (b).

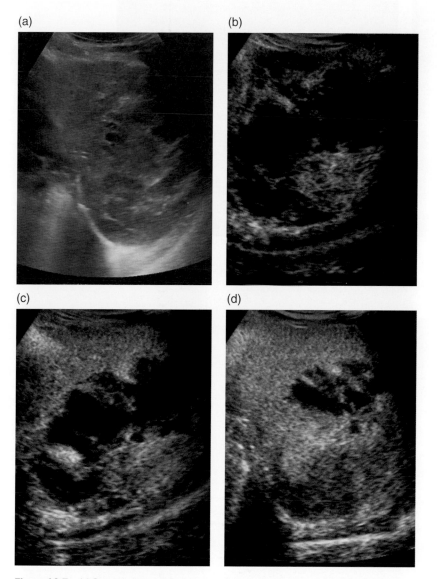

Figure 10.7 (a) B-mode image of a haemangioendothelioma in the left liver lobe. (b–d) Contrast-enhanced ultrasound images demonstrate nodular peripheral enhancement post contrast injection at 10 seconds (b) and 17 seconds (c), and incomplete centripetal filling at 35 seconds (d); the unenhanced region may represent haemorrhage or necrosis. No wash-out was seen on delayed images (not shown).

Mesenchymal Hamartoma

Mesenchymal hamartoma is the second most common benign liver tumour in children. Typically it presents as an asymptomatic abdominal mass. It appears as a cystic mass with multiple thin and thick septa (Figure 10.8), although appearances can vary from a multiseptated cystic mass to a mixed solid and cystic and even a solid-appearing mass. The solid components are generally hypovascular and only demonstrate feeble blood flow on colour Doppler of the solid stromal component and septa [29]. CEUS shows isoenhancement of the solid areas and non-enhancement of the cystic areas, but importantly can help determine vessel patency in large lesions that cause mass effect on the portal venous branches and/or hepatic veins [27].

Hepatic Adenoma

Hepatic adenoma is a liver tumour containing benign proliferation of hepatocytes and is very rare in children. Uncomplicated hepatic adenomas generally have a homogeneous echotexture similar to the liver, unless they have intracellular fat or haemorrhage, which will appear hyperechoic compared to normal liver parenchyma. Central vascularity with a venous waveform may be seen on colour Doppler, in contradistinction to FNH, which will show an arterial waveform. CEUS demonstrates mixed or centripetal enhancement with isoenhancement in early and late portal venous phases (Figure 10.9) [21,23]. In some cases delayed vascular washout is also described leading to a diagnostic dilemma and the need eventually for histological confirmation to exclude underlying malignancy (See Chapter 5).

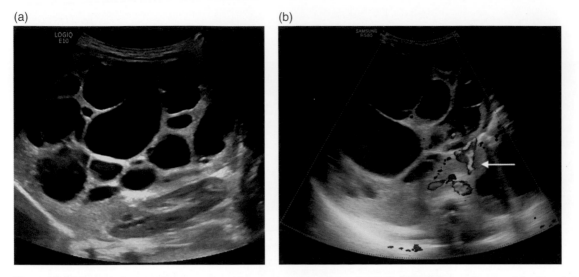

(a)

(b)

Figure 10.8 B-mode image of a mesenchymal hamartoma showing a large multiseptated cystic mass (a) with minimal vascularity in the solid components on colour Doppler (b, arrow) and no vascularity within the cystic spaces (b).

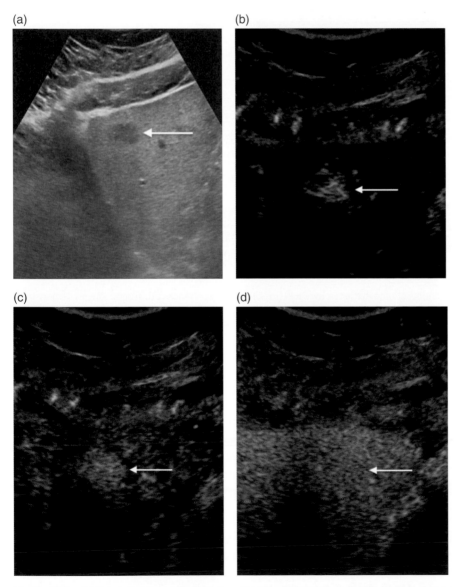

(a)

(b)

(c)

(d)

Figure 10.9 (a) B-mode image of a hepatic adenoma shows a well-demarcated hypoechoic mass in the left liver lobe (arrow). (b–d) Contrast-enhanced ultrasound shows a hypervascular mass at 20 seconds post injection (b, arrow), with centripetal filling at 25 seconds (c, arrow) and no wash-out on the delayed phase at 120 seconds (d, arrow).

Malignant Tumours

Hepatoblastoma

Hepatoblastoma is a malignant neoplasm and the most common primary liver tumour in children, occurring almost exclusively below 5 years of age, although it can present in older children still in the first decade of life mixed with HCC. Patients often present with a distended abdomen, a palpable abdominal mass, anorexia, and weight loss. The majority will show an elevated AFP (90%). Ultrasound features include a well-circumscribed predominantly solid mass, which is hyperechoic to normal liver parenchyma (Figure 10.10) and may contain hypoechoic fibrotic septa; 50% contain coarse calcification [20]. Even though all these patients will undergo cross-sectional imaging to achieve appropriate staging, given its superb spatial resolution ultrasound can assist in defining tumour outlines, in uncertain cases determine if a tumour

has breached the liver capsule, and also assess vessel patency, which are important prognostic factors. CEUS will show early, haphazard enhancement with very early wash-out (Figure 10.10), and can also be of value in the perfusion evaluation of intraluminal vascular thrombi (Figure 10.11).

Hepatocellular Carcinoma

HCC is rare in children under 5 years, but more common in older children. The majority of HCCs occur in children with chronic liver disease or with underlying metabolic disorders (such as tyrosinaemia and glycogen storage disease). HCC can also be associated with an elevated AFP. It can have variable ultrasound features and appears predominantly solid. Focal areas of reduced echogenicity may be due to haemorrhage or necrosis. A tumour capsule may be seen as a hypoechoic halo [30]. Similar to hepatoblastoma,

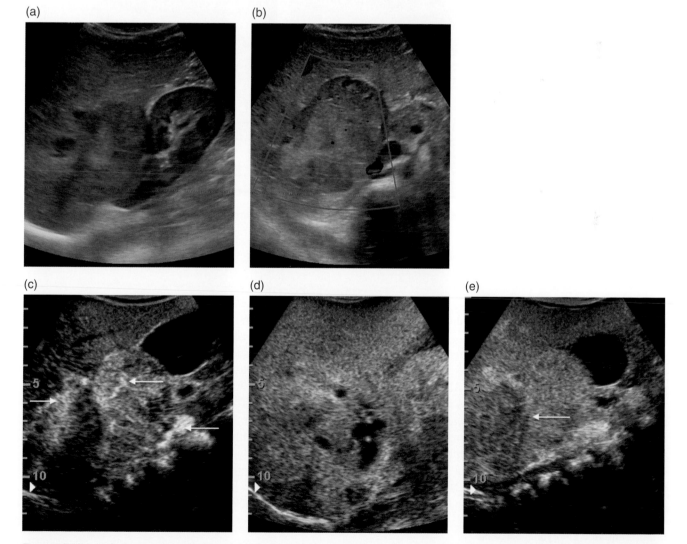

Figure 10.10 (a) B-mode image of a hepatoblastoma showing a heterogeneous solid mass in the right liver lobe displacing the right kidney. (b) Minimally increased vascularity is seen on colour Doppler. (c–e) Contrast-enhanced ultrasound images demonstrate a hypervascular mass with tortuous, irregular arteries at 15 seconds (c, arrows), with wash-out at 45 seconds (d) and 122 seconds (e, arrow).

(a)   (b)

(c)   (d)   (e)

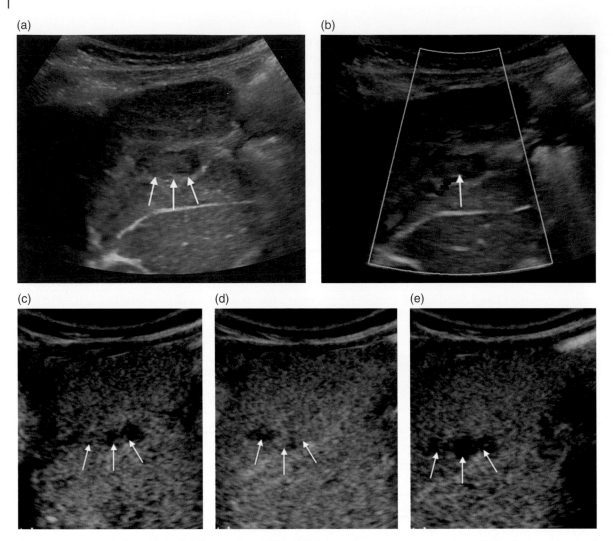

Figure 10.11 (a–e) Post-surgical follow-up in a different patient demonstrates recurrence within the portal vein. B-mode image demonstrates an echogenic solid filling defect in an expanded portal vein (a, arrows), with no vascularity seen on colour Doppler in keeping with complete occlusion (b, arrow). Contrast-enhanced ultrasound demonstrates a malignant enhancement pattern with arterialisation of the portal vein tumour thrombus at 14 seconds (c, arrows), with homogeneous enhancement at 27 seconds (d, arrows) and wash-out at 45 seconds (e, arrows).

HCC tends to invade the portal and hepatic veins (Figure 10.12).

Fibrolamellar HCC is a sub-type presenting mostly in teenagers or young adults. An increase in transcobalamin is reported in these patients, whereas AFP is normal, and FL-HCC presents as a large liver mass in a non-cirrhotic liver. On ultrasound these masses have variable echogenicity and can show a central scar; CEUS may have a theoretical value in assessing the pattern of enhancement of the central scar, which would be delayed in FL-HCC, and therefore in discriminating this from FNH, but there is no published data available to support this.

Undifferentiated Embryonal Sarcoma

Undifferentiated embryonal sarcoma (UES) is a rare mesenchymal tumour that occurs in young children (6–10 years old). AFP is usually normal and presenting symptoms are non-specific, including abdominal mass and pain. A characteristic finding in UES is that it appears predominantly solid (Figure 10.13a) on ultrasound with no significant vascularity (Figure 10.13b) and cystic on CT (Figure 10.13c) and MRI due to its water-containing myxoid stroma. The solid mass is isoechoic to hyperechoic compared to the liver parenchyma, with focal anechoic regions representing necrosis, old haemorrhage, or cystic degeneration [20, 31]. On CEUS the mass shows heterogeneous peripheral enhancement of the solid portions, with complete lack of enhancement of the myxoid stroma. Early wash-out of the solid components can also be demonstrated.

Rhabdomyosarcoma

Rhabdomyosarcoma of the biliary tree is a very rare tumour in children and it is most commonly seen as a

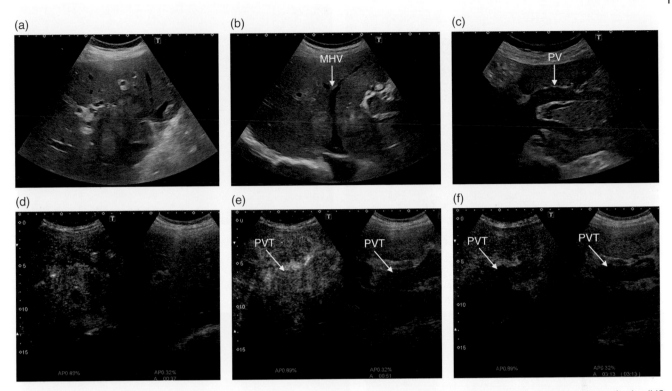

Figure 10.12   (a) B-mode ultrasound shows a large heterorgeneous focal lesion in segment I, IV and VIII that (b) surrounds the IVC compressing the middle hepatic vein, and (c) invades the portal vein that appears filled and stretched by echogenic material. Contrast enhanced ultrasound shows (d) arterial hyperenhancement of the focal lesion and (e) enhancement of the portal venous thrombus (PVT, arrows), both of which washout in the late vascular phase (f). The patient was diagnosed a large hepatocellular carcinoma with compression of the IVC, middle hepatic vein and portal vein invasion. *Source:* Courtesy of Dr Matteo Rosselli.

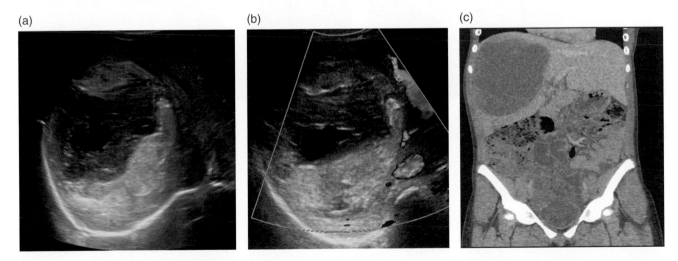

Figure 10.13   (a) B-mode image of a solitary embryonal sarcoma, showing a well-circumscribed and thick-walled cyst, which contains mixed thick and fine echogenic internal material. (b) No cyst wall or internal vascularity is seen on colour Doppler. (c) Coronal computed tomography image demonstrates the cystic nature of the embryonal sarcoma, despite the solid appearance on ultrasound.

heterogeneous mass expanding the common bile duct and infiltrating the intrahepatic bile ducts. It can display internal vascularity on colour Doppler, better demonstrated on CEUS (Figure 10.14).

Hepatic Metastases
Like for adults, the most common malignant hepatic tumour in children is metastatic disease, most commonly from neuroblastoma (Figure 10.15a [greyscale] and b [colour Doppler]) and Wilms' tumour. Metastases show the typical pattern of early arterial enhancement (Figure 10.15c) and portal and delayed phase wash-out (Figure 10.15d,e), as seen in other malignancies [32]. Metastatic neuroblastoma can mimic multifocal haemangioendothelioma, although it would demonstrate elevated urinary catecholamines [33]. Metastases

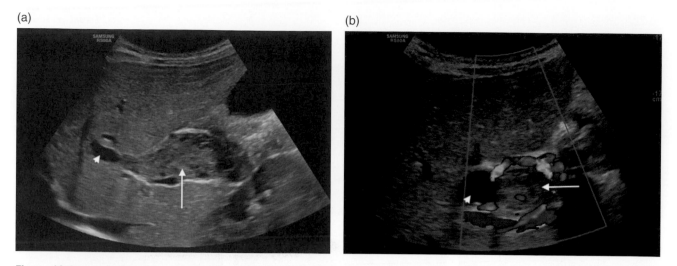

Figure 10.14 (a, b) B-mode ultrasound of a patient with rhabdomyosarcoma, demonstrating a large thickened and expanded extrahepatic bile duct (a, arrow), with minimal internal vascularity in colour Doppler (b, arrow). Both images demonstrate dilated distal intrahepatic bile ducts (arrowheads).

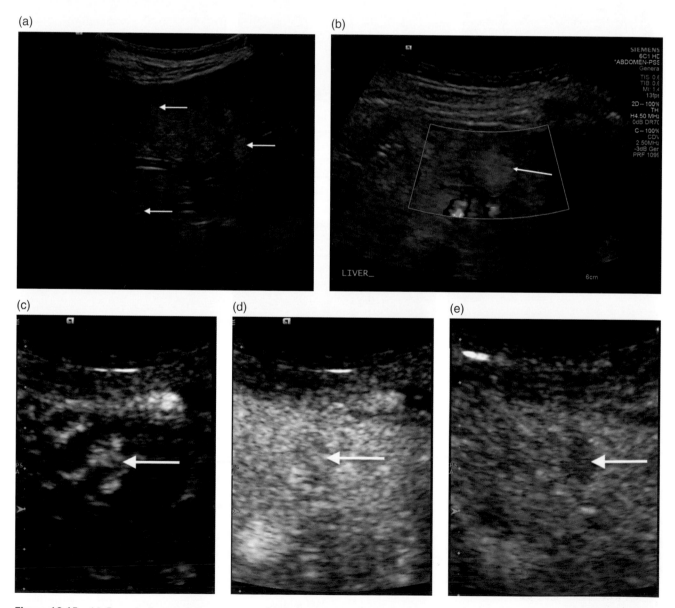

Figure 10.15 (a) B-mode image demonstrates multiple hyperechoic focal lesions in a patients with known neuroendocrine liver metastasis (arrows). (b) Colour Doppler image doesn't reveal any specific vascularity (arrow). (c–e) Contrast-enhanced ultrasound shows early arterial enhancement at 10 seconds (c, arrow), with early wash out at 30 seconds (d, arrow), that is more pronounced during the delayed phase at 200 seconds (e, arrow).

(a) (b)

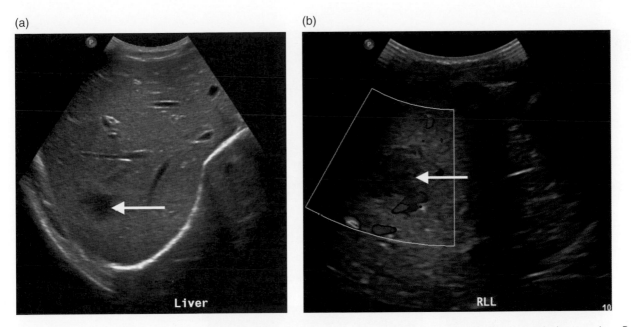

Figure 10.16 Ill-defined hypoechoic mass in the right liver lobe (a, arrow), with minimal peripheral vascularity on colour Doppler (b, arrow) that was found to correspond to a lymphoma metastasis.

can have a variable ultrasound appearance but are predominantly hypoechoic and relatively ill-defined (Figure 10.16).

Key Checkpoints for Emergency/On-Call Scans

Ultrasound plays a major role in screening children presenting acutely with sepsis, abdominal pain, and/or abnormal liver function tests. Correlation with the child's past medical and surgical history and with laboratory findings is paramount, as it can point to a certain cause such as prehepatic, intraparenchymal, or extrahepatic pathology. Key checkpoints of scanning the liver in an unwell child include assessment of the liver parenchyma for diffuse or focal liver disease, biliary duct dilatation and obstruction, hepatic and portal vein flow, and thrombosis. Systemic assessment of the whole abdomen should be done to look for ancillary findings or potential causes of acute liver pathology.

Acute biliary pathology includes cholecystitis, cholelithiasis, choledocholithiasis, cholangitis, and biliary abscesses, some of which may occur in the context of known biliary pathology. Duct dilatation may be due to stones or inspissated bile. Gallbladder calculi more commonly occur in adults, but there is a rising incidence in children. Inspissated bile syndrome is an uncommon cause of jaundice and appears as low-level echoes within the gallbladder, or rarely within a dilated biliary duct, resulting in complete or partial obstruction.

Liver abscess is an uncommon diagnosis in children; nonetheless, it should be considered as a differential diagnosis for focal liver lesions in children who present with elevated liver enzymes and sepsis, especially those who are immunocompromised. A liver abscess can occur as a complication of a pre-existing congenital abnormality of the biliary tree, which can lead to biliary stasis and subsequently bacterial proliferation [34]. On ultrasound, hepatic abscesses can present as poorly demarcated lesion(s) that are predominantly hypoechoic (Figure 10.17a), but with variable echogenicity. There will be an absence of colour flow on colour Doppler. Internal echoes and posterior acoustic enhancement may also be seen. CEUS shows early arterial enhancement (Figure 10.17b–d) and progressive washout on delayed phases of the inflamed tissue; while necrosis or liquefaction, that are usually central to the abscess, will never enhance. Malignant lesions may have a similar appearance, therefore medical history, clinical presentation and eventually neoplastic markers should be considered.

(a)

(b)

(c)

(d)

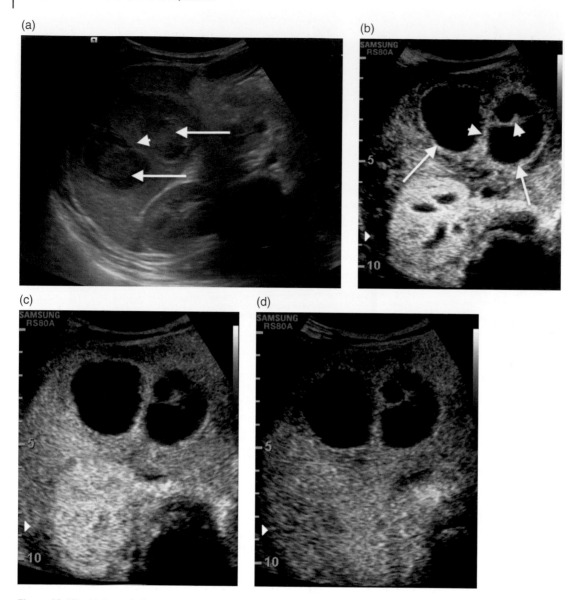

Figure 10.17 (a) B-mode image shows a thick-walled liver abscess (arrow) in the right lobe with septations (arrowhead) and fine internal echogenicity. (b–d) Contrast-enhanced ultrasound demonstrates arterial enhancement of the abscess wall (b, arrows) and internal septations at 10 seconds (b, arrowheads) and 30 seconds (c), with persistent wall enhancement on the venous phase at 60 seconds (d).

Appendicitis can be complicated by portal vein thrombosis and liver abscess formation, therefore the liver should be assessed as a routine checkpoint when scanning for appendicitis. Children with chronic liver disease can present with acute deterioration; haematemesis can be secondary to chronic liver disease and long-standing portal hypertension, therefore the abdomen should be assessed for cirrhosis, portal vein thrombosis, and varices.

References

1 Gubernick, J.A., Rosenberg, H.K., Ilaslan, H. et al. (2000). US approach to jaundice in infants and children. *Radiographics* 20 (1): 173–195.

2 Deganello, A., Sellars, M.E., and Sidhu, P.S.S. Paediatric and neonatal: upper abdomen. In: *Measurement in Ultrasound*, 2e (ed. P.S. Sidhu, W.K. Chong and K. Satchithananda), 237–260. Boca Raton, FL: CRC Press.

3 Choi, S.O., Park, W.H., Lee, H.J. et al. (1996). 'Triangular cord': a sonographic finding applicable in the diagnosis of biliary atresia. *J. Pediatr. Surg.* 31 (3): 363–366.

4 Davenport, M., Savage, M., Mowat, A.P. et al. (1993). Biliary atresia splenic malformation syndrome: an etiologic and prognostic subgroup. *Surgery* 113 (6): 662–668.

5 Shamir, S.B., Kurian, J., Kogan-Liberman, D. et al. (2017). Hepatic imaging in neonates and young infants: state of the art. *Radiology* 285 (3): 763–777.

6 Cho, H.H., Kim, W.S., Choi, Y.H. et al. (2016). Ultrasonography evaluation of infants with Alagille syndrome: in comparison with biliary atresia and neonatal hepatitis. *Eur. J. Radiol.* 85 (6): 1045–1052.

7 Brancatelli, G., Federle, M.P., Vilgrain, V. et al. (2005). Fibropolycystic liver disease: CT and MR imaging findings. *Radiographics* 25 (3): 659–670.

8 Babbitt, D.P. (1969). Congenital choledochal cysts: new etiological concept based on anomalous relationships of the common bile duct and pancreatic bulb. *Ann. Radiol.* 12 (3): 231–240.

9 Todani, T., Watanabe, Y., Narusue, M. et al. (1977). Congenital bile duct cysts. Classification, operative procedures, and review of thirty-seven cases including cancer arising from choledochal cyst. *Am. J. Surg.* 134 (2): 263–269.

10 Singham, J., Yoshida, E.M., and Scudamore, C.H. (2009). Choledochal cysts part 1 of 3: classification and pathogenesis. *Can. J. Surg.* 52 (5): 434–440.

11 van Mourik, I.D.M. (2017). Liver disease in cystic fibrosis. *Paediatr. Child Health (United Kingdom)* 27 (12): 552–555.

12 Akhan, O., Akpinar, E., Karcaaltincaba, M. et al. (2009). Imaging findings of liver involvement of Wilson's disease. *Eur. J. Radiol.* 69 (1): 147–155.

13 Shah, J., Okubote, T., and Alkhouri, N. (2018). Overview of updated practice guidelines for pediatric nonalcoholic fatty liver disease. *Gastroenterol. Hepatol.* 14 (7): 407–414.

14 Di Martino, M., Koryukova, K., Bezzi, M. et al. (2017). Imaging features of non-alcoholic fatty liver disease in children and adolescents. *Children* 4 (8): 73.

15 Maurya, V., Ravikumar, R., Gopinath, M., and Ram, B. (2019). Ultrasound in acute viral hepatitis: Does it have any role? *Med. J. Dr DY Patil Vidyapeeth* 12 (4): 33.

16 Sharma, M.P. and Dasarathy, S. (1991). Gallbladder abnormalities in acute viral hepatitis: a prospective ultrasound evaluation. *J. Clin. Gastroenterol.* 13 (6): 697–700.

17 Sudhamshu, K.C., Sharma, D., Poudya, N. et al. (2014). Acute viral hepatitis in pediatric age groups. *J. Nepal Med. Assoc.* 52 (193): 687–691.

18 Dong, Y., Potthoff, A., Klinger, C. et al. (2018). Ultrasound findings in autoimmune hepatitis. *World J. Gastroenterol.* 24 (15): 1583–1590.

19 Sidhu, P.S., Cantisani, V., Deganello, A. et al. (2017). Role of contrast-enhanced ultrasound (CEUS) in paediatric practice: an EFSUMB position statement. *UltraschallMed.* 38 (1): 33–43.

20 Chung, E.M., Lattin, G.E. Jr., Cube, R. et al. (2011). From the archives of the AFIP: pediatric liver masses: radiologic-pathologic correlation part 2. Malignant tumors. *RadioGraphics* 31 (2): 483–507.

21 Claudon, M., Dietrich, C.F., Choi, B.I. et al. Guidelines and good clinical practice recommendations for contrast enhanced ultrasound (CEUS) in the liver - Update 2012. *Ultraschall Med.* 34 (1): 2013, 11–2029.

22 Franchi-Abella, S. and Branchereau, S. (2013). Benign hepatocellular tumors in children: focal nodular hyperplasia and hepatocellular adenoma. *Int. J. Hepatol.* 2013: 215064.

23 Fang, C., Bernardo, S., Sellars, M.E. et al. (2019). Contrast-enhanced ultrasound in the diagnosis of pediatric focal nodular hyperplasia and hepatic adenoma: interobserver reliability. *Pediatr. Radiol.* 49 (1): 82–90.

24 Ungermann, L., Eliáš, P., Žižka, J. et al. (2007). Focal nodular hyperplasia: spoke-wheel arterial pattern and other signs on dynamic contrast-enhanced ultrasonography. *Eur. J. Radiol.* 63 (2): 290–294.

25 Chung, E.M., Lattin, G.E., Cube, R. et al. (2011). Pediatric liver masses: radiologic-pathologic correlation part 1. Benign tumors. *RadioGraphics* 30: 3. https://doi.org/10.1148/rg.303095173.

26 Piorkowska, M.A., Dezman, R., Sellars, M.E. et al. (2018). Characterization of a hepatic haemangioma with contrast-enhanced ultrasound in an infant. *Ultrasound* 26 (3): 178–181.

27 Chiorean, L., Cui, X.W., Tannapfel, A. et al. (2015). Benign liver tumors in pediatric patients - review with emphasis on imaging features. *World J. Gastroenterol.* 21 (28): 8541–8561.

28 Dong, Y., Wang, W.P., Cantisani, V. et al. (2016). Contrast-enhanced ultrasound of histologically proven hepatic epithelioid hemangioendothelioma. *World J. Gastroenterol.* 22 (19): 4741–4749.

29 Stringer, M.D. and Alizai, N.K. (2005). Mesenchymal hamartoma of the liver: a systematic review. *J. Pediatr. Surg.* 40 (11): 1681–1690.

30 Khanna, R. and Verma, S.K. (2018). Pediatric hepatocellular carcinoma. *World J. Gastroenterol.* 24 (25): 3980–3999.

31 Gabor, F., Franchi-Abella, S., Merli, L. et al. (2016). Imaging features of undifferentiated embryonal sarcoma of the liver: a series of 15 children. *Pediatr. Radiol.* 46 (12): 1694–1704.

32 Ferraioli, G. and Meloni, M.F. (2018). Contrast-enhanced ultrasonography of the liver using sonovue. *Ultrasonography* 37 (1): 25–35.

33 Fernandez-Pineda, I., Sandoval, J.A., and Davidoff, A.M. (2015). Hepatic metastatic disease in pediatric and adolescent solid tumors. *World J. Hepatol.* 7 (14): 1807–1817.

34 Di Serafino, M., Severino, R., Gioioso, M. et al. (2019). Paediatric liver ultrasound: a pictorial essay. *J. Ultrasound* 23 (1): 87–103.

11

Ultrasound in Vascular Liver Diseases

M. Ángeles García-Criado[1] and Annalisa Berzigotti[2]

[1] *Radiology Department, Hospital Clínic i Provincial, University of Barcelona, Barcelona, Spain*
[2] *Department of Visceral Surgery and Medicine, Inselspital, Bern University Hospital, University of Bern, Bern, Switzerland*

Vascular liver diseases (VLDs) – summarised in Table 11.1 – are a heterogeneous group of diseases affecting one or more of the liver vessels, either at micro- or macroscopic level. Many of them are rare or very rare and it is important to note that several VLDs occur in association with, or because of systemic diseases. The latter should therefore be carefully excluded with a VLD diagnosis. The approach and management vary largely according to the type of VLD (see below), ranging from anticoagulation for thrombotic disorders, to interventional radiology techniques (e.g. for large arteriovenous fistulae) and to liver transplantation in selected cases.

Among clinically relevant VLDs, thrombotic diseases of the portal vein and of the hepatic veins constitute the largest proportion. In all patients presenting with signs of portal hypertension, thrombotic diseases should be ruled out since they are the second commonest cause of this syndrome after cirrhosis.

Ultrasound techniques are very useful in identifying and characterising many VLDs and their associations. Ultrasound is the first modality of choice when there is a clinical suspicion of VLD.

This chapter aims to summarise the evidence supporting the use of ultrasound and elastography techniques for the main VLDs.

Portal Vein Thrombosis and Extrahepatic Portal Vein Obstruction

Thrombosis of the portal venous system, or portal vein thrombosis (PVT), is defined by the presence of a clot in the lumen of the vessel at any level (extrahepatic trunk, intrahepatic branches, splenic vein, mesenteric veins), or by the substitution of the vessel with porto-portal collaterals (cavernous transformation) [1]. Cirrhosis and prothrombotic diseases (either congenital or acquired) are risk factors for the onset of PVT. In cirrhosis, cross-sectional studies showed prevalences of up to 20% with an incidence of 5–7% per year, while in the general population the risk of PVT is deemed to be <1% in a lifetime [2]. PVT occurring in subjects without cirrhosis is more correctly termed extrahepatic portal vein obstruction (EHPVO) and should prompt a complete work-up of thrombophilia, including ruling out myeloproliferative neoplasms (JAK2, calreticulin, MPL gene mutations and bone marrow biopsy in selected cases); paroxysmal nocturnal haemoglobinuria (flow cytometry for CD55 and CD59), Behcet's disease; antiphospholipid syndrome; mutations of Factor II, Factor V, ATIII, Protein C and Protein S, human immunodeficiency virus (HIV) infection, coeliac disease autoimmune and inflammatory systemic diseases [2].

Presentation varies from totally asymptomatic cases identified on imaging done for other causes to abdominal pain, to complications of portal hypertension or intestinal ischaemia. These depend on the severity of occlusion, site of occlusion, duration, extension, and comorbidities. These factors are taken into account in a recent anatomical-functional classification [3].

On suspicion of PVT, ultrasound should be used as a first-line technique, since its sensitivity and specificity for thrombosis exceeds 90% [4]. An endoluminal clot or absence of flow or cavernous transformation of at least one of the vessels of the portal system defines PVT. The clot can have an echogenic or hypoechogenic component, and can completely or partially (Figure 11.1) occupy the lumen. The clot is better visualised on greyscale ultrasound but colour and spectral Doppler can help characterise the degree of occlusion (complete/partial with residual flow) [4]. By using the

Table 11.1 Main vascular liver disorders and role of ultrasound and elastography.

Portal vein system	Portal vein thrombosis/extrahepatic portal vein obstruction	• Ultrasound/Doppler ultrasound rules out or confirms thrombosis with good accuracy and identifies cavernous transformation and porto-systemic collaterals • Contrast-enhanced ultrasound (CEUS) is useful to differentiate bland thrombosis from tumour invasion of the portal vein in hepatocellular carcinoma and intrahepatic cholangiocarcinoma • Liver stiffness can help in characterising whether thrombosis occurred on cirrhosis or if the liver is non-cirrhotic • Spleen stiffness is high (confirming portal hypertension) and could be an additional prognostic tool
	Congenital porto-systemic shunts	• Ultrasound allows the malformation(s) to be visualised • Spectral Doppler provides data on flow direction and characteristics • Role of elastography currently unknown, but potentially useful (cirrhosis vs. no cirrhosis)
Liver sinusoids	Porto-sinusoidal vascular disorder (idiopathic portal hypertension)	• On greyscale ultrasound the aspect of the liver can mimic cirrhosis in long-lasting porto-systemic disease • Liver stiffness is usually normal or near normal; spleen stiffness is high (confirming portal hypertension)
	Sinusoidal obstruction syndrome	• Low specificity of the single reported signs: reversal of portal venous flow, reduced phasicity of hepatic venous flow, gallbladder wall oedema, increased resistive indices of the hepatic artery, ascites • Liver stiffness potentially useful (case series)
Diseases affecting the hepatic veins	Budd–Chiari syndrome	• Ultrasound/Doppler ultrasound/CEUS (difficult cases) rules out or confirms by direct signs (thrombosis of one or more liver veins or IVC) or more frequently by pointing out indirect signs (see text) • Identification of the likely cause in secondary Budd–Chiari syndrome (tumours; trauma; alveolar Echinococcosis) • Role of elastography unclear: congestion of the liver increases liver stiffness, which improves after transjugular intrahepatic portosystemic shunt; prognostic role possible
Hepatic artery	Hepatic artery diseases (aneurysm, thrombosis, stenosis)	• Ultrasound/Doppler ultrasound rules out or confirms • No role for elastography
	Arteriovenous fistulae	• Ultrasound/Doppler ultrasound can confirm if directly visualised or can orient the diagnosis if indirect signs are present (reversal of flow in a branch of the portal vein) • Role of elastography unlikely
Congenital vascular malformations and hereditary haemorrhagic telangiectasia		• Ultrasound/Doppler ultrasound rules out or confirms • In hereditary haemorrhagic telangiectasia: grading of liver involvement (see text) • Role of elastography unknown but potential (cirrhosis vs. no cirrhosis)

(a)

(b)

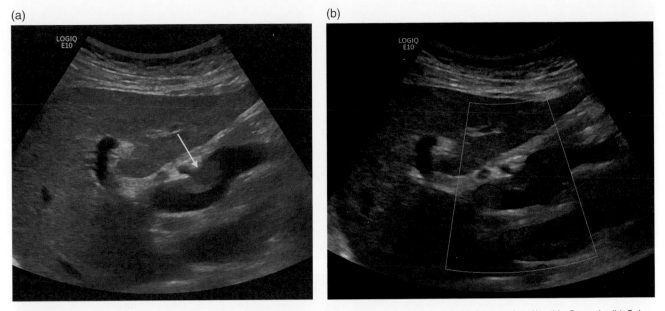

Figure 11.1 Partial portal vein thrombosis in a patient without cirrhosis. (a) Note that the clot is better visualised in B-mode. (b) Colour Doppler further confirms the presence of residual flow in the lumen.

latter techniques, attention should be paid to using the lowest possible scale to avoid false positives owing to slow flow (e.g. in decompensated cirrhosis or in patients on non-selective beta-blockers). The cavernous transformation of the portal vein is identified by porto-portal tortuous collateral vessel substituting (surrounding or within) the thrombosed vessel (Figure 11.2). It can occur at any level of the portal venous system (intra- or extrahepatic).

In addition, ultrasound not only detects the presence of PVT, but also provides information on factors that may predict its recanalisation with anticoagulation therapy, as well as clinical outcomes [4]. These can be summarised as follows:

- *Absence/presence of cirrhosis*: cirrhosis represents per se a risk factor for PVT. An active search for signs of cirrhosis (e.g. nodular liver surface; heterogeneous parenchyma; caudate and left lobe hypertrophy, splenomegaly, and recanalised paraumbilical vein) should be performed [5]. Since long-lasting thrombosis can alter the liver shape, mimicking cirrhosis, the use of elastography can be very helpful in diagnosing cirrhosis in this setting, since liver stiffness is markedly increased only in patients with cirrhosis and not in patients with EHPVO [6]. Spleen stiffness is elevated in both conditions, and is not helpful in the differential diagnosis.
- *Duration of thrombosis*: a well-recognisable vessel with hypoechoic material in the lumen can suggest recent thrombosis in patients who have developed symptoms. On the other hand, the presence of calcifications in the

thrombus or in the walls of the involved vessels is considered a sign of long-lasting thrombosis. Other signs, such as large splenomegaly or degree of porto-systemic and porto-portal collateralisation, cannot be considered specific of long-lasting thrombosis owing to the many confounders that can be encountered in patients with PVT (e.g. myeloproliferative diseases leading per se to splenomegaly; cirrhosis leading to porto-systemic collaterals previous to PVT, etc.), and due to the fact that cavernous transformation has a very early onset (within days/weeks from the acute thrombotic episode) (Figure 11.3).

- *Presence of vessels that can allow interventions*: the presence and size of a remnant portal vein, and/or the dominant vessel within the cavernoma, and the patency of the splenic vein and superior mesenteric vein are key pieces of information to select patients in whom a transjugular intrahepatic porto-systemic shunt (TIPS) or recanalisation procedures can be attempted. For a detailed mapping of the extension of the thrombosis and of the anatomy of the existing collaterals, cross-sectional contrast-enhanced imaging methods (contrast-enhanced computed tomography, CECT, or contrast-enhanced magnetic resonance, CEMR) should be preferred. These methods can also provide information on the presence of extrahepatic malignancies or inflammatory foci.
- *Nature of thrombosis (benign; neoplastic vascular invasion)*: PVT in patients with hepatocellular carcinoma or cholangiocellular carcinoma and patients in whom both a liver tumour and PVT are detected simultaneously represents a diagnostic challenge, since both bland

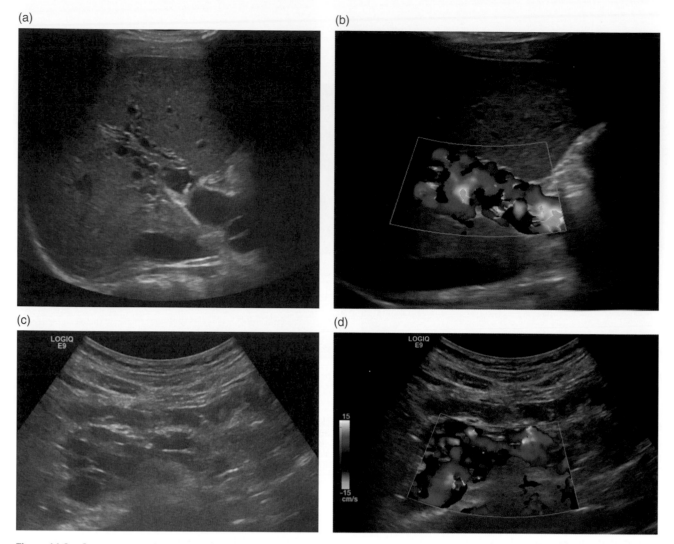

Figure 11.2 Cavernous transformation of the portal vein. (a) The right intrahepatic portal vein is substituted by hyperechoic (fibrous) tissue, around which small tortuous anechoic channels are visible. (b) Colour Doppler confirms that these are vessels with hepatopetal flow, typical of cavernous transformation. (c, d) A case of cavernous transformation of the extrahepatic portal vein (transversal view in epigastrium).

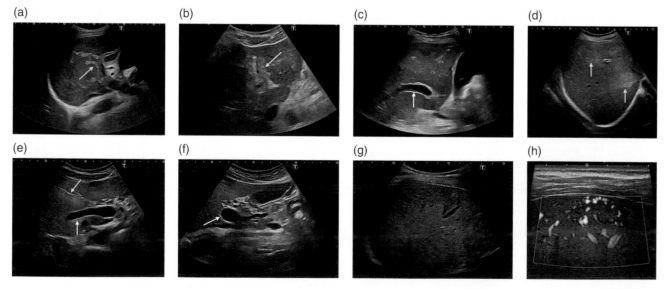

Figure 11.3 These images focus on the vascular changes occuring in the acute (a–d) and chronic phase (e–h) of a portal venous thrombotic event. Acute portal vein thrombosis of the anterior right branch and left branch of the portal vein (a, b yellow arrows). The posterior branch is patent (c, white arrow). Disperfusional changes can be seen within the right liver lobe as subtle ill-defined hyperechoic areas (d, yellow arrows). The second sequence of images shows the vascular changes occured in the right liver lobe at 3 months from the onset (e–h). The posterior right branch has maintained its patency (e, f white arrow), while the anterior branch is now a fibrotic remnant (e, yellow arrow) and proximal cavernous transformation has taken place (e, f red arrows). Note is made of the appearance of small intrahepatic shunts to bypass low perfusion areas (g, h). *Source:* Courtesy of Dr Matteo Rosselli.

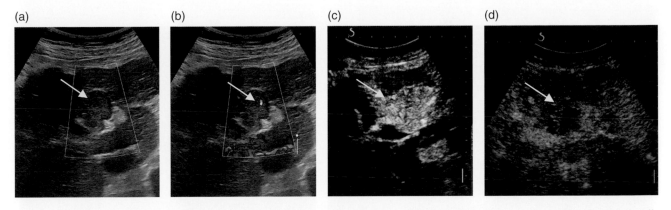

Figure 11.4 Neoplastic complete invasion of the left branch of the portal vein. (a) Note the expansive aspect and the disrupted walls, as well as (b) the presence of signs of arterial flow within the clot. (c) Contrast-enhanced ultrasound shows enhancement of the thrombus in the arterial phase and in continuity with a large tumour (not visible in B-mode) and (d) wash-out in the portal phase, further confirming neoplastic invasion of the portal vein and excluding bland thrombosis.

thrombosis and neoplastic vascular invasion should be considered, and macroscopic vascular invasion in patients with hepatocellular carcinoma (HCC) identifies an advanced stage of the disease, currently not suitable for curative treatment options [7]. On ultrasound, the following signs suggest neoplastic vascular invasion: expansive aspect (>2 cm) of the vessel, interruption of the walls, and presence of signs of arterial perfusion in the thrombus. The latter can sometimes be identified by colour Doppler and pulsed Doppler (arterial flow with high resistance index). The use of contrast-enhanced ultrasound (CEUS) improved the accuracy of ultrasound to diagnose neoplastic invasion of the portal vein, demonstrating wash-in in the arterial phase and wash-out in the late phase (usually quicker than the primary tumour) (Figure 11.4) [8].

- *Presence of portal biliopathy*: this is characterised by gallbladder and biliary duct abnormalities, leading to cholestasis due to the cavernous transformation [9]. While magnetic resonance cholangiopancreatography (MRCP) is the reference standard method to diagnose and stage this complication, the dilatation of biliary ducts can often be seen on ultrasound and should be reported.

Intrahepatic Non-cirrhotic Portal Hypertension

Porto-sinusoidal Vascular Disorder/Idiopathic Portal Hypertension

The term 'porto-sinusoidal vascular disorder' (PSVD) has been proposed recently [10] to designate a group of conditions that present histological alterations that involve the portal venules and/or sinusoids without the presence of cirrhosis. It may or may not be associated with portal hypertension. This term groups entities such as idiopathic portal hypertension, idiopathic portal fibrosis, obliterative portal venopathy, hepatoportal sclerosis, incomplete septal cirrhosis, and nodular regenerative hyperplasia (NRH). Specific causes of VLDs are not included in the term.

The pathogenesis of PSVD is unknown, but in around 50% of patients it is associated with haematological diseases, immunological disorders, drug exposure, abdominal infections, or congenital defects.

Doppler ultrasound is the first step in the imaging evaluation of PSVD, although there are no specific sonographic features that allow the diagnosis to be established. The most frequent findings are those secondary to portal hypertension: dilated spleno-portal axis, splenomegaly, and porto-systemic collaterals. Although the morphology of the liver can be normal, it is frequent to find architectural changes corresponding to a hypertrophy of the caudate lobe and segment IV, with atrophy of the right lobe. In advanced stages, the liver surface could become irregular and it can be indistinguishable from liver cirrhosis (Figure 11.5). It has been reported that the ultrasound contrast Sonazoid could be helpful in the differential diagnosis of both entities because PSVD shows delayed periportal enhancement [11], but more studies would be necessary to confirm this. Elastography may be helpful in differentiating the disease from cirrhosis [10]. The liver of patients with PSVD exhibits only slightly higher stiffness than healthy livers, but is significantly lower compared to cirrhotic patients. The spleen stiffness is high because of portal hypertension, thus the spleen/liver stiffness ratio increases [12]. Low liver stiffness in a patient with portal hypertension requires further testing to rule out PSVD.

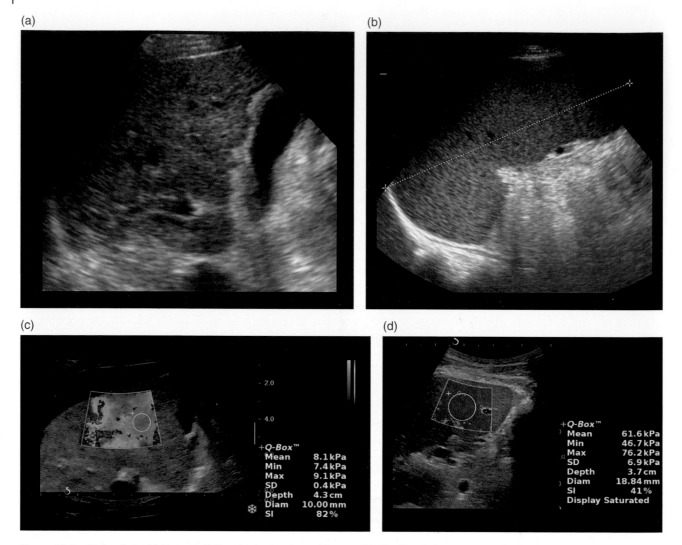

Figure 11.5 Porto-sinusoidal vascular disorder in an advanced stage. (a) The liver is heterogeneous with irregular surface mimicking a cirrhotic liver, and (b) the patient shows a massively enlarged spleen. (c) On 2D shear wave elastography liver stiffness is moderately increased and not compatible with cirrhosis (8.1 kPa), while (d) spleen stiffness is markedly increased (61.6 kPa), confirming portal hypertension (PH). The ratio between the two strongly suggests a non-cirrhotic cause of PH.

Sometimes changes related to periportal fibrosis are translated into thickening and increased echogenicity of the portal tracts. Moreover, the distal portal branches become thin and a sudden narrowing or cut-off of intrahepatic second- and third-degree portal vein branches ('withered tree appearance') could also be present [13].

The incidence of PVT in PSVD is higher than in cirrhosis [10]. Until now, a patent portal vein was a prerequisite in establishing the diagnosis of PSVD in order to prevent confusion with PVT-related findings, but this criterion impedes the diagnosis of primary PSVD with secondary thrombosis. In chronic thrombosis the development of cavernous transformation that could be associated with portal biliopathy is frequent. An increase of the arterial flow on Doppler studies has also been reported.

Occasionally, it is possible to see the hepatic veins running peripherally near the edge of the liver [13]. This is not a frequent finding, but it is strongly characteristic of the disease owing to peripheral parenchymal atrophy from the reduced portal venous blood supply.

As in other VLDs, there is an increased frequency of benign hepatocellular nodules, which are focal nodular hyperplasia (FNH)-like, although the incidence is lower than in Budd–Chiari syndrome (BCS). Usually these nodules are isoechoic and are frequently undetected on sonographic studies [13].

Sinusoidal Obstruction Syndrome

Sinusoidal obstruction syndrome (SOS) is caused by damage and detachment of the sinusoidal endothelial cells thus causing hepatic venous outflow obstruction and liver congestive injury, but the large hepatic veins remain patent [14]. It is a known complication after haematopoietic stem cell transplantation, but it has also been related to a large number of drugs and toxins.

The most frequent ultrasound findings are hepatomegaly and splenomegaly, thickened gallbladder wall and ascites [15, 16]. Reduced phasicity of hepatic venous flow and increased hepatic artery resistive indices have also been described [16]. A reduction of portal flow, and even reversal of portal flow in extreme cases, may be found as a consequence of the increase in sinusoidal pressure. Patchy liver enhancement after CEUS [15], in the same way as CT or MRI, has also been described, but all these imaging findings are non-specific and crucially, require correlation with an appropriate medical history and onset of clinical presentation in order to establish the diagnosis.

Similar to BCS, liver stiffness in SOS is elevated [15, 17]. Its reduction after treatment has been reported and the use of elastography has been proposed for follow-up.

Sinusoidal Dilatation and Peliosis Hepatis

Non-obstructive sinusoidal dilatation is not a totally understood condition [18]. It consists of sinusoidal dilatation, but in the absence of post-sinusoidal outflow block. The term peliosis has been used to describe the severe sinusoidal dilatation, but it is really a different condition characterised by lobular cystic blood lakes with rupture of the reticulin fibres, which are not found in sinusoidal dilatation [18, 19].

The entity is associated with acute inflammatory or infectious diseases such as inflammatory bowel diseases, rheumatoid arthritis, pyelonephritis, or cholecystitis. Toxic agents like oxaliplatin-based chemotherapy can also cause sinusoidal changes, including sinusoidal dilatation, peliosis, and SOS. The condition has also been associated with regular oral contraceptives or anabolic androgen steroids, but this has not been unequivocally demonstrated.

There are no specific ultrasonic features. Patients with sinusoidal dilatation or peliosis can be asymptomatic, but hepatomegaly and portal hypertension–related signs can also be found. Like SOS, a mosaic enhancement pattern has been described on CT or MRI [19, 20], thus it would be possible to have a similar finding with CEUS, although this has not been demonstrated.

Peliosis hepatis are rare lesions and are predominantly heterogeneously hypoechoic on B-mode. In one of the larger CEUS series of this condition, the lesions demonstrated hyperenhancement in the arterial phase and the majority showed mild washout in the portal venous and late phases [21].

Fontan-Associated Liver Disease

Fontan-associated liver disease (FALD) is a liver disease caused by haemodynamic changes following Fontan surgery [22]. The Fontan operation is corrective surgery for patients with single-ventricle physiology consisting of diverting the systemic venous return to the pulmonary arterial system [22]. FALD is the result of an increase in venous pressure with the consequent decrease in portal venous inflow, associated with an arterial hypoperfusion owing to the reduced cardiac output. It has been speculated that the continuous increase in the venous pressure associated with Fontan physiology provokes greater damage than the pulsatile increases that may occur in some valvular diseases [22]. The reduction of lymphatic drainage contributes to the sinusoidal dilatation.

Once again, the ultrasound findings are not specific for the disease. They are related to the congestive hepatopathy: hepatomegaly and portal hypertension signs such as splenomegaly, dilation of the portal vein, low portal flow, or increased resistance index of the hepatic artery [23]. These findings are associated with dilated hepatic veins and loss of the triphasic Doppler waveform secondary to the surgical procedure. Over time, fibrosis develops and the liver may become nodular and heterogeneous. The development of venous–venous communicants is also frequent [23].

Liver stiffness is generally increased, especially when fibrosis has developed, but elastography is unable to distinguish congestion from fibrosis [23]. Recent data from a multicentric study in Spain suggested that values of liver stiffness >21 kPa using vibration-controlled transient elastography are invariably associated with significant fibrosis on liver biopsy.

It could be clinically helpful to determine the trend of the stiffness over time; however, the results are divergent with respect to the change in elastography values.

The arterialisation of the hepatic blood flow increases the incidence of benign nodules that are similar to those of BCS. They are usually isoechoic or hypoechoic on B-mode ultrasound and they show uptake of contrast in the arterial phase. Considering that some case series of hepatocellular carcinoma have recently been reported, the differential diagnosis between benign and malignant lesions is a challenge, as happens in BCS. Currently, there is no consensus regarding surveillance of the hepatic nodules in these patients [24].

Budd–Chiari Syndrome

BCS is the obstruction of the hepatic venous outflow at the level of the hepatic veins or cava vein [25, 26]. The obstruction may be directly related to thrombosis or secondary to tumours, abscesses, parasitic diseases such as alveolar echinococcosis, or trauma. Ultrasound allows to identify the cause of obstruction in these secondary conditions. The primary form in Western countries is usually from thrombosis related to a thrombophilic disorder, but in Eastern countries it is more frequently secondary to a congenital membrane in the inferior vena cava (IVC) [2]. The diagnosis is made on the basis of the detection of thrombosis or the absence of flow in these vessels by imaging techniques. For this purpose, Doppler ultrasound is the first-line diagnostic technique, with a sensitivity of more than 75% [27].

Several ultrasound findings have been described, but they vary over the course of the disease [28].

Acute Budd–Chiari Syndrome

In acute BCS it is possible to detect a thrombus within the vein. Recent thrombus could be hyperechogenic, making it easy to diagnose on greyscale ultrasound. However, in the acute phase the thrombus is frequently hypoechoic, making its detection more complicated (Figure 11.6a,b). In these situations the diagnosis is established by proving the absence of hepatic venous flow with colour Doppler. If the diagnosis is

still unclear, CEUS yields even higher diagnostic accuracy to confirm or exclude the patency of the vessel (Figure 11.6c,d).

The acute obstruction of venous outflow provokes a parenchymal congestion that is reflected in hepatomegaly and heterogeneity with a smooth liver contour. Liver stiffness in this situation is very high despite the absence of fibrosis, which could be noticed with elastography.

In addition, the liver congestion increases the resistance to portal flow, thus manifesting as a reduction in velocity on Doppler studies. In severe cases, ascites may also be present.

Chronic Budd–Chiari Syndrome

Occasionally in the chronic form, the thrombus is still seen within the vein, but usually the vein is totally or partially replaced by a hyperechoic fibrous band or it vanishes completely. In this situation, the diagnosis is based on the non-visibility of a normal hepatic vein or normal IVC [29].

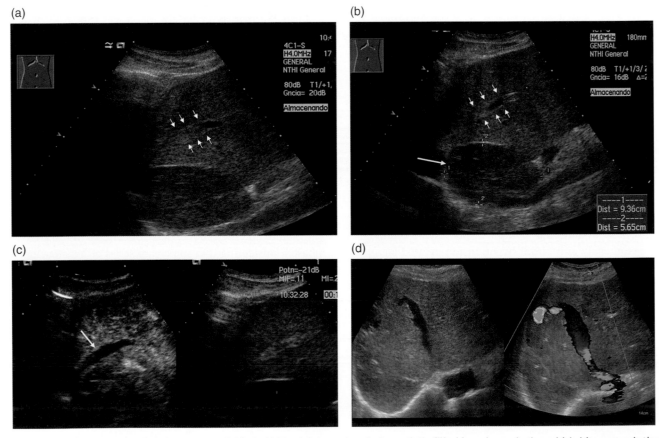

Figure 11.6 Acute Budd–Chiari syndrome (BCS). (a, b) The left hepatic vein is partially filled by echogenic thrombi (white arrows); the patient had a large hypertrophic caudate lobe (yellow arrow). (c) Contrast-enhanced ultrasound demonstrates that the thrombosis is complete (white arrow). (d) In some patients, large veno–venous collaterals form to allow an outflow; here the abnormal anatomy of the vein suggests a collateral secondary to BCS.

In order to improve the outflow, veno–venous collaterals develop over time in the majority of patients (Figures 11.7 and 11.8) [29]. Intrahepatic collateral veins shunt blood from the occluded to the non-occluded segment of the vein, to a non-occluded hepatic vein, or directly to the IVC. These newly formed vessels could follow a similar trajectory to the normal hepatic vein, but should not be confused with a patent vein. The presence of tortuous and multiple vessels instead of a normal hepatic vein should raise suspicion of BCS [29]. The syndrome must also be suspected when the flow within the hepatic vein is inverted, because this would suggest a distal obstruction of the vein and drainage via collaterals.

The development of sub-capsular and extrahepatic collaterals (azygos and hemiazygos pathway, abdominal wall, phrenic collaterals) are also frequent [29, 30], as are porto-systemic collaterals with the same distribution as in cirrhotic patients.

In chronic BCS, liver congestion diminishes and morphological changes appear. The edges become nodular, there is atrophy of segments not adequately drained, and hypertrophy of the caudate lobe is very frequent. In around 50% of patients this is accompanied by the presence of a caudate vein, which is one of the most specific indirect signs of the disease.

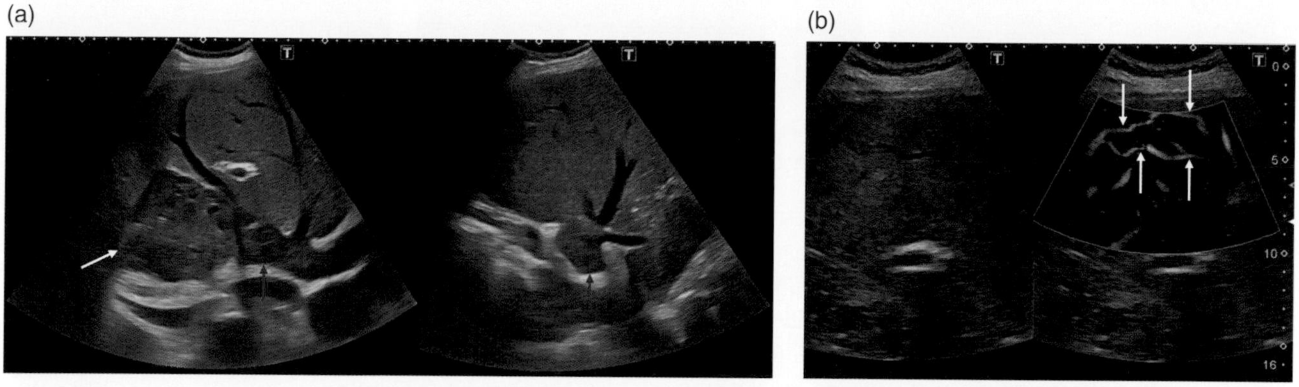

(a) (b)

Figure 11.7 There is a large lesion originating from the right adrenal gland (a, white arrow) with invasion of the IVC (red arrows) causing neoplastic Budd-Chiari syndrome. Note is made of the development of veno-venous shunts between the right and medium hepatic vein (b, white arrows). *Source:* Courtesy of Dr Matteo Rosselli.

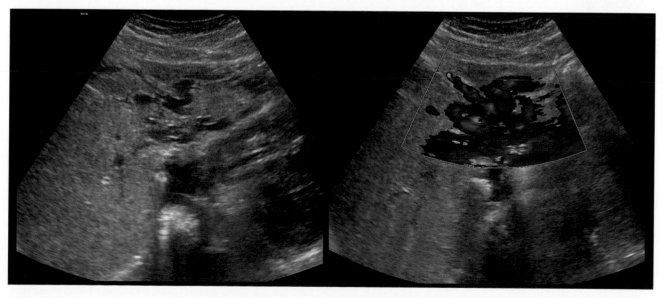

Figure 11.8 Intrahepatic collateral veins in a patient with chronic Budd-Chiari syndrome.

(a) (b) (c)

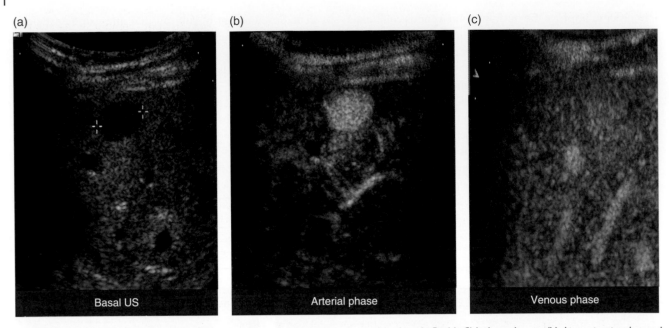

Basal US Arterial phase Venous phase

Figure 11.9 (a) Focal nodular hyperplasia–like liver nodule in a patient with chronic Budd–Chiari syndrome. (b) At contrast-enhanced ultrasound the lesion shows arterial hyperenhancement and (c) subsequent isoenhancement in the late vascular phase, with no wash-out.

The elevation of liver stiffness present in patients with BCS is related to liver congestion [31, 32] and may be a prognostic factor. However, it must be taken into account that interpreting elastography values may be problematic, because it is not possible to distinguish hepatic congestion from fibrosis. A reduction in stiffness after hepatic venous recanalisation has been reported, so elastography may be useful in monitoring patients' outcomes after treatment.

Vascular liver diseases are often associated with the development of benign FNH-like nodules, which are present in more than 50% of patients with established BCS [25, 33]. Frequently, the nodules are multiple and vary in size, from a few millimetres up to sizable lesions of several centimetres. The B-mode sonographic appearance are typically isoechoic, which is hard to differentiate from liver parenchyma, but may also be hypoechoic. On CEUS, the nodules often show arterial hyperenhancement with isoenhancement in the late vascular phase, with no wash-out (Figure 11.9). Occasionally, it is possible to see centrifugal replenishment, which helps to confirm the diagnosis. An increased incidence of HCC in patients with chronic BCS has been described, especially when the outflow obstruction is due to a congenital membrane within the IVC. It is less frequent in thrombosis of the hepatic vein, which is the commonest cause of BCS. It can be difficult to distinguish HCC from benign hypervascular nodules on ultrasound and also with other imaging modalities [33].

Vascular Malformations

Intrahepatic Aneurysms of the Hepatic Artery and Arteriovenous Fistulae

Aneurysms of the hepatic artery at the intrahepatic level are rare (20% of hepatic artery aneurysms) and mostly observed in the context of abnormalities of the connective tissue (Ehlers–Danlos syndrome; vasculitis such as panarteritis nodosa); more recently, long-term oral amphetamine intake has been suggested as a possible cause that should be investigated. On greyscale ultrasound, aneurysms are seen as well-defined, rounded anechoic masses and on Doppler sonography demonstrate arterial, pulsatile hepatopedal flow, which confirms the diagnosis.

Arteriovenous fistulae can occur between the hepatic artery and the portal venous system (arterio-portal fistula, APF) or between the hepatic artery and the hepatic vein system. APF are most of time secondary to trauma, malignant tumours (e.g. HCC), or iatrogenic causes (e.g. liver biopsy, surgery), and their relevance is mostly due to the possible occurrence of portal hypertension and its consequences. Importantly, large APF are a treatable cause of portal hypertension, and should be carefully excluded in patients devoid of other possible causes. On greyscale ultrasound, APF are usually rounded or oval-shaped anechoic focal lesions and on colour Doppler ultrasound they typically show a 'yin-yang' sign associated with spectral

Doppler changes such as high velocity, turbulent flow, with reversed flow direction in the portal vein branches close to the fistula. The reversal of flow in the portal venous system can be complete in large APFs and the portal venous flow shows an arterialised, pulsatile component.

Hereditary Haemorrhagic Telangiectasia (Rendu–Weber–Osler Disease)

Liver vascular malformations in hereditary haemorrhagic telangiectasia (HHT) occur between the liver veins and portal veins, between the hepatic artery and liver veins, and between the hepatic artery and portal vein. As a consequence, liver involvement in HHT [34] can lead to portal hypertension and its complications (gastrointestinal bleeding and ascites), high-output heart failure, intestinal and biliary ischaemia owing to a 'steal' phenomenon [35]. Ultrasound allows the identification and grading of liver involvement in patients with HHT and for their follow-up. On ultrasound, the first vessel showing changes in the early stages of liver involvement is the hepatic artery, which increases in size and shows increase in flow velocity and reduction of resistance and pulsatility index, owing to the decrease in vascular resistance opposed by the intrahepatic shunts (Figures 11.10 and 11.11). Later on, the intrahepatic artery becomes tortuous and can be as large as the portal vein. At this stage, small telangiectasias can be observed as subcapsular 'spots' of signal on colour Doppler, best detected with a high frequency probe. In the later stages, the portal vein and liver veins progressively dilate and signs of portal hypertension and subclinical or clinically evident heart failure can appear. At this stage, patients should be assessed for liver transplantation. Focal liver lesions, mostly FNHs, can be observed similarly to other VLDs.

Buscarini et al. proposed an ultrasound classification of liver involvement in HHT based on five stages, which parallels the clinical progression of the disease (Table 11.2) [36].

In the authors' opinion, CEUS can be used in selected cases to better characterise rare complications such as intrahepatic PVT or ischaemic biliary abscesses, which can occur in HHT.

Currently, there is no role for elastographic techniques in HHT.

Congenital Porto-systemic Shunts (Intra- and Extrahepatic)

Spontaneous/congenital porto-systemic shunts [37] can be identified on ultrasound as anechoic structures that on colour Doppler and spectral Doppler show venous hepatofugal flow (Figures 11.12 and 11.13). The most important form of congenital shunts corresponds to the so-called Abernethy malformation, which is a rare congenital disorder characterised by the presence of congenital extrahepatic porto-systemic (CEPS) communications, which can either occur in the absence of intrahepatic portal veins (type I: Ia if the superior mesenteric and splenic vein drain separately into the IVC; Ib if the superior mesenteric and splenic vein join into a common trunk that drains into the IVC); or in the presence of an intrahepatic portal vein (type II). The clinical spectrum varies from totally asymptomatic cases to mild hepatic dysfunction and hepatic encephalopathy owing to shunting. CEPS are usually identified in childhood during an ultrasound examination performed for other causes. In addition, ultrasound can help in the classification of CEPS (presence/absence of intrahepatic portal veins) and in screening for the presence of focal liver lesions. CEPS are in fact associated with a high prevalence of FNHs and adenomas, and are considered risk factors for the onset of HCC. Even if CEUS can be used to characterise focal liver lesions in patients with CEPS, the exact accuracy in this particular context is unknown.

(a)   (b)

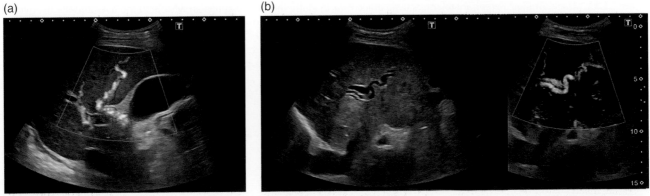

Figure 11.10 (a) Tortuous dilatation of the hepatic artery with (b) intrahepatic 'double channel' aspect in a patient with haemorrhagic hereditary telangiectasia and liver involvement. *Source:* Courtesy of Dr Matteo Rosselli.

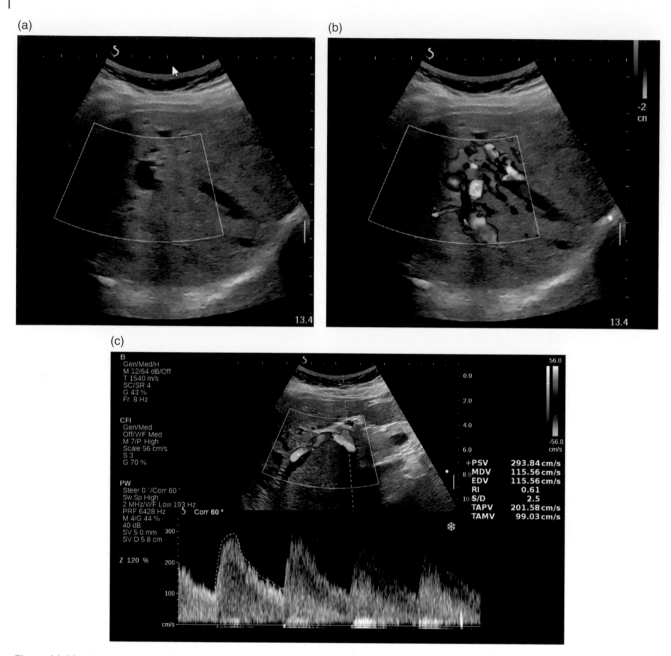

Figure 11.11 Haemorrhagic hereditary telangiectasia grade 3. (a, b) Multiple malformations are visible in the liver and the liver veins are dilated. (c) The hepatic artery is severely dilated and shows a peak systolic velocity of about 3 m/s.

Table 11.2 Ultrasound stages of hepatic involvement in hereditary haemorrhagic telangiectasia, according to Buscarini et al. [36].

Stage	Findings on ultrasound and Doppler ultrasound
0+	Common hepatic artery: • diameter 5–6 mm and/or • systolic peak velocity >80 cm/s and/or • resistance index <0.55 and/or • intrahepatic peripheral hypervascularity
1	Common hepatic artery: • diameter >6 mm and/or • systolic peak velocity >80 cm/s and/or • resistance index <0.55
2	Extrahepatic and intrahepatic dilatation of hepatic artery with 'double channel' aspect and • common hepatic artery with systolic peak velocity >80 cm/s • possibly associated with moderate flow abnormalities in hepatic artery and portal vein
3	Complex changes in hepatic artery and its branches (tortuous) with marked changes in flow associated with: • moderate dilation of hepatic veins and/or portal vein • and/or moderate flow abnormality in hepatic veins and/or portal vein
4	Decompensation of arteriovenous shunts with: • marked dilation of hepatic veins and/or portal vein • and/or marked flow abnormality in all vessels

(a) (b)

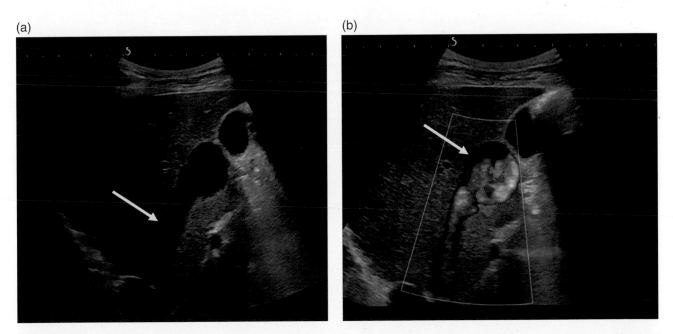

Figure 11.12 Large congenital intrahepatic porto-systemic shunt. Note (a) the dilated liver vein receiving the outflow from the shunt (arrow) and (b) the 'yin-yang' sign within the shunt (arrow).

(a)

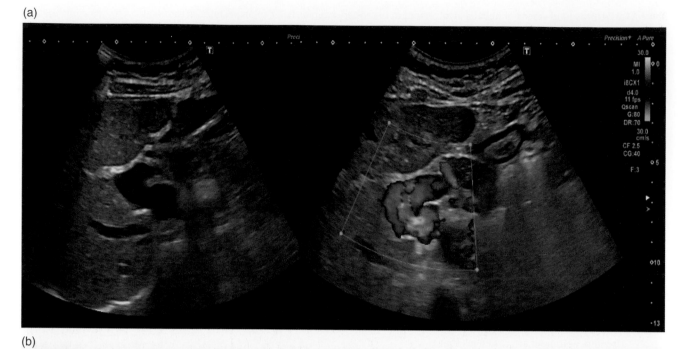

(b)

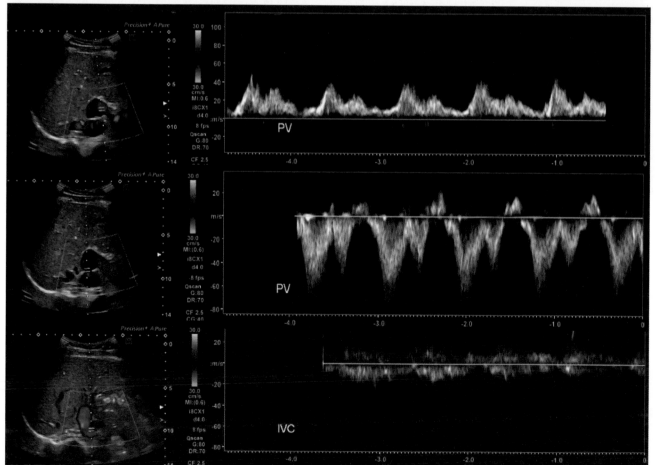

Figure 11.13   (a) Transverse image of a congenital shunt of the right branch of the portal vein (PV) draining into the inferior vena cava. (b) Doppler flow analysis shows the pronounced interference of the central venous pressure and heart flow usually seen in the hepatic veins, which is now observed in the PV as a result of this vascular malformation. *Source:* Courtesy of Prof Adrian K.P. Lim.

Acknowledgement

The two authors of this publication are members (MAGC full member; AB collaborative partner) of the European Reference Network for Hepatological Diseases (ERN RARE-LIVER).

References

1 Rodrigues, S.G., Maurer, M.H., Baumgartner, I. et al. (2018). Imaging and minimally invasive endovascular therapy in the management of portal vein thrombosis. *Abdom. Radiol.* 43: 1931–1946.

2 Hernandez-Gea, V., De Gottardi, A., Leebeek, F.W.G. et al. (2019). Current knowledge in pathophysiology and management of Budd-Chiari syndrome and non-cirrhotic non-tumoral splanchnic vein thrombosis. *J. Hepatol.* 71: 175–199.

3 Sarin, S.K., Philips, C.A., Kamath, P.S. et al. (2016). Toward a comprehensive new classification of portal vein thrombosis in patients with cirrhosis. *Gastroenterology* 151 (574–577): e573.

4 Berzigotti, A., Garcia-Criado, A., Darnell, A., and Garcia-Pagan, J.C. (2014). Imaging in clinical decision-making for portal vein thrombosis. *Nat. Rev. Gastroenterol. Hepatol.* 11: 308–316.

5 Berzigotti, A., Piscaglia, F., and EFSUMB Education and Professional Standards Committee (2012). Ultrasound in portal hypertension—part 2—and EFSUMB recommendations for the performance and reporting of ultrasound examinations in portal hypertension. *Ultraschall Med.* 33: 8–32. quiz 30-31.

6 Berzigotti, A., Seijo, S., Reverter, E., and Bosch, J. (2013). Assessing portal hypertension in liver diseases. *Expert Rev. Gastroenterol. Hepatol.* 7: 141–155.

7 Forner, A., Reig, M., and Bruix, J. (2018). Hepatocellular carcinoma. *Lancet* 391: 1301–1314.

8 Piscaglia, F., Gianstefani, A., Ravaioli, M. et al. (2010). Criteria for diagnosing benign portal vein thrombosis in the assessment of patients with cirrhosis and hepatocellular carcinoma for liver transplantation. *Liver Transpl.* 16: 658–667.

9 Llop, E., de Juan, C., Seijo, S. et al. (2011). Portal cholangiopathy: radiological classification and natural history. *Gut* 60: 853–860.

10 De Gottardi, A., Rautou, P.E., Schouten, J. et al. (2019). Porto-sinusoidal vascular disease: proposal and description of a novel entity. *Lancet Gastroenterol. Hepatol.* 4: 399–411.

11 Maruyama, H., Ishibashi, H., Takahashi, M. et al. (2009). Effect of signal intensity from the accumulated microbubbles in the liver for differentiation of idiopathic portal hypertension from liver cirrhosis. *Radiology* 252: 587–594.

12 Seijo, S., Reverter, E., Miquel, R. et al. (2012). Role of hepatic vein catheterisation and transient elastography in the diagnosis of idiopathic portal hypertension. *Dig. Liver Dis.* 44: 855–860.

13 Arora, A. and Sarin, S.K. (2015). Multimodality imaging of primary extrahepatic portal vein obstruction (EHPVO): what every radiologist should know. *Br. J. Radiol.* 88: 20150008.

14 Deleve, L.D. (2008). Sinusoidal obstruction syndrome. *Gastroenterol. Hepatol.* 4: 101–103.

15 Dietrich, C.F., Trenker, C., Fontanilla, T. et al. (2018). New ultrasound techniques challenge the diagnosis of sinusoidal obstruction syndrome. *Ultrasound Med. Biol.* 44: 2171–2182.

16 Lassau, N., Leclere, J., Auperin, A. et al. (1997). Hepatic veno-occlusive disease after myeloablative treatment and bone marrow transplantation: value of gray-scale and Doppler US in 100 patients. *Radiology* 204: 545–552.

17 Colecchia, A., Ravaioli, F., Sessa, M. et al. (2019). Liver stiffness measurement allows early diagnosis of veno-occlusive disease/sinusoidal obstruction syndrome in adult patients who undergo hematopoietic stem cell transplantation: results from a monocentric prospective study. *Biol. Blood Marrow Transplant.* 25: 995–1003.

18 Marzano, C., Cazals-Hatem, D., Rautou, P.E., and Valla, D.C. (2015). The significance of nonobstructive sinusoidal dilatation of the liver: Impaired portal perfusion or inflammatory reaction syndrome. *Hepatology* 62: 956–963.

19 Brancatelli, G., Furlan, A., Calandra, A., and Dioguardi Burgio, M. (2018). Hepatic sinusoidal dilatation. *Abdom. Radiol.* 43: 2011–2022.

20 Elsayes, K.M., Shaaban, A.M., Rothan, S.M. et al. (2017). A comprehensive approach to hepatic vascular disease. *Radiographics* 37: 813–836.

21 Dong, Y., Wang, W.P., Lim, A. et al. (2021). Ultrasound findings in Peliosis hepatis. *Ultrasonography* 40: 546–554.

22 Daniels, C.J., Bradley, E.A., Landzberg, M.J. et al. (2017). Fontan-associated liver disease: proceedings from the American College of Cardiology Stakeholders Meeting, October 1 to 2, 2015, Washington DC. *J. Am. Coll. Cardiol.* 70: 3173–3194.

23 Tellez, L., Rodriguez-Santiago, E., and Albillos, A. (2018). Fontan-associated liver disease: a review. *Ann. Hepatol.* 17: 192–204.

24 Rychik J, Atz AM, Celermajer DS, Deal BJ, Gatzoulis MA, Gewillig MH, Hsia TY, et al. Evaluation and management of the child and adult with Fontan circulation: a scientific statement from the American Heart Association. *Circulation* 2019;140:e234–e284.

25 Valla, D.C. (2003). The diagnosis and management of the Budd-Chiari syndrome: consensus and controversies. *Hepatology* 38: 793–803.

26 DeLeve, L.D., Valla, D.C., Garcia-Tsao, G., and American Association for the Study Liver Diseases (2009). Vascular disorders of the liver. *Hepatology* 49: 1729–1764.

27 European Association for the Study of the Liver (2016). EASL clinical practice guidelines: vascular diseases of the liver. *J. Hepatol.* 64: 179–202.

28 Bargallo, X., Gilabert, R., Nicolau, C. et al. (2006). Sonography of Budd-Chiari syndrome. *Am. J. Roentgenol.* 187: W33–W41.

29 Buckley, O., O' Brien, J., Snow, A. et al. (2007). Imaging of Budd-Chiari syndrome. *Eur. Radiol.* 17: 2071–2078.

30 Cura, M., Haskal, Z., and Lopera, J. (2009). Diagnostic and interventional radiology for Budd-Chiari syndrome. *Radiographics* 29: 669–681.

31 Dajti, E., Ravaioli, F., Colecchia, A. et al. (2019). Liver and spleen stiffness measurements for assessment of portal hypertension severity in patients with Budd Chiari syndrome. *Can. J. Gastroenterol. Hepatol.* 2019: 1673197.

32 Mukund, A., Pargewar, S.S., Desai, S.N. et al. (2017). Changes in liver congestion in patients with Budd-Chiari syndrome following endovascular interventions: assessment with transient elastography. *J. Vasc. Interv. Radiol.* 28: 683–687.

33 Van Wettere, M., Purcell, Y., Bruno, O. et al. (2019). Low specificity of washout to diagnose hepatocellular carcinoma in nodules showing arterial hyperenhancement in patients with Budd-Chiari syndrome. *J. Hepatol.* 70: 1123–1132.

34 Sabba, C. and Pompili, M. (2008). Review article: the hepatic manifestations of hereditary haemorrhagic telangiectasia. *Aliment. Pharmacol. Ther.* 28: 523–533.

35 Garcia-Tsao, G. (2007). Liver involvement in hereditary hemorrhagic telangiectasia (HHT). *J. Hepatol.* 46: 499–507.

36 Buscarini, E., Danesino, C., Olivieri, C. et al. (2004). Doppler ultrasonographic grading of hepatic vascular malformations in hereditary hemorrhagic telangiectasia – results of extensive screening. *Ultraschall Med.* 25: 348–355.

37 Alonso-Gamarra, E., Parron, M., Perez, A. et al. (2011). Clinical and radiologic manifestations of congenital extrahepatic portosystemic shunts: a comprehensive review. *Radiographics* 31: 707–722.

12

Point-of-Care Ultrasound in Liver Disease

Matteo Rosselli[1,2] and Robert de Knegt[3]

[1] *Department of Internal Medicine, San Giuseppe Hospital, USL Toscana Centro, Empoli, Italy*
[2] *Division of Medicine, Institute for Liver and Digestive Health, University College London, Royal Free Hospital, London, UK*
[3] *Department of Gastroenterology and Hepatology, Erasmus MC University Medical Centre, Rotterdam, The Netherlands*

Ultrasound is an imaging technique that has the great benefit of providing a dynamic image of anatomy, physiology, and pathology in real time. The extension of physical examination by directly correlating images with a patient's signs and symptoms [1] is called echoscopia, meaning literally 'to look into with the use of ultrasound' (Figure 12.1). This medical approach, known as point-of-care ultrasound (POCUS), was employed initially to detect free intraperitoneal fluid in multitrauma patients (focused assessment sonography of trauma or FAST) [2, 3]. With time POCUS has developed, proving to be a life-saving medical tool for clinicians through the stages of diagnosis, resuscitation, surgery, and post-operative critical care [4]. However, although it finds immediate applications in specialties such as emergency, acute, and intensive care medicine, it is clear that many medical fields can benefit from its use [1]. This chapter describes the technical aspects and practicalities of liver POCUS examination and its use in different clinical scenarios, such as in acute presentations of liver pathology, rapid assessment of chronic liver disease (CLD), post-procedural findings, and finally an overview of the importance of POCUS in the critically ill patient, highlighting the differences that might be found in cirrhosis.

In this chapter a lot of emphasis has been given to the ultrasound assessment of haemodynamic instability and respiratory failure, since both can be a cause and consequence of severe liver dysfunction and are thus important sequelae and findings to recognise and assimilate with the whole patient clinical scenario.

Basics of POCUS and Training Requirements

POCUS should provide information on the anatomical site that is the object of a clinical inquiry, as well as on the interactions between organs that are anatomically close and physiologically linked. It is a quick, problem-solving assessment tool for improving patient management in a timely manner. POCUS does not differ from 'regular' ultrasound, although it is more goal directed and driven by the most likely clinically diagnosis. As such, training for 'regular' and 'point-of-care' ultrasound should not be different. Most clinicians using POCUS as part of 'regular' sonography will have had full training according to the guidelines of national or international ultrasound societies. Changes in epidemiology or the occurrence of new diseases might attract those with 'regular' ultrasound experience to opt for POCUS or focused ultrasound. An important example today is the increasing use of ultrasound in patients with Covid-19 pulmonary disease [5]. However, at the present time scientific or professional societies do not offer POCUS training, since it is considered always embedded in general sonography. Selective POCUS training is currently only being offered by commercial institutions and mostly lacks accreditation, and it seems that those with POCUS experience only might be valuable in screening situations or when searching for a specific finding (e.g. screening for aortic aneurysms, free fluid in trauma patients, biliary obstruction in patients with jaundice), whereas in the clinical setting full training is to be preferred.

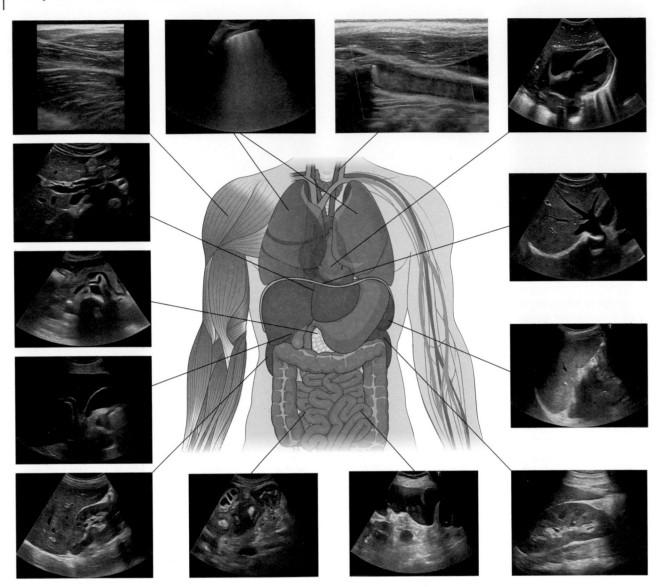

Figure 12.1 The ultrasound beam is able to penetrate by 'looking through' the superficial tissues, revealing deeper structures, organs, and eventually underlying pathological findings in real time.

POCUS Examination Technique

The general scanning technique should follow the standard operating procedure used to image the hepato-biliary system, the spleen, and the splanchnic circulation (Chapter 3). What changes is the approach and the clinical and physiopathological integration that comes with POCUS, including the haemodynamic as well as respiratory assessment, especially useful in clinically unstable patients. With regard to haemodynamic assessment, cardio-hepatic interactions are a cornerstone of POCUS

assessment. This is evident if one considers that the inferior vena cava (IVC) before terminating in the right atrium crosses the liver, receiving the blood drained from the hepatic veins. The examination technique requires the use of a curvilinear transducer or phase array transducer (usually used by cardiologists or intensive care physicians) that is placed just below the xiphoid process with a sagittal orientation, in order to obtain a longitudinal view of the left liver lobe and the retrohepatic IVC. Measurements are performed in B-mode or M-mode, approximately 2–3 cm from the atrio-caval junction. For completion a transverse subcostal approach will ensure visualisation of the hepatic veins draining into the IVC, and by tilting the probe upwards a more panoramic four-chamber view of the heart can be obtained. This approach is particularly useful when right heart dysfunction and a pericardial effusion need to be ruled out. In case of overlying bowel gas or when a certain pressure needs to be exerted with the risk of external IVC compression, it is preferable to use a coronal transhepatic approach by scanning the patient intercostally along the mid-axillary line (Figure 12.2) [6]. In normal individuals the absolute anteroposterior diameter of the IVC is 1.5–2.5 cm. During spontaneous breathing the IVC collapses in inspiration, because the negative intrathoracic pressure favours venous return [7]. The calibre and the respiratory collapsibility of the IVC have been shown to correlate with right atrium pressure and hence central venous pressure (CVP). As a general rule, an inspiratory collapse ≤50% of the maximal expiratory diameter is physiological; an IVC collapse at end inspiration >50%, especially in the case of normal or narrow IVC, correlates with low CVP; while a collapse <50% in the case of a wide IVC is associated with high atrial pressure and hence increased CVP (Figure 12.3) (Video 12.1) [6].

A detailed description of lung ultrasound scanning technique is beyond the scope of this text, which will rather refer to the interpretation of different sonographic patterns and clinical scenarios related to respiratory failure. The air–fluid interaction between the pleura and the lung parenchyma provides the necessary information to differentiate between pleural effusion, pulmonary oedema, interstitial as well as lobar pneumonia, and other pathological findings [8]. It is important to highlight that in order to assess lung pathology sonographically, at least part of the process causing respiratory failure must be in contact with the pleura. In fact, the interposition of ventilated lung between the ultrasound beam and an area of consolidation, for example, will cause an acoustic barrier, giving a false-negative result or underestimating the severity of an underlying condition. This is surely a limitation of lung ultrasound that should be kept in mind. Among the different findings of lung ultrasound the one we wish to highlight is related to B-lines as an expression of fluid that replaces air within the lung interstitium and eventually alveoli that can be an expression of fluid overload, but also inflammatory changes. B-lines are related to long laser-like hyperechoic lines that arise from the pleura and move sincroniously with the lung. The more fluid is accumulated withing the lung, regardless of its cause, the more confluent the B-lines will be.

In general, the assessment of a patient with respiratory failure should always include both lung fields, since monolateral and bilateral findings can have different pathological and diagnostic implications. In addition, the IVC calibre and its collapsibility should also be assessed, since the interpretation of 'cardio–respiratory' interaction has a high accuracy in distinguishing respiratory failure with high CVP from respiratory failure with low CVP, which has a completely different physiopathological background and clinical management. In this respect the differential diagnosis between cardiogenic pulmonary oedema and respiratory distress syndrome seen in sepsis is an excellent example of the importance of POCUS clinical application.

As a basic ultrasound scanning approach, basolateral lung fields can be evaluated by imaging the costophrenic recess, which is found by following the upper-posterolateral margins of both liver and spleen while the patient is lying in supine or lateral position. In normal conditions this space is dynamically covered by the 'lung curtain' related to the expansion of air-filled lung parenchyma (Figure 12.4) (Video 12.2). In the presence of pleural effusion, the fluid fills the costophrenic space and the lung parenchyma is compressed and displaced proportionally to the amount and nature of the effusion itself (Figures 12.5–12.7) (Video 12.3). To evaluate the extension of the pleural effusion as well as other findings such as lobar pneumonia, atelectasis, or interstitial involvement, the operator should continue scanning upwards until the higher postero-lateral lung fields are assessed. Although the posterior lung fields are better evaluated with the patient sitting up or in lateral position, an overdiaphragmatic lung consolidation/effusion can also be visualised by using a subcostal approach while the patient is supine. Due to the liver's larger size, this approach usually favours right-sided findings (Figures 12.6 and 12.7). The anterior lung fields should also be evaluated, especially in cases of pulmonary cardiogenic oedema, adult respiratory distress syndrome (ARDS), and suspected pneumothorax. Features of pneumonia include hepatisation of lung parenchyma in case of alveolar lobar pneumonia (Figure 12.8) (Video 12.4), while interstitial pneumonia is usually visualised as a combination of diffuse bilateral B-lines in conjunction with pleural irregularities and clear hypoechoic subpleuric areas of different sizes (Figure 12.9) (Video 12.5). A mixed pattern is characterised by signs of consolidation and diffuse thick B-lines, usually adjacent to the areas of alveolar involvement (Figure 12.10). Of note is that the sonographic appearance of lung disease,

(a)

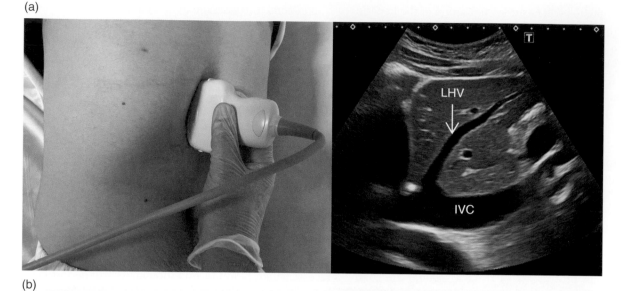

(b)

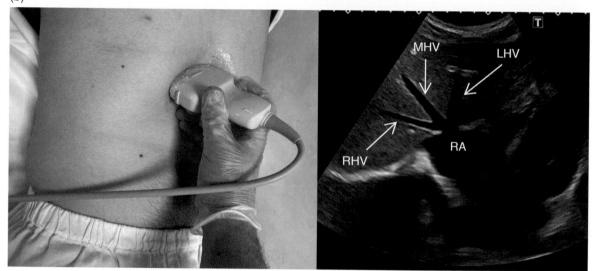

(c)

Figure 12.2 The retrohepatic inferior vena cava (IVC) crosses the liver, receiving the blood from the hepatic veins before terminating in the right atrium. The IVC can be visualised using a sagittal (a) or subcostal approach (b). The subcostal approach grants a more panoramic view of the three hepatic veins draining into the IVC. In addition, by tilting the probe upwards the IVC can be seen draining into the right atrium. In case of overlying bowel gas or other technical limitations, the IVC can be imaged by using an intercostal coronal approach (c). LHV, left hepatic vein; MHV, medium hepatic vein; RHV, right hepatic vein; RA, right atrium.

(a)

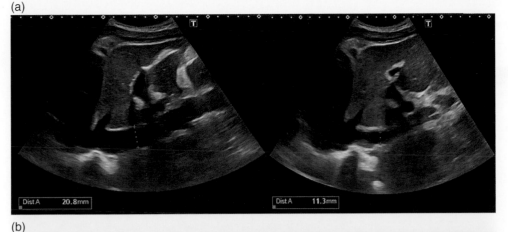

Dist A   20.8mm   Dist A   11.3mm

(b)

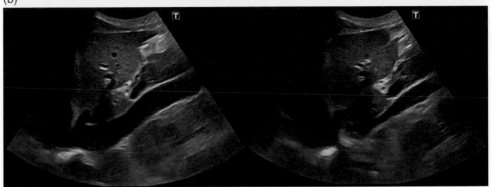

(c)

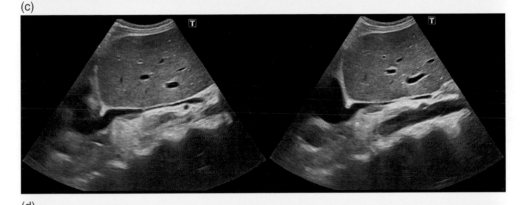

(d)

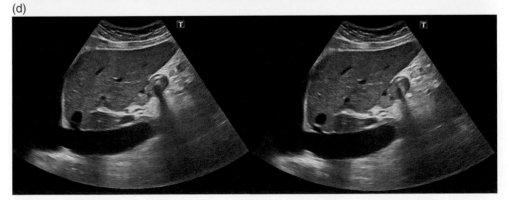

Figure 12.3 Although constitutional variability has been described, in normal conditions during respiration the inferior vena cava (IVC) has a diameter of approximately 1.5–2.5 cm, and its collapsibility is approximately 50%. A calibre <1.5 cm with a collapsibility >50% is associated with hypovolemia and low central venous pressure (CVP); a diameter >2.5 cm with a collapsibility <50% is an expression of increased CVP. Four pairs of images are explicatory examples. The left image of each pair represents the retrohepatic IVC calibre at the end of expiration, the right image the retrohepatic IVC calibre at the end of inspiration. (a) The IVC has a normal calibre of 20 mm and at end inspiration it is 11 mm, therefore showing a reduction in calibre of approximately 50%. (b) A similar case is shown where a normal IVC calibre is initially observed, with subsequent significant calibre reduction during inspiration. (c) The IVC is almost collapsed in both respiratory phases as a sign of severe hypovolemia. (d) The IVC is distended in both respiratory phases with no modification of its calibre during inspiration, in keeping with increased CVP that in this case was secondary to severe pulmonary hypertension (Video 12.1).

(a)

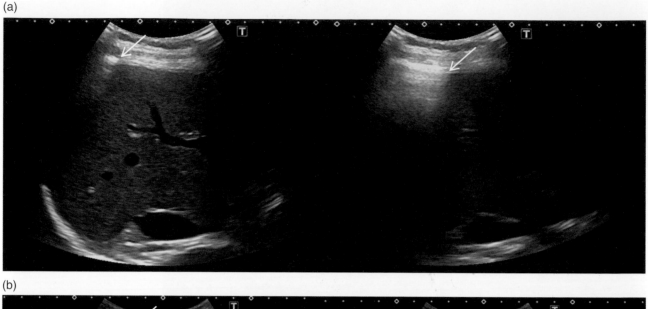

(b)

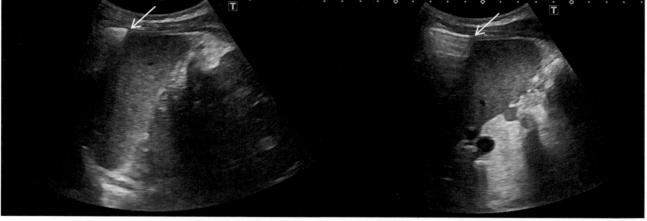

Figure 12.4 During inspiration the diaphragm lowers, allowing lung expansion. On ultrasound the normal ventilated lung parenchyma corresponds to a 'lung curtain' that dynamically fills the costophrenic recess during respiration. The white arrows point to the interface between the expanding ventilated lung and the liver (a) and spleen (b) parenchyma (Video 12.2).

(a)   (b)   (c)

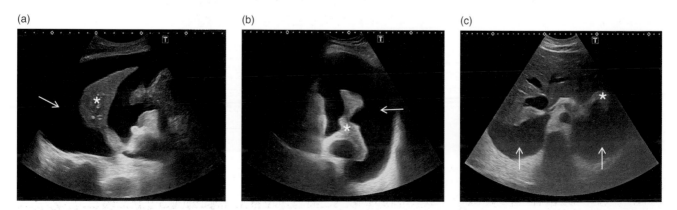

Figure 12.5 (a) Right pleural effusion (arrow) with complete atelectasis of the right lung base (asterisk). (b) Large left pleural effusion (arrow) with complete left lung collapse (asterisk). (c) Subcostal transverse view showing bilateral pleural effusion (arrows) and left lung base atelectasis (asterisk).

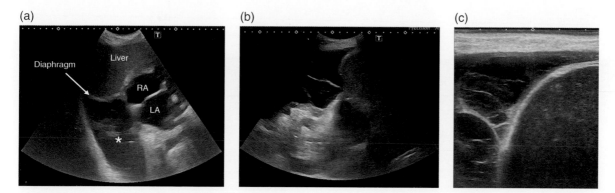

Figure 12.6 (a) Oblique transverse subcostal view showing a large right pleural effusion (asterisk), right and left atrium and liver. (b) Intercostal approach revealing septations within the effusion that are further confirmed at higher magnification with a linear transducer (c). Features in keeping with multiloculated pleural effusion caused by a Streptococcus pneumoniae infection. RA, right atrium; LA, left atrium.

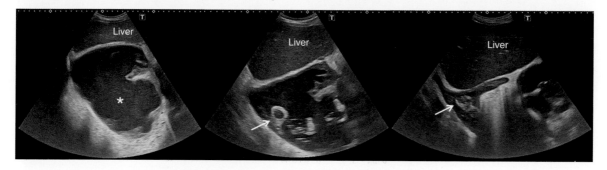

Figure 12.7 Subcostal transverse view revealing large echogenic right pleural effusion (asterisk). A 14 F pigtail drain was positioned (arrow), with progressive drainage of what appeared to be a large empyema. The sequence of images shows reduction of the effusion and decompression of the right liver lobe.

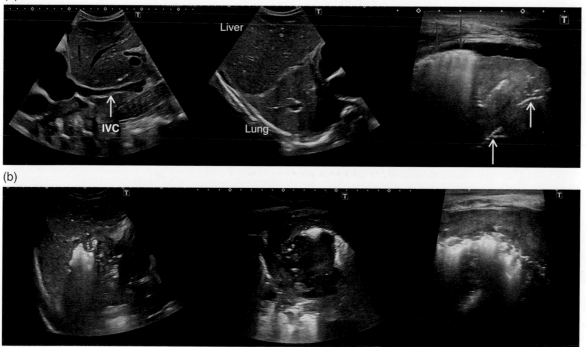

Figure 12.8 Patient with respiratory failure and sepsis. Point-of-care ultrasound reveals severe hypovolemia as demonstrated by a threaded IVC with complete collapse during inspiration (a, left side image). There are features of diffuse right lung hepatisation (a, middle image). Note is made of air bronchogram (a, right side image, white arrows) and interstitial involvement of the ventilated parenchyma (a, right side image, red arrows). There is evidence of air-fluid filled cavity within the lung compatible with lung abscess (b) (Video 12.4).

(a)

(b)

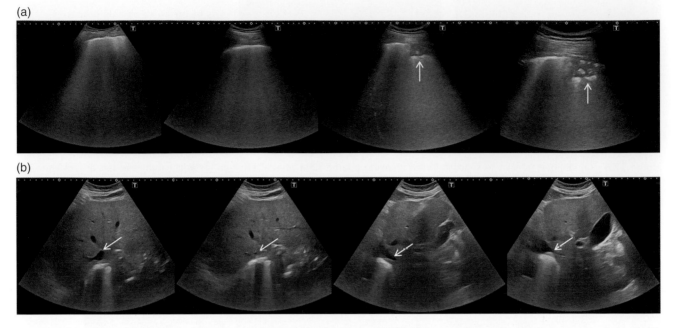

Figure 12.9   (a) Bilateral B-lines and sub-pleuric lung consolidation (arrow). (b) There is threading of the inferior vena cava (arrow) with complete collapse during inspiration. Findings in keeping with interstitial pneumonia and severe hypovolemia.

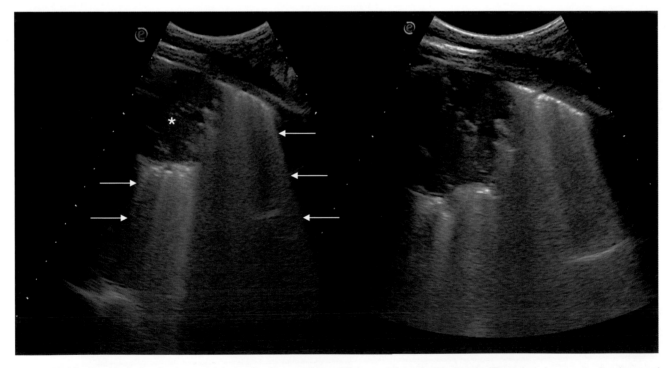

Figure 12.10   A mixed alveolar-interstitial pattern in a patient with severe fungal pneumonia. There is a large sub-pleuric round parenchymal consolidation (asterisk) surrounded by diffuse interstitial lung involvement (arrows).

especially in acute processes, may vary considerably during its development as well as in response to treatment, and this is why POCUS is such a useful tool due to its repeatability, cost-effectiveness, and no radiation exposure.

Confounding Factors and Co-existing Pathologies

It is important to bear in mind that one or more physiopathological conditions might co-exist, sometimes making ultrasound findings difficult to interpret unless appropriate integration of all the necessary information and organ interactions is considered.

Thoracic/Respiratory Factors

Since the change in size of the IVC depends on intrathoracic pressure variations, which occur during respiration, the magnitude of the respiratory effort represents a crucial but not quantifiable variable [9]. Regardless of the volaemic state, the respiratory effort might lead to collapse of the IVC in conditions of euvolaemia, while patients with superficial respiration might have poor IVC collapsibility even in cases of hypovolaemia.

Increased CVP as an expression of pulmonary hypertension is often found in chronic obstructive pulmonary disorder (COPD) and asthma, two conditions that are characterised by positive intrathoracic pressure, especially during expiratory exertion, making IVC-volaemic assessment not always reliable (see Video 12.6).

It is of note that during positive pressure ventilation the respiratory shifts of the IVC will be the opposite to those in spontaneous breathing.

Cardiac Factors

Right-sided heart failure, severe tricuspid regurgitation, pulmonary hypertension, cardiac tamponade, and constrictive pericarditis lead to IVC distension and thus a challenging haemodynamic/volaemic status assessment (Figures 12.11 and 12.12) (Videos 12.7–12.9). Table 12.1 summarises the sonographic findings of POCUS assessment in respiratory failure. Haemodynamic interactions are also considered.

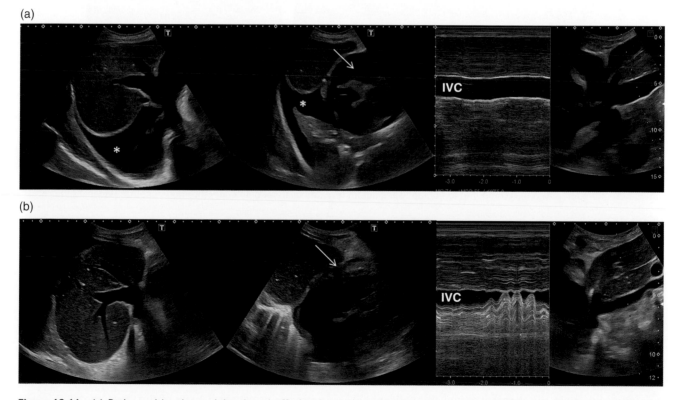

Figure 12.11 (a) Patient with a large right pleural effusion (asterisk) and tamponading pericardial effusion (white arrow). M-mode section of the inferior vena cava (IVC) shows no respiratory variation in keeping with increased central venous pressure (CVP). (b) Point-of-care ultrasound assessment after pericardial and pleural effusion drainage. There is persistent distension of the hepatic veins, the IVC is also distended at the end of expiration; however, it almost completely collapses during inspiration in keeping with significant decreased CVP. M-mode highlights the dynamic changes of the IVC calibre during respiration (red arrows). The arrow in (a) shows the pericardial space occupied by the effusion and collapse of the right heart cavities; the white arrow in (b) shows heart re-expansion after drainage of the pericardial effusion (Video 12.7).

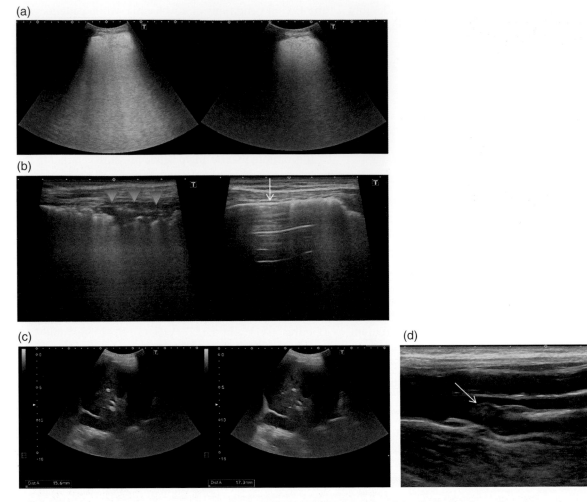

Figure 12.12 An example of the interference of confounding factors and the usefulness of extending point-of-care ultrasound examination in a patient with severe respiratory failure and sepsis. (a) Lung ultrasound shows bilateral thick and confluent B-lines ('white lung'). (b) At higher magnification with a linear transducer, there is evidence of interstitial consolidation (arrowheads) and skip areas of ventilated lung (arrow). (c) The inferior vena cava (IVC) assessed intercostally is distended, with a very small inspiratory shift suggesting increased central venous pressure, although the patient was hypotensive. Usually a lung ultrasound showing these features is compatible with septic interstitial involvement, but the IVC is usually reduced in calibre. (d) For completion, a Doppler ultrasound scan of the lower limbs was performed showing bilateral deep vein thrombosis of the femoral veins (arrow). The white arrow points to a thrombus at the level of the bifurcation of the femoral vein. A computed tomography angiogram revealed bilateral pulmonary thromboembolism (Video 12.9).

Abdominal Factors

Obesity, ileus, and tense ascites are causes of technical, constitutional, and physiopathological interference. Since the IVC is a retroperitoneal structure, in case of abdominal distension the operator might need to exert significant pressure, potentially influencing it's calibre; moreover, ileus might be associated with air-filled distended bowel loops with acoustic shadowing. Therefore under these conditions an intercostal coronal approach is recommended. However, it should be kept in mind that elevated intra-abdominal pressure leads to a complete loss of the relationship between IVC size, collapsibility, and fluid responsiveness. An important example can be seen in cirrhosis with tense ascites. In this case the IVC can have a variable calibre and can even be quite narrow, since often these patients are relatively hypovolaemic. However, minimal or no-calibre variations are seen during respiration due to both increased intra-abdominal pressure and reduced thoracic expansion secondary to diaphragmatic splinting (Figure 12.13) (Video 12.10) [10, 11]. In other circumstances upstream dilatation can be observed in IVC stenosis due to structural vascular or parenchymal abnormalities (Figure 12.14), or after interventional procedures such as in liver transplant, where the stenosis is usually at the site of the anastomosis. It is also possible that extrinsic IVC compression occurs, secondary to oedema of the graft, fluid collections, haematomas, or abscesses (Figure 12.15). In all these cases IVC calibre and collapsibility will not be a reliable index of CVP.

Table 12.1 Different causes of respiratory failure with lung sonographic pattern and inferior vena cava (IVC) appearance.

Respiratory failure	Ultrasound findings	IVC pattern
Cardiogenic pulmonary oedema	Bilateral lung diffuse continuous B-lines	Distended IVC Reduced IVC collapsibility
Adult respiratory distress syndrome (ARDS)/sepsis	Discontinuous bilateral B-lines with signs of scattered lung consolidation with interstitial involvement Ultrasound findings of septic source (e.g. liver abscess, infective colitis, pyelonephritis, pneumonia)	Collapsed or narrowed IVC
Lobar pneumonia	Monolateral or bilateral lung consolidation with air bronchogram	Usually narrowed IVC, unless pre-existing pulmonary hypertension or co-existing pathologies that increase central venous pressure (CVP)
Interstitial pneumonia	Usually bilateral B-lines with irregular distribution and sub-pleural lung consolidations	IVC calibre varies according to the presence of sepsis, hypovolaemia, or other underlying causes that interfere, increasing or decreasing CVP
Pulmonary embolism	Negative lung ultrasound or monolateral or bilateral small wedged sub-pleural hypoechoic areas or larger atelectasic lung areas surrounded by effusion Ultrasound findings of deep vein thrombosis have a high diagnostic positive predictive value for pulmonary embolism in case of suspicious clinical presentation and respiratory failure	Distended IVC as an expression of pulmonary hypertension
Pneumothorax	M-mode barcode sign, in the majority of cases monolateral	IVC calibre varies according to the extension of pneumothorax, respiratory rate, hypovolaemia, the presence of tension pneumothorax with reduced venous return, and increased CVP
Pleural effusion	Monolateral or bilateral: anechoic, echogenic, or multiloculated according to the nature of the pleural effusion (transudate, exudate, haemorrhagic, neoplastic, empyema) Adjacent lung parenchyma is usually collapsed and might present changes related to underlying pathology (e.g. infectious, neoplastic)	IVC might be narrow in case of hypovolaemia, but it also can be distended in case of congestive heart disease or co-existing pathologies associated with pulmonary hypertension such as chronic obstructive pulmonary disorder

Figure 12.13 Coronal view with M-mode evaluation of the inferior vena cava (IVC) in a patient with cirrhosis, tense ascites, and diaphragmatic splinting. The patient is severely intravascularly depleted, as shown by an IVC calibre of 8.3 mm, and there is tense ascites. Hypovolemia is responsible for the narrowed IVC. However, both increased intra-abdominal pressure and poor respiratory expansion (because of tense ascites) do not allow a significant respiratory IVC calibre shift (0.9 mm), thus influencing the evaluation of fluid responsiveness in this clinical scenario (Video 12.10).

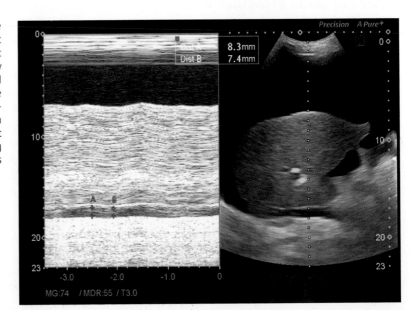

(a)

(b)

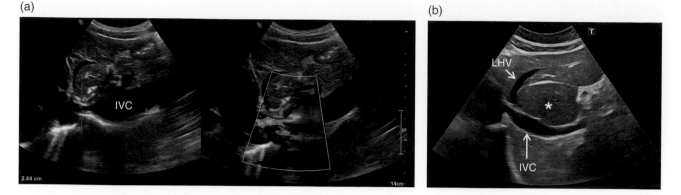

Figure 12.14 (a) Patient with periportal fibrosis and non-cirrhotic portal hypertension. The caudate lobe is small, but its anatomy is distorted, leading to a stenosis of the atrio-caval junction and upstream inferior vena cava (IVC) dilatation with turbulent flow, as revealed by colour aliasing. Although these findings initially raised concerns regarding outflow obstruction, there was no apparent liver impairment and flow in the hepatic veins was normal. (b) A patient with cirrhosis and large hypertrophy of the caudate lobe (asterisk) bulging against the retrohepatic IVC. In both cases, because of the influence of the distorted anatomy it is difficult to use the IVC as a surrogate marker of volume depletion, central venous pressure estimation, and fluid responsiveness. LHV, left hepatic vein.

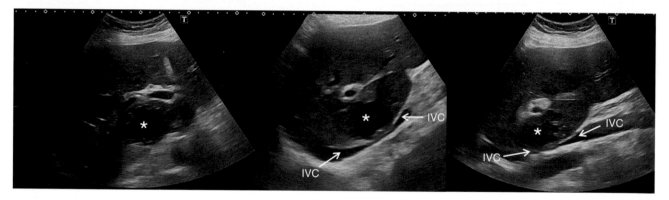

Figure 12.15 A large hypoechoic lesion known to be a hepatic abscess (asterisk) can be identified within the caudate lobe, bulging against and compressing the retrohepatic inferior vena cava (IVC).

POCUS in Acute Presentation of Liver Dysfunction

Acute presentation of liver dysfunction, elevated liver enzymes, and right upper quadrant pain in patients with no related past medical history includes a broad variety of pathological conditions ranging from diffuse and focal liver disease to biliary pathology and vascular disease. The presenting signs and symptoms as well as biochemistry help to narrow the differential diagnosis and guide the ultrasound examination. However, there might be situations in which no specific sonographic abnormality is able to justify the clinical or biochemical picture. Often these are situations in which there is a diffuse acute parenchymal process. Alternatively, biochemical abnormalities might precede anatomical changes and a repeat scan or second-level imaging might be warranted in the case of a first diagnostic discrepancy. In the presence of acutely

elevated liver enzymes with a cholestatic picture and jaundice with or without abdominal pain, the presence of biliary pathology must be ruled out [12]. Regardless of the underlying aetiology and excluding non-hepatic causes, jaundice can be roughly distinguished into obstructive and hepatocellular. The first question therefore will be related to the presence of biliary obstruction, including a rapid assessment of the gallbladder. The recognition of features compatible with cholecystitis should be followed by the description of its content, the integrity of the wall, and the presence of fluid collections (Videos 12.11 and 12.2). Indirect signs of perforation can be evaluated by the presence of intraperitoneal fluid, often with an organised/loculated appearance, which can be appreciated in the Morrison pouch, around the gallbladder, the liver, duodenum, the round and/or falciform ligament, or surrounding the spleen and accumulating in the pelvis (Figure 12.16). The presence of biliary duct obstruction leads to upstream dilatation (Figure 12.17). The site and underlying cause

(a)

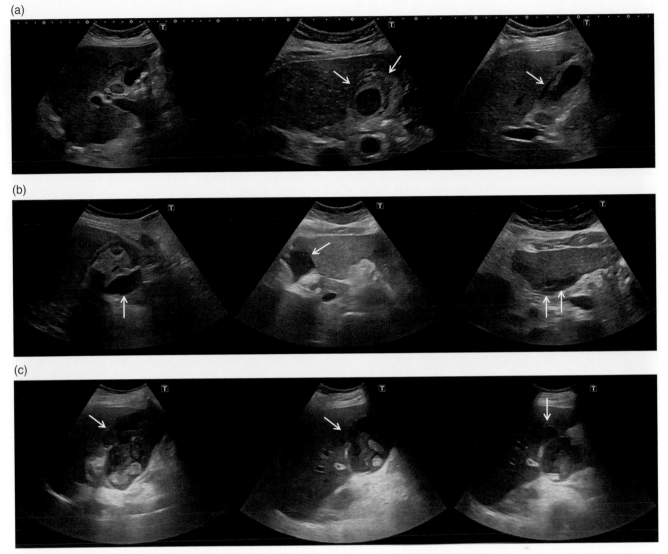

(b)

(c)

Figure 12.16 Three cases of cholecystitis are described. (a) Acute lithiasic cholecystitis (left image, red arrow) characterised by gallbladder (GB) wall thickening and a rim of fluid within the thickened wall (middle and right side image, arrows). (b) Another case of acute lithiasic cholecystitis with perihepatic loculated collections (arrows). On ultrasound there was no clear evidence of perforation, although the presence of fluid collection can be an indirect sign and in this context should yield immediate second-level imaging. Contrast-enhanced ultrasound and computed tomography scan showed features of gangrenous cholecystitis with GB wall perforation. (c) Gangrenous cholecystitis with clear discontinuation of the GB wall and adjacent collection (arrow) (Video 12.11).

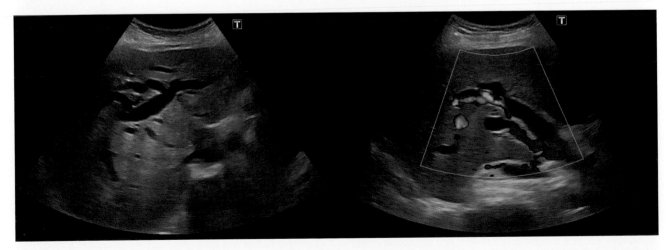

Figure 12.17 Patient admitted with painless jaundice. Point-of-care ultrasound immediately revealed pronounced and extensive dilatation of the whole biliary tree. No gallbladder pathology. Magnetic resonance cholangiopancreatography and endoscopic retrograde cholangiopancreatography revealed cholangiocarcinoma of the distal common bile duct.

can sometimes be identified by POCUS. Nevertheless in other cases, especially when the obstruction is proximal to the duodenum such as in choledocholithiasis, second-level imaging may be necessary for diagnostic completion, management planning, and follow-up. In the absence of any evidence of biliary obstruction and gallbladder pathology, the presence of jaundice associated with signs of liver injury is secondary to a diffuse hepatocellular involvement. In acute hepatitis ultrasound findings are generally non-specific and can range from a completely normal-looking liver to features that include slightly hypoechoic parenchyma, heterogeneous echotexture, and pseudo-cirrhotic appearance, when the

inflammatory process is so severe that it might lead to submassive/massive necrosis with a clinical picture that ranges from acute to subacute liver failure (Figures 12.18 and 12.19). It is of note that often in acute hepatitis reactive thickening of the gallbladder walls mimicking acute acalculous cholecystitis can be observed (Figure 12.20).

Patency of the hepatic vasculature should be part of the POCUS assessment checklist. Although rare, portal vein thrombosis and Budd–Chiari syndrome are both a cause of acute onset of abdominal pain and deranged liver function tests and can be easily diagnosed on POCUS (Figures 12.21–12.23) [13]. Moreover, ultrasound assessment not only is accurate but is very important in specific

(a)

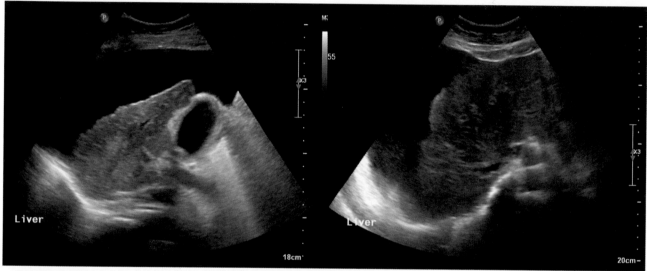

(b)

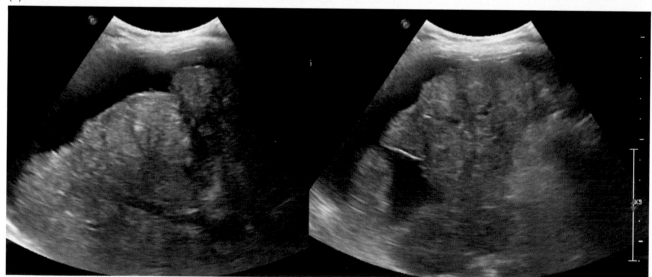

Figure 12.18 (a) Patient with rapid onset of malaise, jaundice, and abdominal distention. Point-of-care ultrasound revealed a shrunken liver with irregular outline and heterogeneous echotexture surrounded by abundant ascites. These features were highly suspicious of decompensated cirrhosis. However, clinical presentation and patient's history suggested an acute pathogenetic process. A transjugular liver biopsy showed sub-massive necrosis and sinusoidal collapse. This patient had severe drug-induced liver injury (DILI) leading to massive necrosis and subacute liver failure. The sonographic findings can be indistinguishable from advanced cirrhosis (see also Chapter 8). (b) Liver parenchymal distortion surrounded by abundant ascites in another patient with subacute liver failure secondary to severe DILI.

(a)

(b)

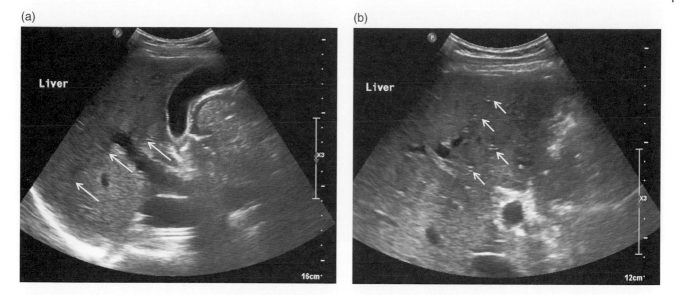

Figure 12.19 A case of acute liver failure secondary to autoimmune hepatitis. (a) The first liver ultrasound was negative, the patient was reassessed on the ward after one week from admission with bedside point-of-care ultrasound highlighting an ill-defined hypoechoic area (white arrows) demarcated from the rest of the liver parenchyma. This aspect is not pathognomonic, but integrated with the clinical presentation and rapid progression is in keeping with parenchymal inflammatory/necrotic changes, which were proven on liver biopsy. (b) Bright portal tracts stand out against the hypoechoic background (arrows).

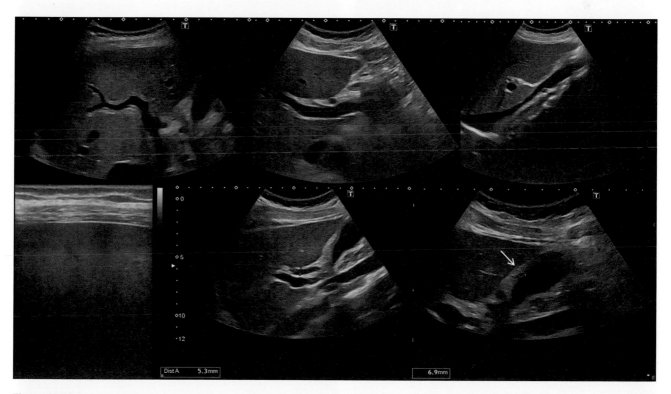

Figure 12.20 Patient with acute hepatitis B presenting with jaundice, malaise, and right upper quadrant pain. There is no parenchymal abnormality (the echotexture is homogeneous and the outline smooth) or bile duct dilatation (the common bile duct diameter is 5.3 mm). Of note is reactive gallbladder wall thickening (6.9 mm) that sometimes might be misinterpreted as acute acalculous cholecystitis (white arrow).

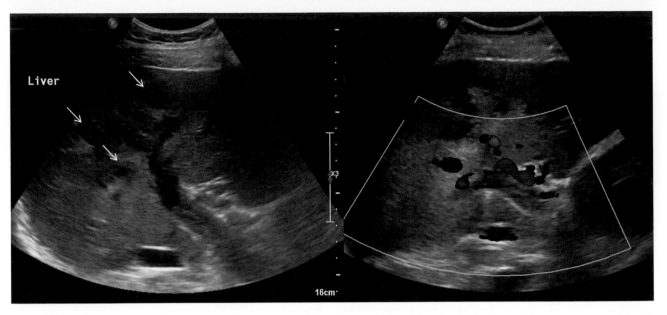

Figure 12.21 Liver point-of-care ultrasound in a patient with a five-day history of abdominal pain and fever revealed portal vein thrombosis and multiple hypoechoic lesions, suspicious of liver abscesses (white arrows). Colour Doppler confirmed the absence of flow in the portal vein. A computed tomography scan with contrast confirmed the diagnosis, highlighting a diverticular abscess of the descending colon as the cause of the sepsis and related pylephlebitis.

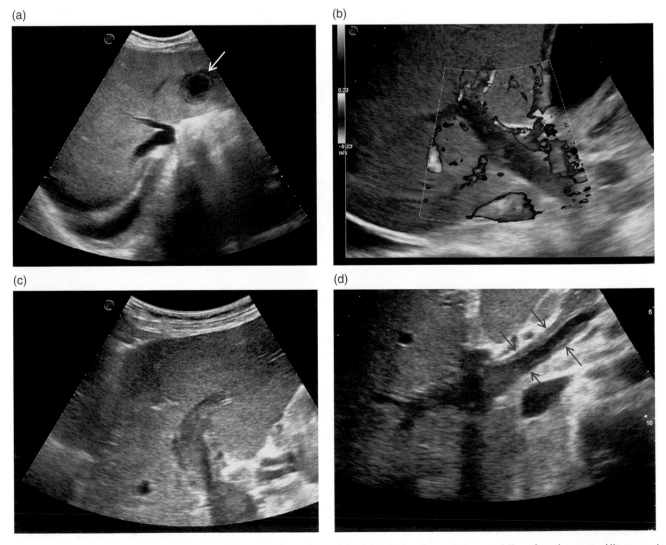

Figure 12.22 Liver point-of-care ultrasound in a septic patient with abdominal pain and abnormal liver function tests. Ultrasound revealed a hepatic abscsess (a, white arrow) and portal vein thrombosis (b–d). Second level imaging revealed features compatibile with pancreatitis and an infected pseudocyst as the source of infection/inflammation and cause of hepatic abscesses and portal vein thrombosis. Of note the pronounced thickening of the portal vein walls (d, red arrows) as a distinctive feature of thrombophlebitis.

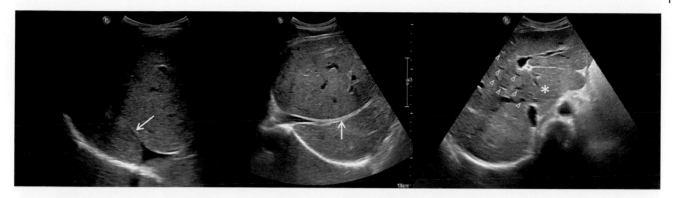

Figure 12.23 A 34-year-old woman who presented after three months of abdominal distension and discomfort. On point-of-care ultrasound hepatic veins were characterised by fibrotic remnants (arrows), the liver structure was grossly distorted and increased in volume, with a large caudate lobe (asterisk) and multiple serpiginous small venous–venous collaterals (arrowheads) scattered throughout the liver parenchyma. Features in keeping with Budd–Chiari syndrome.

categories of patients, such as pregnant or post-partum women who can be prone to thrombophilia [14]. Both portal vein thrombosis and Budd–Chiari syndrome can lead to acute liver ischaemia and liver failure or have a more indolent course. In the latter case variceal bleeding might be the consequence of severe non-cirrhotic portal hypertension in patients with portal vein thrombosis and cavernous transformation, while abdominal discomfort and ascites are more frequent in late presentation of Budd–Chiari syndrome.

Abdominal pain associated or not with jaundice or abnormal liver function tests can be related to the presence of liver lesions detectable with POCUS. Non-traumatic complications of focal liver lesions include different scenarios according to their nature, size, location, number, bleeding, and eventually infection [15]. The ultrasound assessment performed to integrate the clinical examination in an acute/emergency scenario may vary from finding a single and often large focal lesion with compression and invasion of the vascular structures, metastatic cancer, infected cysts, bleeding from benign or malignant focal liver lesions, as well as obstructive jaundice. Abdominal pain and elevated liver enzymes might be the first presentation of an unfortunate catastrophic diagnosis such as metastatic cancer or large multifocal hepatocellular carcinoma (HCC) (Figures 12.24 and 12.25). The presence of a liver lesion, particularly if sub-capsular, abdominal free fluid, haemoglobin drop, and hypotension should suggest active bleeding from the lesion (Figure 12.26) (Video 12.13). Solid focal lesions, especially HCC or large metastasis, might be complicated by an infection, especially when part of the lesion becomes necrotic. Necrosis/liquefaction is suspected on ultrasound by the appearance of a hypoechoic or anechoic area usually central to the lesion compatible with fluid component (Figure 12.27) that might be associated with the presence of gas, suggesting anaerobe gas-producing bacterial infection. Integration with laboratory analysis and clinical presentation as well as comparison with previous imaging are very important. Infection of simple liver cysts can present with fever, abdominal pain, and raised inflammatory markers. Infective complication might occur in a single large cyst or in the context of other pathologies such as polycystic liver disease or hydatid disease. On ultrasound, infected cysts may present with an echogenic content and debris. Simple cysts can develop multiple thin septations and loculations, which are a consequence of the proteinaceous content or intracystic bleeding associated with the development of an exudate (Figure 12.28). IVC compression, right atrium involvement, and clinical instability might occur as a consequence of a large hepatic cyst, more often found in polycystic liver disease. Cystic echinococcosis (Figure 12.29) can also cause outflow venous obstruction or biliary obstruction as well as rupture of a cyst within the biliary system. Solid benign or more often malignant lesions can also cause vascular compression, invasion, or biliary obstruction. In the latter case the lesion will compress the system, with upstream dilatation of the biliary ducts involved. The vessels might be compressed and displaced by the lesion. The presence of intravascular echogenic material adjacent to a lesion will instead suggest vascular invasion (Figure 12.30).

(a)

(b)

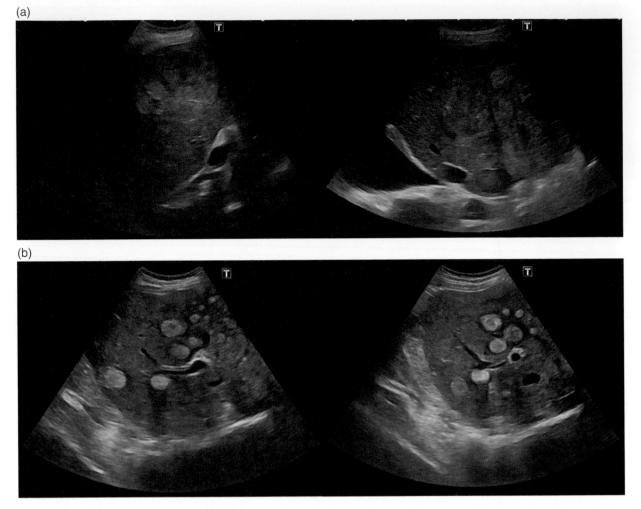

Figure 12.24 (a) Large focal liver lesion with satellite lesions in an 80-year-old woman with no previous history of chronic liver disease. Presenting symptoms were abdominal pain and distension together with mild transaminase increase. Alpha-fetoprotein of 8000 ng/mL together with imaging yielded a diagnosis of multifocal hepatocellular carcinoma. (b) A patient presenting with abdominal pain and weight loss, with ultrasound features of diffuse liver metastasis.

(a) (b) (c)

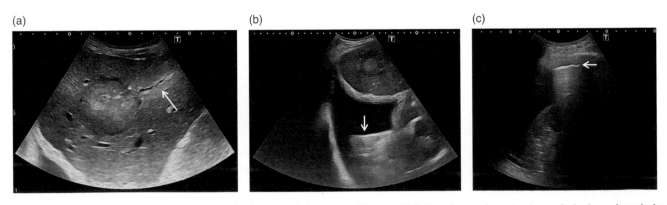

Figure 12.25 A patient admitted with abdominal pain and shortness of breath. (a) Point-of-care ultrasound revealed a large isoechoic right liver lobe lesion and signs of adjacent biliary duct dilatation (arrow). (b, c) A subcostal and intercostal scan view showed signs of right hydro-pneumothorax. The arrows point to the air–fluid interface within the hydropneumothorax. Second-level imaging revealed underlying lung cancer with liver metastasis, as confirmed by histology.

(a)

(b)

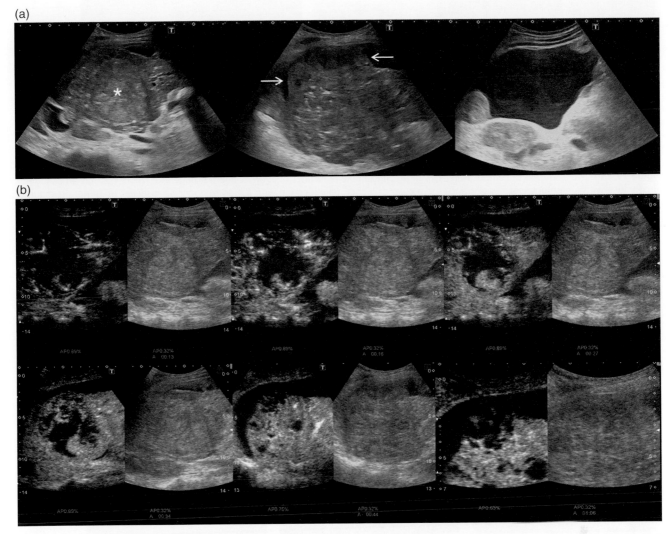

Figure 12.26 A patient with hepatitis C–related cirrhosis was admitted with liver failure and severe anaemia. The patient was severely jaundiced and encephalopathic, and there was no sign of gastrointestinal bleeding. (a) Point-of-care ultrasound showed features of known cirrhosis with a large right liver lobe lesion (asterisk). An ill-defined echogenic band can be seen between the liver capsule and the peritoneum (arrows). There is evidence of echogenic ascites with 'smoke' artefacts in the lower abdominal quadrants, a feature that is highly suspicious for intraperitoneal bleeding, especially in this clinical context (right side image). (b) Contrast-enhanced ultrasound (CEUS) was carried out showing inhomogeneous arterial enhancement of the lesion and ill-defined areas of non-enhancement, compatible with intralesional necrosis and parenchymal lacerations. Finally CEUS identified the site of rapture of the liver capsule (lower middle and right image) just below the intraperitoneal echogenic band, which corresponded to a large clot covering blood extravasation from the ruptured lesion (Video 12.13).

Figure 12.27 A large right lobe isoechoic lesion with a central ill-defined anechoic core containing debris. Findings are in keeping with central necrotic liquefaction of a large colorectal metastasis.

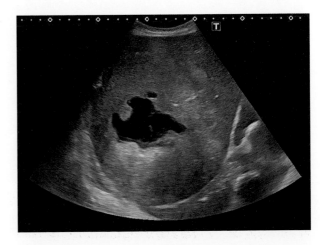

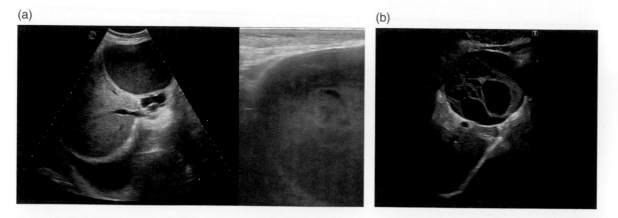

Figure 12.28 Two examples of complicated cysts. In (a) an example of intralesional cystic haemorrhage. The whole cyst has an echogenic appearance with a heterogeneous appearance more clear at higher magnification with a high frequency transducer. In (b) note is made of the presence of multiple intracystic septations as a consequence of superimposed infection as demonstrated by percutaneous aspiration.

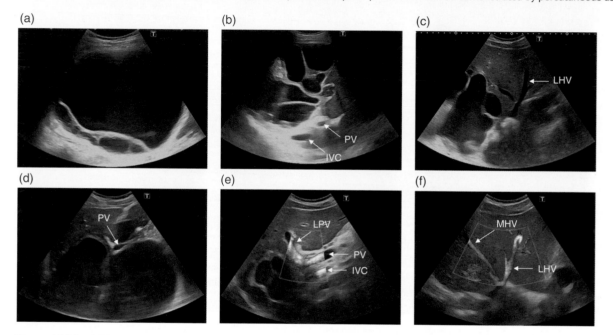

Figure 12.29 A 30-year-old man with abdominal distension and right upper quadrant tenderness. Point-of-care ultrasound revealed diffuse right liver lobe involvement of multiple large cysts with thickened walls compatible with extensive cystic echinococcosis (a–d). The right portal vein and hepatic vein were not visible because of their complete displacement (b–d). Left portal vein and left and medium hepatic vein were clearly visible, with good flow (c, e, f). Cystic echinococcosis can be a rare cause of secondary Budd–Chiari syndrome. Computed tomography scan revealed the patency of the hepatic vasculature and drainage into the inferior vena cava. Liver function tests were unremarkable. The patient was started on albendazole and elective surgery was scheduled.

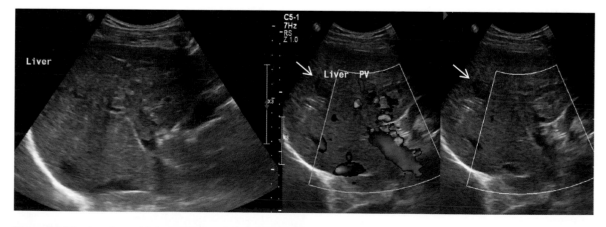

Figure 12.30 A patient with hepatitis B–related cirrhosis who complained of malaise, weight loss, and worsening liver function. Point-of-care ultrasound revealed an occluded portal vein with signs of sudden vascular amputation and the presence of a hypoechoic lesion (arrow), which was proven to be hepatocellular carcinoma with neoplastic vascular invasion.

Post-procedural Interventional Complications

POCUS is an excellent tool for rapidly evaluating patients who have undergone an interventional procedure and show signs of a possible complication, such as haemodynamic instability, anaemia, pain, or sepsis. The presence of post-procedural free abdominal fluid in a patient who has undergone a liver biopsy is compatible with intraperitoneal bleeding (Figure 12.31). Other biopsy-related complications are biliary leakage, intraparenchymal or sub-capsular haematoma, or arteriovenous fistula. Ultrasound is also very useful in post-surgical follow-up (Figures 12.32 and 12.33) (Video 12.14), infective post-interventional complications such as liver abscesses (Figure 12.34), or in case of biliary stent placement and follow up (See Chapter 6).

POCUS in Liver Trauma

Ultrasound has revolutionised the management of trauma patients thanks to its accuracy in detecting signs of haemorrhage in the peritoneum, pleural, and pericardial space [6]. Its use has been extended to evaluate the volaemic state and guide resuscitation, as well as exclude signs of pneumothorax and parenchymatous organ injuries. The sonographic appearance of liver injury can vary depending on the type and extent of the traumatic wound as well as on the time since the event. A large contusion can be recognised as an echogenic parenchymal heterogeneity in which lacerations appear as branching hypoechoic band-like areas. Alternatively it can also appear as an ill-defined subtle hyperechoic area, sometimes almost indistinguishable from the surrounding intact parenchyma [16]. Intraparenchymal haematomas, depending on the size, blood extravasation,

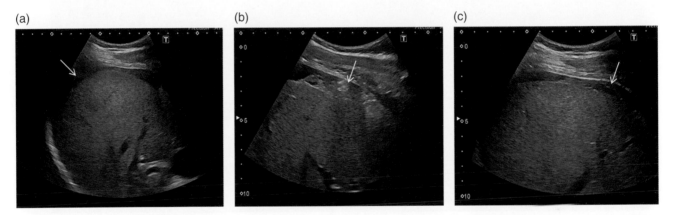

Figure 12.31 (a) Perihepatic fluid (arrow) seen shortly after a percutaneous liver biopsy is compatible with intraperitoneal bleeding. (b) Bedside follow-up showed the appearance of an echogenic heterogeneous layer between the liver capsule and the peritoneum (arrow), compatible with clotting. (c) Further follow-up showed reduction of the fluid and echogenic layer (arrow). Findings were confirmed by computed tomography scan with contrast. The patient remained haemodynamically stable with no significant blood loss, and had a spontaneous recovery with no need for intervention.

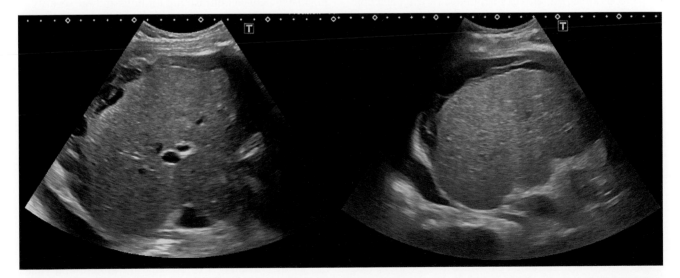

Figure 12.32 Post-surgical follow up in a patient who underwent laparotomy for bowel perforation. Point-of-care ultrasound reveals loculated fluid surrounding the liver as a consequence of intraperitoneal bleeding.

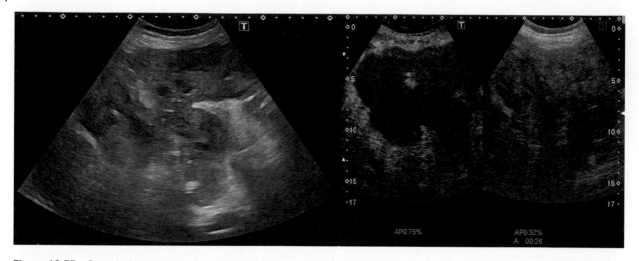

Figure 12.33 Post-cholecystectomy large haemorrhagic collection. Contrast-enhanced ultrasound allows to better define the large extrahepatic collection (right side) (Video 12.14).

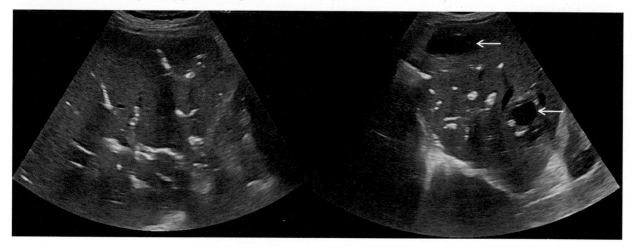

Figure 12.34 Liver point-of-care ultrasound in a patient who developed severe sepsis post endoscopic retrograde cholangiopancreatography reveals aerobilia and two right liver lobe hypoechoic fluid-filled focal lesions, compatible with hepatic abscesses (arrows).

and pooling, can appear as hypoechoic, anechoic, or heterogeneous areas, sometimes surrounded by a hyperechoic subtle ill-defined halo. Sub-capsular haematomas can be visualised as a hypoechoic, anechoic, hyperechoic, or heterogeneous rim around the liver parenchyma depending on the chronicity of the haemorrhage. The size of the haematoma can range from a few millimetres to a significant size, large enough to displace the hepatic parenchyma (Figure 12.35). Although the presence of these signs is highly specific in this clinical context, B-mode ultrasound accuracy is low for hepatic injuries and solid organ injuries in general [17, 18]. In fact, a negative ultrasound scan is not infrequent, since deep organs and sub-diaphragmatic injuries are difficult to assess. In addition, the sonographic aspect of early post-traumatic injuries can be subtle or overlooked, considering that the first assessment might be carried out with limited time contemporarily with life-saving procedures. In trauma patients the presence of free abdominal fluid, even in the absence of ultrasound signs of parenchymal abnormalities, is always compatible

with blood extravasation. Therefore, due to the possible mismatch between ultrasound findings and the severity of traumatic injuries, computed tomography (CT) scan with contrast should always follow for grading purposes and follow-up, since management can require surgery or embolisation.

Ultrasound has an even more important role at a later stage in apparently stable patients who are moved to the ward, where they undergo a careful clinical, biochemical, and sonographic follow-up. The purpose of ultrasound in this phase is to highlight the appearance of free fluid or its increase, to focus on the areas of injuries initially identified and defined by CT scan, and to exclude complications that might occur in a second phase, such as infection of post-traumatic collection or pseudoaneurysms requiring embolisation. The follow-up of trauma patients surely benefits from contrast-enhanced ultrasound (CEUS), which has all the advantages of portable ultrasound and yields similar results to contrast CT (Figures 12.36–12.38) (Videos 12.15 and 12.16) [19].

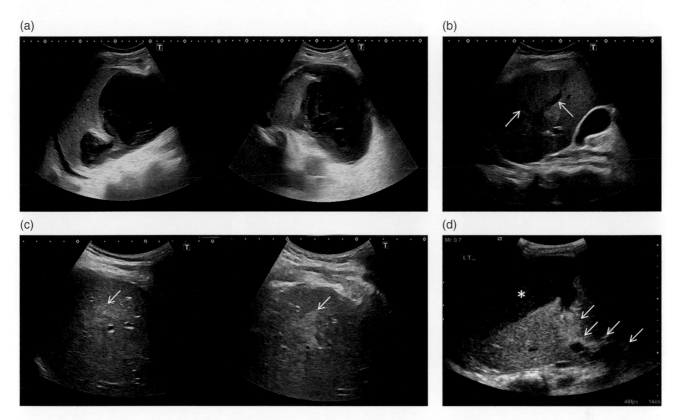

Figure 12.35 (a) Large intraparenchymal haematoma. (b) Liver contusion with lacerations defined by hypoechoic band-like irregularities (arrows). (c) Liver contusion with subtle intraparenchymal haemorrhage (arrows). (d) A case of hepatic laceration and large subcapsular haematoma. In this case the line of laceration is seen on ultrasound as a thick, ill-defined hyperechoic line (arrows) that runs across the liver parenchyma. Note is made of an anterior large subcapsular haematoma with a hypoechoic heterogeneous appearance asterisk). *Source:* Courtesy of Dr Annamaria Deganello.

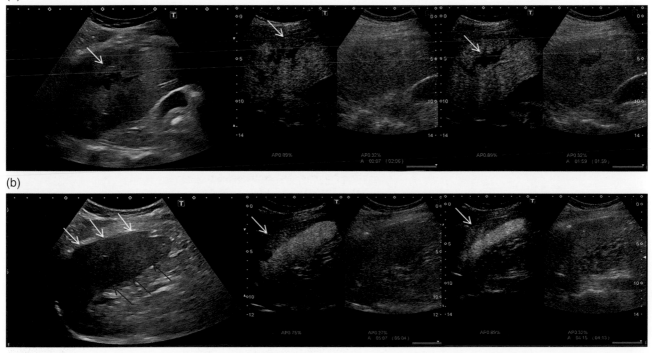

Figure 12.36 (a) On B-mode ultrasound an ill-defined heterogenic area is compatible with liver contusion as a consequence of blunt abdominal trauma (arrow) (Video 12.15). Contrast-enhanced ultrasound (CEUS) clearly defines liver parenchymal lacerations within the area of contusion as hypo-unenhancing areas (arrows). (b) Anterior to the spleen a subtle crescent area can be seen on B-mode suspicious for sub-capsular haematoma (white arrows point to the crescent area, while red arrows point to the spleen). CEUS shows enhancement of the area, which is compatible with an elongated left liver lobe, in keeping with an anatomical variant 'sliver liver' (see Chapter 3).

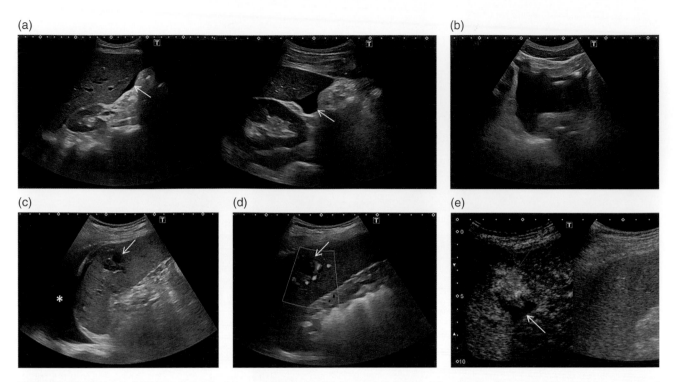

Figure 12.37 Patient with blunt abdominal trauma. Point-of-care-ultrasound detected free intraperitoneal fluid in the Morrison pouch (a, arrows) and in the pelvis (b). (c) There is an ill-defined heterogeneous hypoechoic area within the spleen, and presence of perisplenic fluid (red arrow) as well as a left pleural effusion (asterisk). (d) On colour Doppler the signal is highly suspicious for a splenic pseudoaneurysm. (e) Contrast enhanced ultrasound confirmed the diagnosis showing rapid arterial hyperenhancement of the suspected post-traumatic vascular complication (red arrow) and an adjacent unenhancing area compatibile with parenchymal laceration (white arrow).

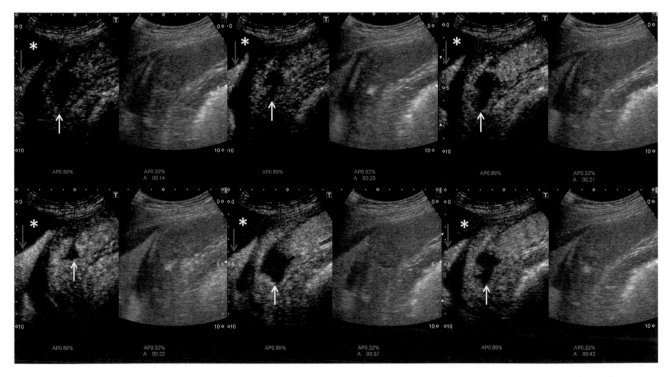

Figure 12.38 Contrast-enhanced ultrasound is repeated after embolisation of the pseudoaneurysm. The resulting infarcted areas are seen as unenhancing splenic areas (white arrows). An elongated left liver lobe can be seen surrounding the spleen (red arrows). Note is made of left pleural effusion (asterisk) and atelectasic left lung base (blue arrows) (Video 12.16).

POCUS in Cirrhosis

POCUS in cirrhosis has the objective of identifying specific hallmarks of advanced CLD. Heterogeneous echotexture and coarse echopattern are expressions of the architectural distortion that occurs as a consequence of collagen deposition and nodular regeneration, which makes the liver outline irregular and sometimes grossly nodular. The right liver lobe is often hypotrophic, with compensatory hypertrophy of the left and caudate lobes. The sonographic sequelae of clinically significant portal hypertension that can be assessed easily with POCUS are splenomegaly, ascites, the presence of portal venous flow inversion, and/or porto-systemic collateral shunts (recanalisation of umbilical and/or paraumbilical veins, splenorenal shunts, paracolic shunts; Table 12.2 and Figure 12.39). There are some considerations that require further attention and a more thorough evaluation that go beyond a rapid POCUS assessment, and these are discussed in Chapter 8.

Table 12.2 Ultrasound signs of cirrhosis and clinically significant portal hypertension.

Parenchyma	Portal hypertension
Heterogenic echotexture	Splenomegaly
Irregular/nodular outline	Ascites
Caudate lobe hypertrophy	Increased portal vein calibre
	Porto-systemic shunts/portal venous flow inversion

POCUS in Cirrhosis and Worsening Liver Function

Hepatic dysfunction in cirrhosis might occur as a consequence of the progression of its natural history, or it might be triggered by a specific cause that leads to a sudden and sometimes unexpected functional decline. A rapid assessment including blood tests, clinical examination, and ultrasound is the first-line diagnostic approach. Keeping in mind that often causes such as toxins, drugs, dehydration, nutrition, and bleeding can be responsible for tipping the edge of a precarious balance, POCUS assessment is aimed at identifying hepatic as well as extrahepatic/indirect causes (Table 12.3).

Table 12.3 Hepatic and extrahepatic causes that should be excluded with point-of-care ultrasound in a patient with cirrhosis and worsening liver function.

Hepatic causes	Extrahepatic causes
Biliary obstruction, cholecystitis	Infections
Liver abscesses	Urinary outflow obstruction
Neoplasia (especially hepatocellular carcinoma–related parenchymal extension with biliary obstruction or vascular invasion)	Heart failure (left heart failure, congestive heart disease)
	Respiratory failure
	Renal failure
Portal vein thrombosis	
Ascites; hepatorenal syndrome; spontaneous bacterial peritonitis	

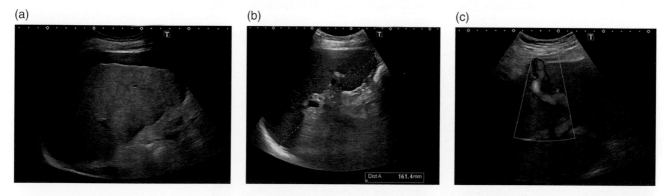

(a) (b) (c)

Figure 12.39 Obvious ultrasound features of cirrhosis complicated by clinically significant portal hypertension: (a) heterogenic echotexture, irregular outline, and ascites; (b) splenomegaly; (c) recanalisation of the umbilical vein.

POCUS in these scenarios is used with a two-step approach: investigation of the underlying pathophysiological process and identification of its direct cause [20, 21].

Distributive shock found in sepsis is typically associated with reduced CVP, correlating with a narrowed and hypercollapsible IVC [22]. POCUS will need to rule out intrahepatic causes such as cholecystitis, biliary obstruction with or without cholangitis, or hepatic abscesses

(Figures 12.40 and 12.41) (Video 12.17). In the case of hypovolemic shock due to intraperitoneal bleeding, the abdominal free fluid is usually visualised on ultrasound as echogenic with a 'smoke-like' appearance (Figure 12.26). It may be very difficult to ascertain the cause of active bleeding on ultrasound unless the source is a parenchymal organs such as liver (Figure 12.26), spleen (Figure 12.37) or kidneys. Nevertheless these are always conditions that

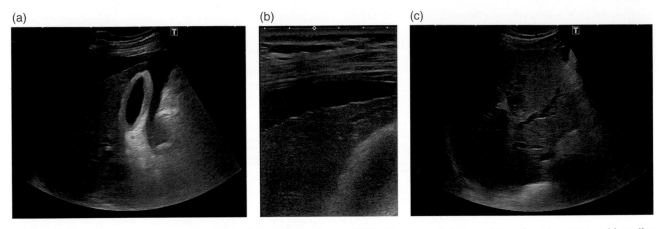

Figure 12.40 A 71-year-old man with advanced liver disease was admitted because of abnormal liver function tests and jaundice. (a, b) Point-of-care ultrasound showed features in keeping with cirrhosis (irregular outline, heterogeneous echotexture, ascites, thickened gallbladder wall) and (c) biliary duct dilatation. Magnetic resonance imaging with contrast revealed findings suspicious for cholangiocarcinoma.

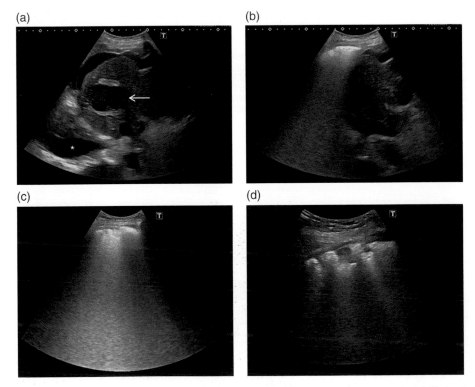

Figure 12.41 A patient with cirrhosis and multiorgan failure secondary to sepsis. (a) Cirrhotic-looking liver surrounded by ascites and a large right lobe hypoechoic lesion corresponding to a hepatic abscess (arrow). Note is made of a right pleural effusion (asterisk). (b, c) Inflammatory lung interstitial involvement, as proven by diffuse confluent B-lines. (d) Note is made of multiple small sub-pleural consolidations (Video 12.17).

need CT imaging with contrast for completion. Otherwise loculations can be seen as a consequence of fibrin deposition, although this is usually found in the subacute phase of bleeding (Figure 12.32). Haematic collections can be seen as heterogeneous, ill-defined areas (Figure 12.33). In the presence of gastroesophageal variceal bleeding ultrasound is useful to rule out the presence of portal vein thrombosis in cirrhosis as a trigger for worsening portal hypertension, haemorrhage, and worsening liver function overall (Figure 12.42) (Video 12.18).

Extrahepatic causes can generally be related to infections complicated by sepsis, respiratory failure with hypoxaemia, and haemodynamic instability with liver ischaemia. All these processes can lead to liver injury with synthetic dysfunction even in a healthy liver, although a fibrotic or a cirrhotic liver, especially if complicated by clinically significant portal hypertension, is surely more prone to damage and functional impairment.

Extrahepatic causes of sepsis should exclude pneumonia, empyema, pyelonephritis with or without urinary tract obstruction, endocarditis, or soft tissue infection (Figures 12.43 and 12.44) (Videos 12.19 and 12.20), as well as the presence of bowel obstruction and severe infective/ischaemic enterocolitis, which can be associated with distended fluid-filled bowel loops, air within the bowel wall, and eventually visualisation of air within the portal venous system (Figure 12.45). It is of note that hepatic portal venous gas can be found in different circumstances, some of which are not purely pathological [23, 24]. Nevertheless its presence, supported by clinical suspicion, is highly specific and should warrant urgent referral and second-level imaging [24–26].

Finally, an important extrahepatic cause of abnormal liver function, as well as liver failure in CLD, is liver congestion as a consequence of heart failure, pulmonary hypertension with or without associated pulmonary embolism, tricuspid regurgitation, and pericardial effusion/constriction.

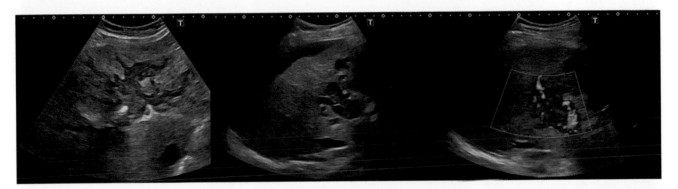

Figure 12.42 Rapidly progressive liver failure in a patient with known hepatitis B–related cirrhosis and evidence of extensive portal vein thrombosis as a cause of worsening liver function and acute variceal bleeding. The expansion of the thrombus within the portal vein as well as its vascularisation seen on colour Doppler were highly suspicious for neoplastic portal vein thrombosis. Diagnosis was confirmed with both contrast-enhanced ultrasound (See Chapter 5, Figure 5.27) and computed tomography with contrast.

(a) (b) (c)

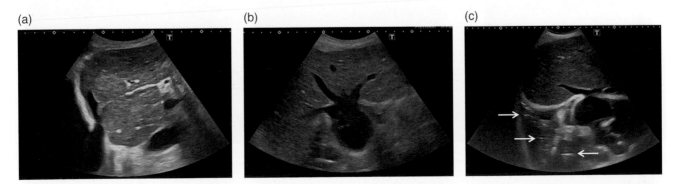

Figure 12.43 (a) Patient with sepsis, and respiratory and liver failure. Point-of-care ultrasound revealed heterogeneous liver echotexture, irregular outline, and hypertrophy of the caudate lobe, all features in keeping with cirrhosis. (b) There is pronounced distension of the inferior vena cava and hepatic veins compatible with right-sided heart failure, and (c) a large right echogenic pleural effusion with hyperechoic focuses and ring-down artefact compatible with pleural empyema secondary to gas-producing bacteria (Video 12.19).

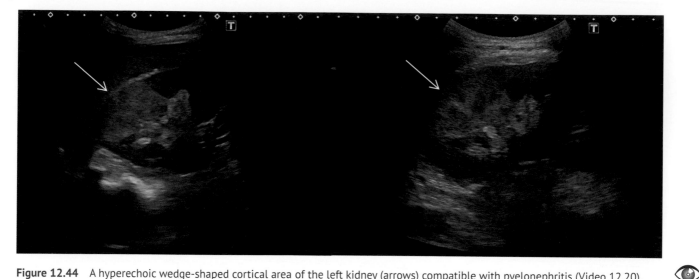

Figure 12.44 A hyperechoic wedge-shaped cortical area of the left kidney (arrows) compatible with pyelonephritis (Video 12.20).

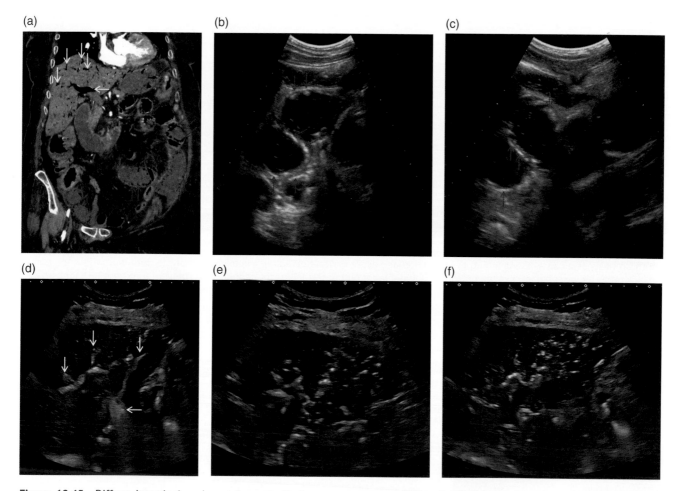

Figure 12.45 Diffuse intestinal and portal pneumatosis as a consequence of severe bacterial necrotising enterocolitis in an immunecompromised patient. The extensive gastrointestinal necrotic process led to accumulation of gas in the bowel wall that reached the liver through the enterohepatic circulation. (a) On CT the air can clearly be seen in the gastric and bowel wall (red arrows) as well as in the whole portal venous system (yellow arrows). On ultrasound intestinal pneumatosis can be seen as echogenic spots within the bowel wall (b and c, red arrows). Portal venous gas is identified as a diffuse hyperechoic signal that in this case follows the main portal vein and its more proximal branches (d, yellow arrows). Air in the distal portal venous branches is seen as diffuse parenchymal scattered hyperechoic foci (e, f).

The most common cause is severe congestive heart failure, which is usually chronic and can clinically precipitate in case of worsening left ventricular function, leading to liver failure as a consequence of ischaemia (acute cardiogenic liver injury [27]). POCUS is extremely useful to diagnose congestive hepatopathy and its haemodynamic consequences on portal flow, since the IVC is typically distended and motionless during respiration, the hepatic veins are grossly distended, and the portal venous flow is pulsatile and in severe cases inverted as a consequence of increased post-sinusoidal portal pressure (Figures 12.46 and 12.47) (Videos 12.21 and 12.22). Finally, the spectral wave form analysis of the hepatic veins can yield important clues to the underlying cause of outflow obstruction, bearing in mind that the presence of cirrhosis has been described as a cause of dampening of the Doppler signal [28, 29].

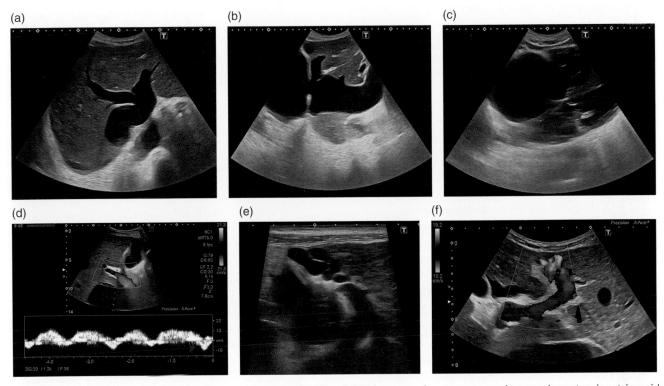

Figure 12.46 (a, b) Extreme inferior vena cava and hepatic veins distension secondary to severe pulmonary hypertension, tricuspid insufficiency, and right atrial enlargement (c). (d) Pulsatile portal venous flow as a sign of severe increase of central venous pressure and post-sinusoidal portal hypertension. (e, f) Recanalised umbilical vein reveals portal-systemic shunting as a sign of clinically significant portal hypertension (Video 12.21).

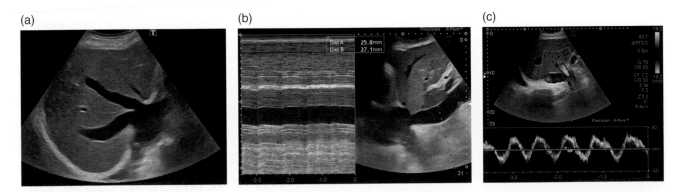

Figure 12.47 (a) Pronounced distension of inferior vena cava (IVC) and hepatic veins ('starfish-like' appearance) in a patient with liver failure and known severe pulmonary hypertension. (b) Longitudinal view of the retrohepatic IVC (M-mode) reveals almost absent IVC respiratory shifts as a sign of increased central venous pressure. (c) Pulsatile inverted portal flow is a sign of severe post-hepatic pressure that is transmitted to the portal venous system through the sinusoids (Video 12.22).

Basic Principles of POCUS in Liver Disease

- Always consider the clinical scenario, medical history, and presenting signs and symptoms.
- Focus the ultrasound examination using a rule-in/rule-out approach to answer the clinical query following a 'scanning checklist'.
- If the patient is not known to have CLD but the clinical and biochemical picture does suggest it, keep in mind the sonographic hallmarks of cirrhosis and portal hypertension.
- In patients with cirrhosis and worsening liver function, ultrasound examination should focus on excluding hepatic and extrahepatic causes.
- POCUS in a patient with liver dysfunction and clinical instability should provide answers on the potential cause and systemic involvement, such as haemodynamics and respiratory apparatus. This will help to add information for the interpretation of a sometimes complex clinical scenario in which liver impairment can be the consequence of a systemic process such as sepsis or heart failure.
- Consider the pathophysiological changes that occur in cirrhosis and other related conditions that might interfere with the interpretation of sonographic results. Two or more pathologies might co-exist, making diagnostic interpretation more complex.

Videos

Videos for this chapter can be accessed via the companion website: www.wiley.com/go/LiverUltrasound.

References

1 Moore, C.L. and Lobel, J. (2011). Point of care ultrasonography. *N. Engl. J. Med.* 364: 749–757.

2 Abu-Zidan, F.M., Zayat, I., Sheikh, M. et al. (1996). Role of ultrasonography in blunt abdominal trauma: a prospective study. *Eur. J. Surg.* 162: 361–365.

3 Goldberg, B.B. (1976). Ultrasonic evaluation of intraperitoneal fluid. *JAMA* 235 (22): 2427–2430.

4 Abu-Zidan, F.M. and Cevik, A.A. (2018). Diagnostic point-of-care ultrasound (POCUS) for gastrointestinal pathology: state of the art from basics to advanced. *World J. Emergency Surg.* 13 (47): 1–14.

5 Smith, M.J., Hayward, S.A., Innes, S.M., and Miller, A.S.C. (2020). Point-of-care lung ultrasound in patients with COVID-19 – a narrative review. *Anaesthesia* 75: 1115–1116.

6 Wongwaisayawan, S., Suwannanon, R., Prachanukool, T. et al. (2015). Trauma ultrasound. *Ultrasound Med. Biol.* 41: 2543–2561.

7 Goldflam K, Saul T, Lewiss R. (2011). Inferior vena cava ultrasound. *ACEPNow*, 1 June. www.acepnow.com/article/inferior-vena-cava-ultrasound/4.

8 Lichtenstein, D.A. (2014). Lung ultrasound in the critically ill. *Ann. Intensive Care* 4: 1.

9 Scott, J. (2019). Millington ultrasound assessment of the inferior vena cava for fluid responsiveness: easy, fun, but unlikely to be helpful. *Can. J. Anesth.* 66: 633–638.

10 Iwatsuki, S. and Reynolds, T.B. (1973). Effect of increased intraabdominal pressure on hepatic hemodynamics in patients with chronic liver disease and portal hypertension. *Gastroenterology* 65: 294–299.

11 Wachsberg, R.H. (2000). Narrowing of the upper abdominal inferior vena cava in patients with elevated intra-abdominal pressure: sonographic observations. *J. Ultrasound Med.* 19: 217–222.

12 Jain, A., Mehta, N., Secko, M. et al. (2017). History, physical examination, laboratory testing, and emergency department ultrasonography for the diagnosis of acute cholecystitis. *Acad. Emerg. Med.* 24: 281–297.

13 Wells, D. and Brackney, A. (2017). Acute portal vein thrombosis diagnosed with point-of-care ultrasonography. *Clin. Pract. Cases Emerg. Med.* 1 (1): 50–52.

14 Blanco, P. and Abdo-Cuza, A. (2019). Point-of-care ultrasound in the critically ill pregnant or postpartum patient: what every intensivist should know. *Intensive Care Med.* 45: 1123–1126.

15 Caremani, M., Tacconi, D., and Lapini, L. (2013). Acute non traumatic liver lesions. *J. Ultrasound* 16: 179–186.

16 Glaser, K., Tschmelitsch, J., Klingler, P. et al. (1994). Ultrasonography in the management of blunt abdominal and thoracic trauma. *Arch. Surg.* 129: 743–747.

17 McGahan, J.P., Rose, J., Coates, T.L. et al. (1997). Use of ultrasonography in the patient with acute abdominal trauma. *J. Ultrasound Med.* 16: 653–662. quiz 63–64.

18 Rothlin, M.A., Naf, R., Amgwerd, M. et al. (1993). Ultrasound in blunt abdominal and thoracic trauma. *J. Trauma* 34: 488–495.

19 Catalano, O., Lobianco, R., Raso, M.M., and Siani, A. (2005). Blunt hepatic trauma: evaluation with contrast-enhanced sonography. Sonographic findings and clinical application. *J. Ultrasound Med.* 24: 299–310.

20 Denault, A., Vegas, A., and Royse, C. (2014). Bedside clinical and ultrasound-based approaches to the management of hemodynamic instability—part I: focus on the clinical approach: continuing professional development. *Can. J. Anaesth.* 61: 843–864.

21 Vegas, A., Denault, A., and Royse, C. (2014). A bedside clinical and ultrasound-based approach to hemodynamic instability—part II: bedside ultrasound in hemodynamic shock: continuing professional development. *Can. J. Anaesth.* 61: 1008–1027.

22 Denault, A., Canty, D., Azzam, M. et al. (2019). Whole body ultrasound in the operating room and intensive care unit. *Korean J. Anesth.* 72: 413–428.

23 Wong, M.-F. and Lien, W.-C. (2014). Hepatic portal venous gas in a COPD patient. *J. Med. Ultrasound* 22: 106–109.

24 Maher, M.M., Tonra, B.M., Malone, D.E., and Gibney, R.G. (2001). Portal venous gas: detection by gray-scale and Doppler sonography in the absence of correlative findings on computed tomography. *Abdom. Imaging* 26: 390–394.

25 Strote, S.R., Caroon, L.V., and Reardon, R.F. (2012). Identification of portal venous air with bedside ultrasound in the emergency department. *J. Emerg. Med.* 43: 698–699.

26 Liang, K.-W., Huang, H.-H., Tyan, Y.-s., and Tsao, T.-F. (2018). Hepatic portal venous gas. Review of ultrasonographic findings and the use of the 'meteor shower' sign to diagnose it. *Ultrasound Q.* 34 (4): 268–271.

27 Xanthopoulos, A., Starling, R.C., Kitai, T., and Triposkiadis, F. (2019). Heart failure and liver disease. *J. Am. Coll. Cardiol.* 7 (2): 87–96.

28 McNaughton, D.A. and Abu-Yousef, M.M. (2011). Doppler US of the liver made simple. *RadioGraphics* 31: 161–188.

29 Kim, M.Y., Baik, S.K., Park, D.H. et al. (2007). Damping index of Doppler hepatic vein waveform to assess the severity of portal hypertension and response to propranolol in liver cirrhosis: a prospective nonrandomized study. *Liver Int.* 27: 1103–1110.

13

Liver Transplantation

Thomas Puttick and Paul S. Sidhu

Department of Radiology, King's College Hospital, London, UK

Orthotopic liver transplantation was introduced in 1963 and has been continually modified to improve patient outcome [1]. Liver transplantation is performed when there is end-stage liver damage that has failed conservative medical and surgical treatments. The ultrasound assessment of the pre-transplant patient is limited, with important areas of surveillance including underlying hepatocellular carcinoma (HCC) detection and the status of portal vein blood flow. The traditional orthotopic liver transplantation is the preferred technique, but with the shortage of cadaveric livers, both split-liver transplantation and living donor liver transplantation are becoming more common [2]. Following transplantation, ultrasound plays a vital role. The introduction of bedside ultrasound, with colour and spectral Doppler techniques, was a milestone in the post-operative care of these patients [3]. It is important that ultrasound practitioners understand common surgical techniques, particularly the anastomotic techniques, expected post-operative imaging findings and that they are able to identify complications. Any post-surgical complication, such as a fluid collection, abscess, small bowel ileus or a pleural effusion, will be a possibility following liver transplantation. The unique complications associated with a liver transplant are important too appreciate. The most common complications in the immediate post-operative period are related to the vascular anastomoses and the hepatic artery is crucial; the patent artery is clearly depicted by Doppler ultrasound techniques. This chapter will present an overview of the position of ultrasound in the assessment of the liver transplant patient [4, 5].

Indications for Transplant

Common indications for liver transplantation in the adult population include cirrhosis secondary to chronic hepatitis, acute hepatitis, metabolic disorders, sclerosing cholangitis, and Budd–Chiari syndrome. Widely accepted guidelines for patients with HCC requiring liver transplant are the Milan criteria, which state that no HCC lesion should be larger than 5 cm or up to three lesions equal to or less than 3 cm in diameter [6]. Contraindications for liver transplantation include sepsis, extrahepatic malignancy, severe cardiopulmonary disease, active alcohol or substance misuse, or abnormal anatomy that excludes liver transplantation. Portal vein thrombosis is a relative contraindication that makes surgery challenging with increased morbidity and mortality [7]. The pre-operative ultrasound aspects in the liver transplant candidate are primarily associated with parenchymal change, presence of focal liver lesions, presence of portal hypertension, varices and the state of the portal vein [4].

Surgical Techniques in Liver Transplantation

Surgery for transplantation in the recipient involves hepatectomy, vascularisation of the new liver and biliary reconstruction. The surgical technique can be varied, but whole-liver transplantation involves one biliary and four vascular anastomoses. The biliary anastomosis is an end-to-end anastomosis from the donor common bile duct (CBD) to the recipient common hepatic duct (CHD): a choledo-choledochostomy. If the recipient CHD is diseased or absent, then a choledojejunostomy is formed. In orthotopic liver transplantation, the donor coeliac artery is anastomosed to the recipient hepatic artery via the bifurcation of the hepatic artery or the gastroduodenal artery. If there is a small or diseased hepatic artery or coeliac artery, then a donor iliac artery graft or aorto-hepatic graft can be anastomosed to the recipient aorta. Portal vein connection is via an end-to-end anastomosis. The supra- and infrahepatic vena cava anastomoses are often end-to-end anastomoses [8]. Other surgical techniques include 'piggy-back' transplant with an anastomosis between the donor vena cava at the junction with the hepatic veins directly onto the recipient vena cava, with a remnant blind donor inferior vena cava (IVC); right or left transplants; segmental transplant (in small children); and living donor transplants. Understanding ultrasound segmental liver anatomy using the Couinaud nomenclature is common practice and is essential in segmental transplants [9, 10]. The appearances of the normal vascular anatomy in the post-transplant patient is readily identified on colour and spectral Doppler ultrasound (Figure 13.1) [11].

Post–Liver Transplant Imaging

Imaging is used to identify post-transplantation complications, which are broadly divided into vascular, biliary and other complications associated with the surgical procedure. Identification of normal post-operative appearances is vital to identify complications. Normal post-operative ultrasound assessment would entail an examination on days 1, 3, and 5 following liver transplantation, primarily for the integrity of the vascular component of the transplant and to document any early post-operative collections (haematoma, biloma, or less often infective). Any more frequent imaging with ultrasound or computed tomography (CT) is

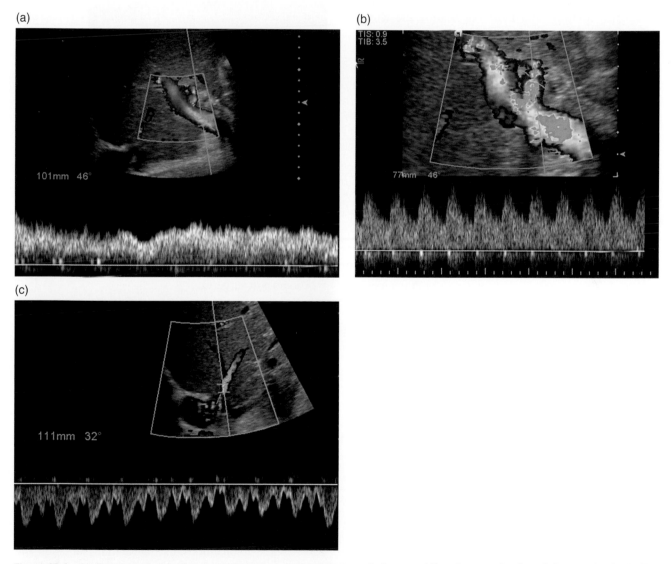

Figure 13.1 (a) The normal post-liver transplantation colour and spectral ultrasound Doppler examination of the portal vein. (b) The normal post-liver transplantation colour and spectral Doppler ultrasound examination of the hepatic artery. (c) The normal post-liver transplantation colour and spectral Doppler ultrasound examination of a hepatic vein.

based on clinical requirements, and when ultrasound is inconclusive. A routine ultrasound examination involves assessment of the liver parenchyma and colour, spectral Doppler ultrasound interrogation of the vessels and assessment of the biliary tree and perihepatic spaces.

There are common expected findings in the postoperative liver transplantation that should resolve within a short time period, which include a small perihepatic haematoma, small right-sided pleural effusion, small-volume ascites and periportal oedema.

Complications following liver transplantation identified with ultrasound include vasculature abnormality, biliary duct changes, liver parenchyma abnormalities and changes in perihepatic spaces. It is important not to take the imaging findings in isolation but to correlate the imaging findings with the liver graft function, biochemical and haematological findings, and most importantly the clinical assessment of the patient.

Rejection is a common cause of hepatic dysfunction following transplantation, which is confirmed on liver biopsy, usually performed under ultrasound guidance. The role of ultrasound is to identify other causes of post-transplantation hepatic dysfunction that can mimic rejection [12].

Vascular Complications

Vascular complications can involve occlusion (arterial or venous thrombosis), stricture (arterial or venous stenosis) and leaking (arterial pseudoaneurysm formation). Vascular thrombosis or stenosis can occur within the hepatic artery, portal vein or less commonly the intrahepatic veins and the IVC. Vascular complications may occur in the immediate post-operative period, prompting initial identification with a bedside ultrasound, which is vital for graft preservation. Once the abnormality is suspected on ultrasound examination and if there is ongoing clinical concern or a suboptimal ultrasound, then contrast-enhanced CT is often performed to confirm a vascular abnormality. The application of contrast-enhanced ultrasound (CEUS) at this stage has also been reported successful [13].

Hepatic Artery

The normal hepatic artery waveform demonstrates a rapid systolic upstroke (<80 m/s, time from end diastole to the first systolic peak) and continuous diastolic flow. The resistive index (RI, peak systolic velocity – peak diastolic velocity/peak systolic velocity) should be between 0.5 and 0.7. The post-transplant hepatic artery should be readily identified on colour and spectral Doppler ultrasound, with

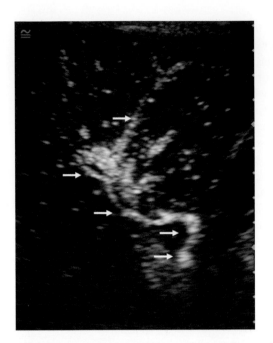

Figure 13.2 A contrast-enhanced ultrasound examination of a 'difficult' hepatic artery not seen clearly on the colour Doppler ultrasound examination. The hepatic artery is clearly patent (arrows), with a short window of opportunity to assess the artery after the ultrasound contrast agent injection, before enhancement of the portal vein and liver parenchyma.

the addition of CEUS to help delineate difficult vessels (Figure 13.2). In the immediate post-transplant period, the hepatic artery may exhibit a high RI with little or no flow seen in diastole which is often due to reperfusion oedema. For this reason, scanning on day 0 post transplant is usually avoided and the initial ultrasound is scheduled for after >24 hours post surgery.

Hepatic Artery Thrombosis

Hepatic artery thrombosis occurs in 3–10% of liver transplantations and accounts for 60% of all post-transplantation complications [14]. Hepatic artery thrombus results in liver parenchyma ischaemia, then infarction, followed by biliary duct stricture and necrosis. If the hepatic artery thrombosis occurs early (within approximately 15 days of transplantation) and prior to the development of arterial collaterals, it can be life threatening (with a 20–60% mortality rate) and requires urgent surgical intervention. Risk factors for early hepatic artery thrombosis include acute rejection, prolonged cold ischaemic time of the donor liver, ABO blood incompatibility, paediatric transplantation and small donor or recipient vessels [15]. The colour Doppler and spectral ultrasound will identify over 90% of patent hepatic arteries, with a spectral Doppler ultrasound trace mandatory to demonstrate the arterial waveform [16]. If there is uncertainty as to the patency of the hepatic artery, a CEUS examination is useful prior to further imaging with CT (Figure 13.3) [17].

In the transplanted liver, the hepatic artery provides the only blood supply to the bile ducts and therefore occlusion of the hepatic artery can result in hepatic failure, delayed biliary leak or bacteraemia clinically. With an 'impending' hepatic artery thrombosis, initial flow on day 1 post transplantation may sometimes be present but compromised; normally an initial high RI (>0.80) is present, indicating increased end-organ resistance. With subsequent imaging there may be dampening of the systolic peak and complete loss of the forward diastolic flow, and an abnormal hepatic waveform. Normally, in the post-operative period an initial high RI returns to a more normal hepatic waveform with good forward diastolic flow and low RI, reflecting improved graft function [18].

If an initial hepatic artery thrombosis is not identified and there is no immediate graft dysfunction, over time there may be collateral vessel formation. This is associated with an intrahepatic arterial waveform that is abnormal, resulting in a tardus-parvus spectral waveform pattern with an increased acceleration time (time from initial systolic upstroke to maximum velocity, measured at >80 msec) and a low RI measured at <0.5. This is more often seen in the paediatric age group and where a hepaticojejunostomy is formed, which allows for neo-vascularisation around an occluded hepatic artery. Colour and spectral Doppler ultrasound has high sensitivity and specificity for hepatic artery thrombosis. Non-visualisation of the hepatic artery can also occur secondary to spasm or low cardiac output [19]. Patient surgical dressings and positioning can also limit proper assessment; a CEUS examination can help improve flow visualisation of the hepatic artery [17, 20].

In patients in whom no flow is detected within the hepatic artery, which requires further imaging, this is usually a contrast-enhanced CT to identify the site of thrombus formation. A hepatic artery thrombosis requires urgent revascularisation to the liver graft, but even with rapid correction up to 60% of cases require retransplantation. Delayed hepatic artery thrombosis can occur years following transplantation and is often associated with chronic rejection or recurrent unexplained sepsis.

Hepatic Artery Stenosis

Hepatic artery stenosis occurs in approximately 11% of liver transplantations, often at the anastomotic site and due to allograft rejection, intimal trauma, clamp injury at the time of surgery or a disrupted vasa vasorum resulting in ischaemia. Median time from transplantation to diagnosis of hepatic artery stenosis is 100 days [21]. This results in biliary ischaemia, causing hepatic dysfunction and ultimately hepatic failure without adequate treatment. The spectral Doppler ultrasound waveform at the site of stenosis shows increased velocity (>200 cm/s) and turbulence distal to the stenosis, which results in a tardus–parvus waveform and

(a)

(b)

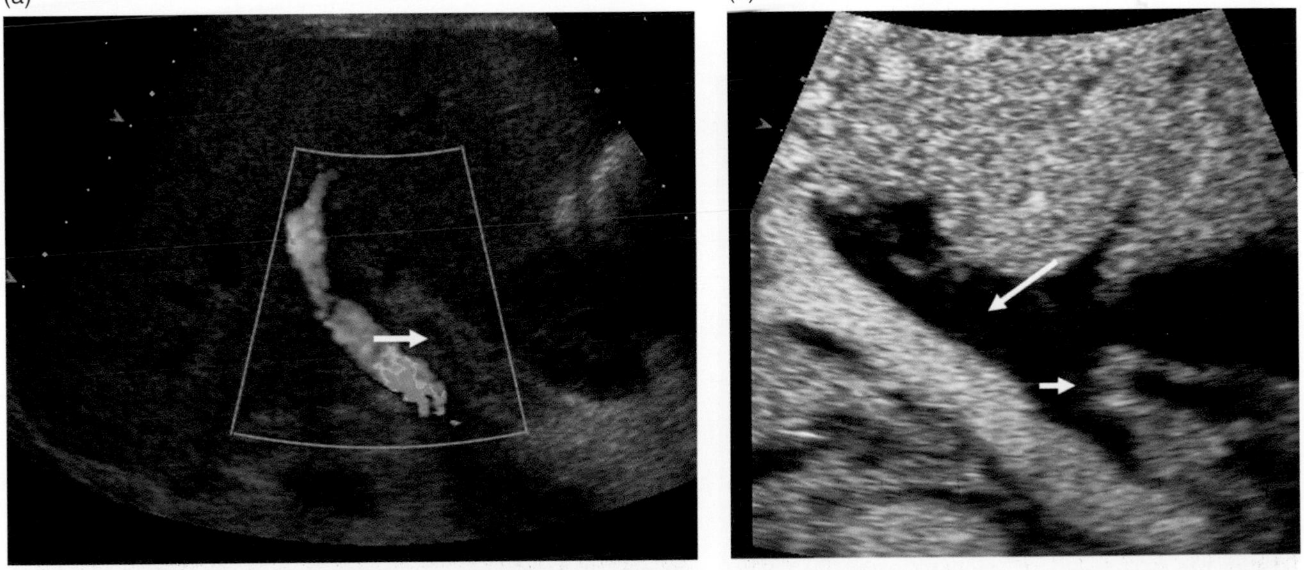

Figure 13.3 A 34-year-old male patient with a day 5 ultrasound examination of a liver transplantation. (a) On the colour Doppler image, the portal vein is clearly depicted with colour flow, but no signal from the expected position of the hepatic artery (arrow) is present. (b) Following the administration of an ultrasound contrast agent, there is flow in the coeliac axis and splenic artery (short arrow) but no flow is present in the hepatic artery (long arrow), consistent with an acute hepatic artery thrombosis.

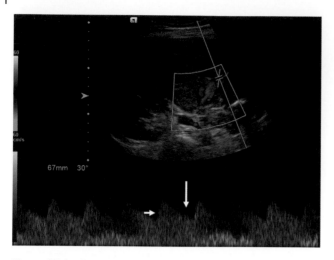

Figure 13.4 A split-liver transplantation in a 21-year-old male patient, with the spectral Doppler ultrasound waveform of the hepatic artery demonstrating a slow upstroke (short arrow) and a high diastolic forward flow (long arrow), the tardus–parvus waveform of a hepatic artery stenosis.

reduced RI (<0.5). Older donor age and a prolonged period of ischaemia are associated with increased hepatic artery resistance (Figure 13.4).

Pseudoaneurysm

A hepatic artery pseudoaneurysm is rare, occurring in <1%, and when present is often mycotic and occurring at the vascular anastomotic site [22]. Some occur in an intrahepatic location, usually following percutaneous intervention or parenchymal infection. Clinically these may present with hepatic failure or haemodynamic compromise if there is rupture of the pseudoaneurysm. A colour Doppler ultrasound assessment often shows a disorganised arterial flow pattern (ying–yang sign) or may demonstrate a tardus–parvus waveform in the affected intrahepatic artery (Figure 13.5) [23]. Surgery or interventional repair is usually performed but prognosis is poor with any extrahepatic pseudoaneurysm, with underlying fungal sepsis the mitigating factor.

Portal Vein Complications

The normal portal vein Doppler ultrasound waveform should be a continuous flow pattern towards the liver, with mild variation induced by inspiration and expiration. Thrombosis and stenosis of the portal vein occur in 1–2% of liver transplants (Figure 13.6). Factors contributing to these portal vein complications include hypercoagulable states, surgical technique, misalignment of vessels, longer vessels or prior portal vein surgery [24]. Clinically the patient may present with portal hypertension, ascites, oedema or hepatic failure. Ultrasound demonstrates portal vein narrowing or echogenic luminal thrombus without colour Doppler ultrasound flow. Acute thrombus can appear anechoic. The colour and spectral Doppler ultrasound assessment also shows colour aliasing with a three- to fourfold increase in velocity at the stenosis relative to the pre-stenotic portal vein. Portal vein thrombus

(a)   (b)

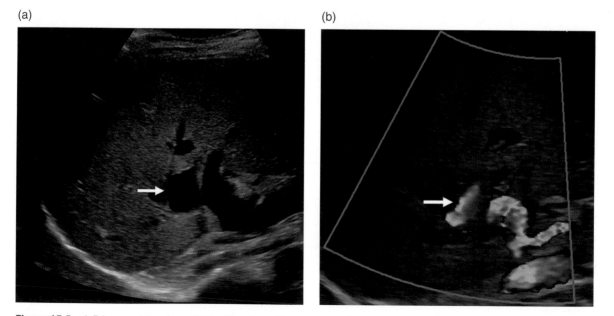

Figure 13.5 A 34-year-old male patient with a hepatic artery pseudoaneurysm. (a) A low-reflective area (arrow) lies adjacent to the posterior aspect of the portal vein in the region of the hepatic artery. (b) The colour Doppler image confirms that this is a vascular structure (arrow), consistent with a hepatic artery pseudoaneurysm.

(a) (b)

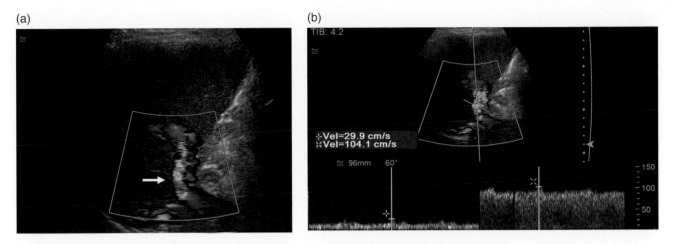

Figure 13.6 A 52-year-old male patient with a recent liver transplantation. (a) There is colour Doppler ultrasound turbulence at the site of the portal vein anastomosis (arrow), indicating the possibility of an underlying portal vein stenosis. (b) On the spectral Doppler ultrasound image, the velocity measurements are suggestive of a velocity increase across the narrowing with an underlying stenosis.

(a) (b)

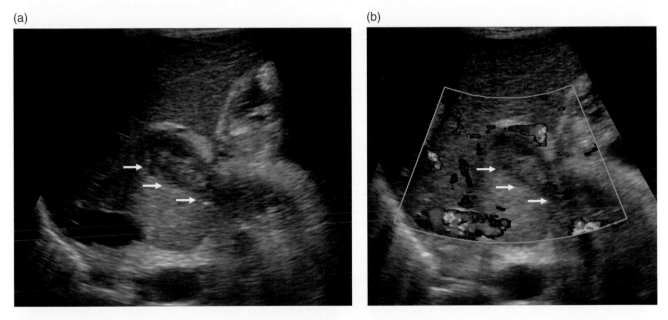

Figure 13.7 A 52-year-old man with a second liver transplantation and an occluded portal vein. (a) On the greyscale image there is expansion of the portal vein, which contains echogenic material (arrows) consistent with a portal vein thrombosis. (b) The colour Doppler ultrasound confirms absence of flow in the portal vein (arrows).

may also demonstrate retrograde or absence of flow on Doppler assessment (Figure 13.7) [25]. Treatment options include surgical correction with thrombectomy, placement of a venous graft, portosystemic shunt creation, balloon angioplasty or thrombolysis.

Inferior Vena Cava Complications

The normal hepatic vein Doppler ultrasound waveform shows a triphasic flow pattern due to changes in flow reflective of the cardiac cycle. Hepatic vein thrombosis and stenosis occur in <1%, predominantly at the anastomosis of the hepatic veins with the IVC, and are usually secondary to retransplantation or with a paediatric patient. Stenosis of the IVC can occur relatively acutely due to anastomotic size discrepancy or suprahepatic vena cava kinking due to rotation of the liver [26]. Ultrasound demonstrates increased velocity through the site of stenosis compared to the pre-stenotic segment if there is severe stenosis. Ultrasound may show reversed flow or absence of phasicity in the hepatic veins. Imaging may also show hepatomegaly, ascites or pleural effusions. Treatment can involve vascular stent placement or balloon angioplasty. With an IVC thrombosis, there may be vessel narrowing or intraluminal echogenic thrombus, and absent colour Doppler ultrasound signal.

Biliary Complications

Biliary complications occur in 25% of liver transplants, with approximately 80% occurring within the first six months following transplantation [27]. Biliary complications can include leaks, stones or sludge, strictures, recurrent disease and sphincter of Oddi dysfunction. Anastomotic strictures occur in 5–14% of patients and are associated with duct-to-duct anastomoses and prolonged graft ischaemia [28]. Biliary leaks can occur and the most common site is the end-to-end biliary anastomosis. Bile leaks allow collections to form in the perihepatic space or in the peritoneal cavity and clinical symptoms may range from non-specific abdominal pain to septic shock. Non-anastomotic strictures are most often caused by occlusion of the hepatic artery. Ultrasound may demonstrate intrahepatic duct dilatation, which may be segmental. In these patients, it is vital to accurately assess the hepatic artery to ensure there is no arterial compromise. Sloughing of biliary epithelium can occur due to necrosis of the biliary tree and this can cause intrahepatic duct dilatation with echogenic material within the ducts [29]. Biliary ischaemia, stricture, dilatation and sloughing can be complicated by sepsis and biliary abscess formation [30].

Neoplastic Disease

Neoplastic disease in the liver transplant patient can be due to recurrent cancer or post-transplantation lymphoproliferative disease (PTLD). Following liver transplantation, previously undiagnosed HCC most commonly presents with lung metastases, followed by multifocal liver lesions in the transplant. Approximately 2–8% of liver transplant patients develop PTLD, which most commonly occurs within 12 months following transplantation; the immunosuppression to prevent liver transplant rejection causes unregulated lymphoid expansion. This may present as a spectrum of manifestations from benign mononucleosis to malignant lymphoma, with both hepatic or extrahepatic abnormalities [22, 31]. PTLD appearances within the liver can vary on ultrasound from multiple foci of decreased echogenicity with increased vascularity to diffuse hepatomegaly or rarely soft tissue within the biliary tree at the porta hepatis causing biliary obstruction (Figure 13.8). Common extrahepatic sites in PTLD include the spleen and small bowel. Nodal disease occurs in approximately 20% of patients, most commonly at the porta hepatis and coeliac axis [32]. Following identification on ultrasound, these findings should be assessed with a staging CT, multidisciplinary discussion and eventual image-guided biopsy confirmation.

Parenchymal Abnormalities

Parenchymal abnormalities can be focal or diffuse. The differential diagnosis for a focal parenchymal abnormality will include an abscess, infarct, biloma, metastatic disease, pre-existing liver disease or PTLD. Hepatic infarction or an abscess will often be associated with abnormalities of the hepatic artery and arterial flow should always be

(a)　　　　(b)

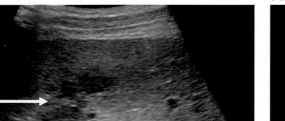

Figure 13.8 A 46-year-old male patient with a liver transplantation of one year, with post-transplant lymphoproliferative disorder. (a) Focal lesions of low reflectivity in the right lobe of the liver (arrow). (b) Multiple sub-hepatic oval-shaped low-reflective lymph nodes (arrows).

assessed. Ultrasound can demonstrate a solid area of abnormality, with a central hypoechoic area due to necrosis and sometimes 'dirty shadowing', which is difficult to distinguish from abscess formation (Figure 13.9). Typically abscesses have thick walls with a central hypoechoic area, which can also contain gas. The differential diagnosis for diffuse parenchymal abnormalities are wide and can include rejection, hepatitis, ischaemia and cholangitis. These will usually require histopathological diagnosis following biopsy.

Perihepatic Complications

Ascites, fluid collections and haematomas are common following liver transplantation [30]. A focal collection or haematoma at the cut surface or bare area of the liver is common and can be demonstrated as a non-specific fluid or complex collection on ultrasound (Figure 13.10). Collections at the porta hepatis are associated with hepatic artery pseudoaneurysm formation (Figure 13.5). Abscess formation outside the liver occurs in 10% of liver transplant patients and can be either bacterial or fungal. These most commonly occur in the sub-phrenic or sub-hepatic spaces and ultrasound assessment is often non-specific. Intrahepatic abscess

formation can occur and can appear either hypo- or hyperechoic due to the presence of gas formation and necrosis. A hepatic abscess increases the suspicion of a biliary stricture or hepatic artery thrombus.

Contrast-Enhanced Ultrasound in Liver Transplant

Contrast-enhanced ultrasound (CEUS) enhances the Doppler and colour signal, making it easier to identify the site of stenosis or thrombus and also to identify collateral formation [13, 17, 33, 34]. The application of CEUS in assessing focal liver lesions and guiding ultrasound interventional procedures is particularly useful [35].

Conclusion

Ultrasound has a vital role in the post-operative care of liver transplantation patients to identify complications. Visualisation of the hepatic vasculature, parenchyma and perihepatic spaces makes ultrasound a reliable initial imaging modality, and CEUS improves sensitivity for detecting hepatic artery occlusion.

(a) (b)

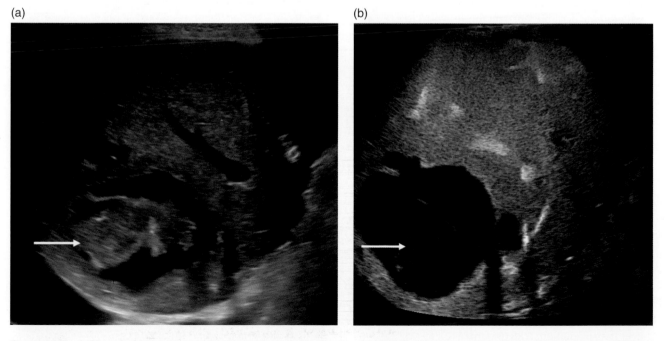

Figure 13.9 A 48-year-old woman post liver transplantation with a known hepatic artery thrombosis. (a) A large mixed-reflective area in the right lobe of the liver (arrow), which may be a biliary abscess. (b) Following administration of a contrast agent, the internal structure of the collection is avascular (arrow), indicating a probable necrotic liver, with no clear evidence of features of an abscess, e.g. rim enhancement or septations, in the collection.

(a) (b)

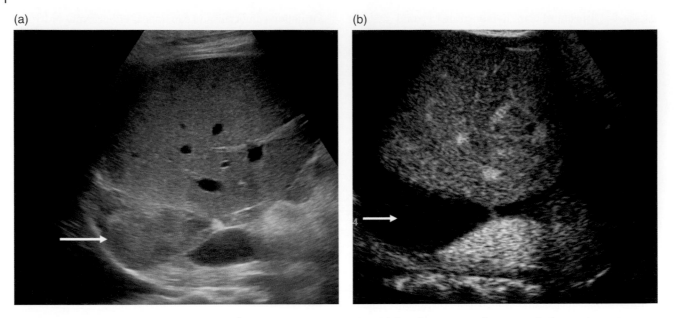

Figure 13.10 A 55-year-old male patient following liver transplantation. (a) Day 5 post-operative greyscale image demonstrates a focal area of iso-reflectivity to the normal transplant liver (arrow). (b) Following the administration of an ultrasound contrast agent, this area is seen to be avascular (arrow) and consistent with a resolving haematoma.

References

1 Starzl, T.E., Marchioro, T.L., Vonkaulla, K.N. et al. (1963). Homotransplantation of the liver in humans. *Surg. Gynecol. Obstet.* 117: 659–676.

2 Keeffe, E.B. (2000). Liver transplantation at the millennium: past, present, and future. *Clin. Liver Dis.* 4 (1): 241–255.

3 Raby, N., Meire, H.B., Forbes, A., and Williams, R. (1988). The role of ultrasound scanning in the management after liver transplantation. *Clin. Radiol.* 39: 507–510.

4 Shaw, A.S., Ryan, S.M., Beese, R.C. et al. (2002). Liver transplantation. *Imaging* 14: 314–328.

5 Ryan, S.M., Sellars, M.E., and Sidhu, P.S. (2011). Liver transplantation. In: *Clinical Ultrasound*, 3e (ed. P.L. Allan, G.M. Baxter and M.J. Weston), 199–224. New York: Elsevier.

6 Gunsar, F. (2017). Liver transplantation for hepatocellular carcinoma beyond the Milan criteria. *Exp. Clin. Transplant.* 15: 59–64.

7 Mazzaferro, V., Regalia, E., Doci, R. et al. (1996). Liver transplantation for the treatment of small hepatocellular carcinomas in patients with cirrhosis. *N. Engl. J. Med.* 334: 693–699.

8 Llado, L. and Figueras, J. (2004). Techniques of orthotopic liver transplantation. *HPB (Oxford)* 6 (2): 69–75.

9 Lafortune, M., Madore, F., and Patriquin, H. (1991). Segmental anatomy of the liver: a sonographic approach to the Couinaud nomenclature. *Radiology* 181: 443.

10 Bowles, M. and Rela, M. (2002). Liver transplantation: surgical techniques. In: *Ultrasound of Abdominal Transplantation* (ed. P.S. Sidhu and G.M. Baxter), 69–75. Stuttgart: Thieme.

11 Ryan, S.M. and Sidhu, P.S. (2002). Early post-operative liver transplant ultrasound. In: *Ultrasound of Abdominal Transplantation* (ed. P.S. Sidhu and G.M. Baxter), 90–104. Stuttgart: Thieme.

12 Oliver, J.H., Federle, M.P., Campbell, W.L., and Zajko, A.B. (1991). Imaging the hepatic transplant. *Radiol. Clin. North Am.* 29: 1285–1298.

13 Berry, J.D. and Sidhu, P.S. (2004). Microbubble contrast-enhanced ultrasound in liver transplantation. *Eur. Radiol.* 14: P96–P103.

14 Di Martino, M., Rossi, M., Mennini, G. et al. (2016). Imaging follow-up after liver transplantation. *Br. J. Radiol.* 89 (1064): 20151025.

15 Jain, A., Reyes, J., Kashyap, R. et al. (2000). Long-term survival after liver transplantation in 4,000 consecutive patients at a single center. *Ann. Surg.* 232: 490–500.

16 Flint, E.W., Sumkin, J.H., Zajko, A.B., and Bowen, A. (1988). Duplex sonography of hepatic artery thrombosis after liver transplantation in the cyclosporin era. *Am. J. Roentgenol.* 151: 481–483.

17 Sidhu, P.S., Shaw, A.S., Ellis, S.M. et al. (2004). Microbubble ultrasound contrast in the assessment of hepatic artery patency following liver transplantation:

role in reducing frequency of hepatic artery arteriography. *Eur. Radiol.* 14: 21–30.

18 Caiado, A.H.M., Blasbalg, R., Marcelino, A.S.Z. et al. (2007). Complications of liver transplantation: multimodality imaging approach. *Radiographics* 27: 1401–1417.

19 Dodd, G.D., Memel, D.S., Zajko, A.B. et al. (1994). Hepatic artery stenosis and thrombosis in transplant recipients: Doppler diagnosis with resistive index and systolic acceleration time. *Radiology* 192: 657–661.

20 Kim, J.S., Kim, K.W., Lee, J. et al. (2019). Diagnostic performance for hepatic artery occlusion after liver transplantation: computed tomography angiography versus contrast-enhanced ultrasound. *Liver Transpl.* 25 (11): 1651–1660.

21 Abbasoglu, O., Levy, M.F., Vodapally, M.S. et al. (1997). Hepatic artery stenosis after liver transplantation - incidence, presentation, treatment, and long term outcome. *Transplantation* 27: 250–255.

22 Marshall, M.M., Muiesan, P., Kane, P.A. et al. (1999). Hepatic artery pseudoaneurysms following liver transplantation: review of radiological features and management. *J. Vasc. Interv. Radiol.* 10: 278–279.

23 Tobben, P.J., Zajko, A.B., Sumkin, J.H. et al. (1988). Pseudoaneurysms complicating organ transplantation: roles of CT, duplex sonography and angiography. *Radiology* 169: 65–70.

24 Lerut, J., Tzakis, A., Bron, K.M. et al. (1987). Complications of venous reconstruction in human orthotopic liver transplantation. *Ann. Surg.* 205: 404–414.

25 Platt, J.F., Rubin, J.M., and Ellis, J.H. (1995). Hepatic artery resistance changes in portal vein thrombosis. *Radiology* 196: 95–98.

26 Karani, J.B. and Heaton, N.D. (1998). Review imaging in liver transplantation. *Clin. Radiol.* 53: 317–322.

27 Klein, A.S., Savador, S., Burdick, J.F. et al. (1991). Reduction of morbidity and mortality from biliary complications after liver transplantation. *Hepatology* 14: 818–823.

28 Stratta, R.J., Wood, R.P., Langnas, A.N. et al. (1989). Diagnosis and treatment of biliary tract complications after orthotopic liver transplant. *Surgery* 106: 675–684.

29 Kok, T., Van der Sluis, A., Klein, J.P. et al. (1996). Ultrasound and cholangiography for the diagnosis of biliary complications after orthotopic liver transplantation; a comparative study. *J. Clin. Ultrasound* 24: 103–115.

30 Shaw, A.S., Ryan, S.M., Beese, R.C., and Sidhu, P.S. (2003). Ultrasound of non-vascular complications in the post-transplant patient. *Clin. Radiol.* 58: 672–680.

31 Wu, L., Rappaport, D.C., Hanbidge, A. et al. (2001). Lymphoproliferative disorders after liver transplantation: imaging features. *Abdom. Imaging* 26 (2): 200–206.

32 Pickhardt, P.J. and Siegel, M.J. (1999). Post transplantation lymphoproliferative disorder of the abdomen: CT evaluation in 51 patients. *Radiology* 213: 73–78.

33 Sidhu, P.S., Marshall, M.M., Ryan, S.M., and Ellis, S.M. (2000). Clinical use of Levovist, an ultrasound contrast agent, in the imaging of liver transplantation: assessment of the pre and post transplant patient. *Eur. Radiol.* 10: 1114–1126.

34 Sidhu, P.S., Ellis, S.M., Karani, J.B., and Ryan, S.M. (2002). Hepatic artery stenosis following liver transplantation: significance of the tardus parvus waveform and the role of microbubble contrast media in the detection of a focal stenosis. *Clin. Radiol.* 57: 789–799.

35 Huang, D.Y., Yusuf, G.T., Daneshi, M. et al. (2018). Contrast-enhanced ultrasound (CEUS) in abdominal intervention. *Abdom. Radiol.* 43 (4): 960–976.

14

Ultrasound in Hepatobiliary Intervention

Neeral R. Patel, James P.F. Burn, and Ali Alsafi

Department of Imaging, Imperial College Healthcare NHS Trust, London, UK

Over the past three decades, ultrasound has become widely available, with increasingly powerful and portable machines at lower cost. Ultrasound is now more accessible across healthcare settings. In addition to its use as a diagnostic modality, guidance on minimally invasive procedures has been adopted widely in interventional radiology as well as other invasive disciplines. This has improved technical success and resulted in a proven reduction in complications. This is most notable in the use of ultrasound for central venous access.

As hepatobiliary intervention becomes ever more complex, with a variety of pathologies being treated in a minimally invasive manner, ultrasound guidance is now indispensable. In this chapter we will discuss the use of ultrasound in some common hepatobiliary interventional procedures.

Patient Preparation

Prior to any interventional procedure, patients' clinical history and previous imaging should be reviewed. Reviewing previous imaging gives the operator the opportunity to assess suitability for ultrasound guidance as opposed to other modalities such as fluoroscopy or computed tomography (CT). Cross-sectional imaging is particularly useful in planning intervention, but is not always necessary. The indications and appropriateness of the procedure should be carefully considered. For intervention in very ill or uncooperative patients, general anaesthesia should be considered.

A comprehensive approach to preparing any patient for an ultrasound-guided procedure can be remembered with the acronym ABCD:

Authorisation from the patient (informed consent)
Blood results and blood thinners
Checklist
Drugs (sedation, analgesia, antibiotics)

Authorisation (Informed Consent)

Written informed consent is imperative in order for the operator to proceed, and should be obtained by explaining to the patient, in lay terms, what the procedure will entail, the risks and the benefits, and alternative options, as well as satisfying any questions or concerns the patient may have. In circumstances where the patient is unable to give informed consent or does not have capacity, local ethical guidance should be applied.

Blood Results and Blood Thinners

Prior to any ultrasound-guided liver procedure, the patient's blood results must be scrutinised, in particular the clotting profile, to minimise the risk of bleeding. The acceptable limit will depend on local guidance and the level of risk of the planned intervention. The majority of ultrasound-guided liver interventions will fall under the moderate-risk category (liver biopsy, drain/aspiration, simple radiofrequency ablation [RFA]), while biliary drainage and complex RFAs are considered high-risk procedures. An example of the recommendations for blood result thresholds and pausing anticoagulants (based on Society of Interventional Radiology [SIR] guidance) when planning ultrasound-guided liver procedures is summarised in Table 14.1 [1].

Checklist

A safety checklist undertaken with all members of staff involved in the procedure is essential to reduce the risk of untoward events [2]. A modified World Health Organization (WHO) surgical checklist, specific to image-guided intervention, may be used [3].

Liver Ultrasound: From Basics to Advanced Applications, First Edition. Edited by Adrian K.P. Lim and Matteo Rosselli.
© 2024 John Wiley & Sons Ltd. Published 2024 by John Wiley & Sons Ltd.
Companion website: www.wiley.com/go/LiverUltrasound

Table 14.1 Guidance on coagulation threshold and pausing anticoagulants based on the bleeding risk of the ultrasound-guided liver intervention being performed.

	Low risk	Moderate risk	High risk
Example cases	Ultrasound-guided abdominal paracentesis	Liver biopsy (targeted and non-targeted) Intrahepatic abscess drain/aspiration Radiofrequency ablation of a liver lesion (simple)	Biliary drainage Radiofrequency ablation of a liver lesion (complex)
Haemoglobin	$>80\,g/L$	$>80\,g/L$	$>80\,g/L$
Platelets	$>50\times10^9/L$	$>80\times10^9/L$	$>80\times10^9/L$
Prothrombin time (PT)	<25 seconds	<24 seconds	<22 seconds
International normalised ratio (INR)	<1.6	<1.5	<1.4
Activated partial thromboplastin time (APTT)	<42 seconds	<41 seconds	<40 seconds
Aspirin	Continue	Continue	Continue
Abciximab	Withhold for 2 days	Withhold for 2 days	Withhold for 2 days
Clopidogrel	Withhold for 5 days	Withhold for 5 days	Withhold for 5 days
Direct thrombin inhibitors (e.g. dabigatran)	Withhold for 2 days	Withhold for 2 days	Withhold for 2 days
Factor Xa inhibitors (e.g. apixaban)	Withhold for 2 days	Withhold for 2 days	Withhold for 2 days
Low molecular weight heparin (e.g. enoxaparin)	Withhold prophylactic dose for 12 hours; therapeutic dose for 24 hours	Withhold prophylactic dose for 12 hours; therapeutic dose for 24 hours	Withhold prophylactic dose for 12 hours; therapeutic dose for 24 hours
Warfarin*	Withhold for 3 days	Withhold for 3 days	Withhold for 5 days

*duration to withhold depends on INR levels prior to biopsy

Drugs

These include prophylactic antibiotics, analgesia, and conscious sedation medication. There is joint Cardiovascular and Interventional Radiological Society of Europe (CIRSE) and SIR guidance on the use of antibiotics in interventional radiology, which includes their use prior to intrahepatic abscess and biliary drainage as well as RFA. The exact antibiotic(s) to be administered will depend on local antibiotic policy and sensitivities. It is important that prophylactic doses are administered within 60 minutes of skin puncture [4].

Liver intervention can be complex and often lengthy. For this reason, conscious sedation and analgesia are used to improve patient tolerance. Titrated doses of midazolam and fentanyl used in combination can provide effective conscious sedation. In procedures such as RFA of liver lesions, where high doses of sedation are likely to be required, some operators prefer the use of general anaesthesia, with the added advantage of reproducible breath holding for accurate needle positioning. Whichever is chosen, the patient must be fasted for at least 4–6 hours prior to the procedure.

Important General Points in Ultrasound-Guided Liver Intervention

- Review of cross-sectional imaging, careful planning, and consideration of the indications and contraindications is imperative.
- Correct coagulopathy prior to intervention.
- Drain any ascitic fluid prior to intervention to reduce the risk of bleeding.
- The liver capsule is well innervated, therefore good infiltration around it is very important to ensure the procedure is tolerable.
- The liver capsule *bleeds*. It is therefore imperative to minimise the number of passes the needle makes across it.

- The needles used should always cross normal liver prior to reaching its target in order to reduce bleeding risk. Abnormal liver (e.g. tumour) is more likely to bleed.
- Avoid using a transpleural/intercostal approach if possible, particularly for drainage procedures, as this can result in a thoracic empyema.
- Never perform a percutaneous biopsy of the liver if there is undrained biliary obstruction. This *will* result in a bile leak.

Liver Biopsies

Percutaneous liver biopsy is the standard procedure for obtaining liver tissue for histopathological assessment, used principally in the diagnosis and management of parenchymal liver diseases ('non-targeted') and in the characterisation of liver lesions ('targeted').

A 'blind' liver biopsy is obtained without imaging during, or immediately prior to, taking the biopsy. This has largely been superseded by image-guided biopsy, with a reduction in major complications, post-biopsy pain, and biopsy failure [5]. The reported risk of a major complication resulting from percutaneous liver biopsy remains 0.6–2%. Ultrasound is the preferred modality, as it provides real-time imaging in a non-conventional plane from skin to lesion.

Pre-procedural Imaging

If a targeted biopsy is intended, CT or magnetic resonance imaging (MRI) within four weeks prior to the biopsy is recommended by the British Society of Gastroenterology. This is essential to assess the exact location of the target lesion, its vascularity, and the distribution of regional vessels and bile ducts, as well as the presence of extrahepatic disease. All of these will influence the risk/benefit assessment in determining whether to proceed with biopsy.

Full ultrasound assessment immediately prior to biopsy is also essential. This will confirm the ongoing presence of a target lesion (e.g. one that may have responded to chemotherapy since prior imaging) and to identify any new preclusive factors, such as intervening bowel loops, large-volume ascites, or biliary obstruction.

Consideration of Contraindications

In addition to uncorrected coagulopathy, the presence of ascites is widely considered a contraindication to liver biopsy. The exact impact of ascites on bleeding risk is not clear [6]. Despite this, given the theoretical risk of uncontrolled bleeding into the ascitic fluid, pre-biopsy paracentesis or a transjugular route is recommended in such instances [7]. The presence of intrahepatic biliary dilatation poses a risk of biliary leak resulting in biloma or biliary peritonitis, with serious complications occurring in up to 4% of cases [8]. It is therefore prudent to consider biliary drainage and transbiliary biopsy when feasible [9].

Technique

Pre-procedural ultrasound is required to plan optimal patient positioning for biopsy. The relationship of the liver to adjacent organs or overlying ribs may be improved from that demonstrated on prior cross-sectional imaging by changing patient positioning, for instance left lateral decubitus of posterior right lobe of the liver lesions.

Once the lesion and a safe approach have been identified (Figure 14.1), the skin is marked, cleaned, and draped in a sterile manner. The skin and deep tissues are infiltrated with local anaesthetic (typically 10–20 mL of 1% lidocaine). It is important to inject a sizeable proportion of the local anaesthetic in the region of the liver capsule, as this is well innervated and a traversing needle can cause significant discomfort to the patient if they are not adequately anesthetised. At the planned site of entry, a small nick is made in the skin with a blade. During the biopsy, respiration may be ceased in order to arrest diaphragmatic and liver movement. Typically this is in end-expiration, both to aid consistent reproducibility of liver position and to ensure maximum elevation of the diaphragm/pleura away from the biopsy site.

The specific technique thereafter varies somewhat according to whether the biopsy is targeted, needle selection, and whether a coaxial technique is employed.

Needle Choice

A variety of needle types are used for liver biopsy, each with its own merits and limitations. While the balance of patient safety and diagnostic yield is paramount, selection of technique may be influenced by operator preference, risk factors for haemorrhage, cost and availability.

Cutting-Type Needles

The Tru-Cut® biopsy needle (Merit Medical, South Jordan, UT, USA) is a disposable needle comprising an obturator with a sharp end and outer sheath integrated into an all-in-one design. The device is advanced up to the margin of the target in the closed position. The obturator is then advanced through the target tissue while holding the outer cutting sheath steady. Finally, the sheath is advanced to cut the liver and the whole assembly is withdrawn.

The Tru-Cut biopsy needles have been superseded by automatic and semi-automatic variants, which are spring-loaded devices. Automatic needles trigger a rapid-firing side-notched Tru-Cut–type biopsy needle, while in semi-automatic devices the obturator is advanced manually as an isolated action before triggering the rapid-fire outer sheath. The latter has the advantage of allowing real-time assessment of the full length of the needle, with the ability to readjust position prior to firing. This is particularly important when the deep margin of the lesion poses a risk. This method is favoured by the authors.

More recently, an end-cut full-core needle such as the Biopince™ (Argon Medical, Athens, TX, USA) spring-loaded

(a)

(b)

(c)

(d)

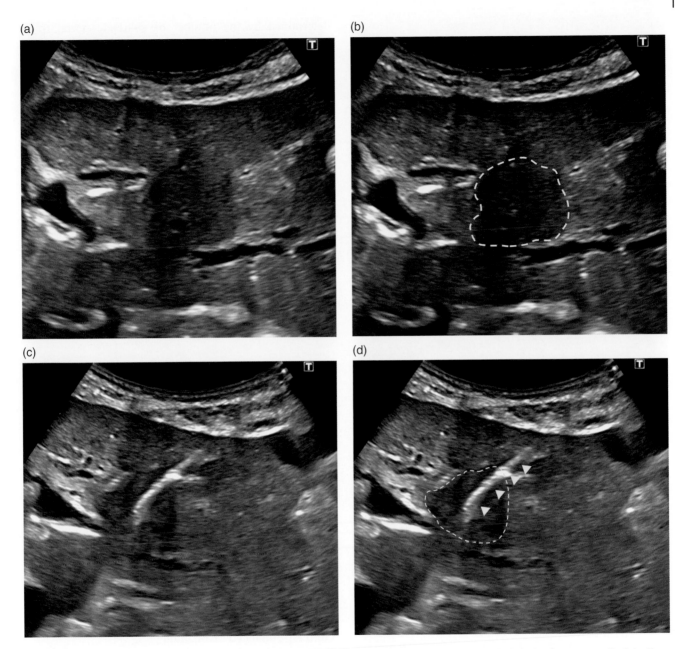

Figure 14.1 (a, b) Pre-procedure ultrasound with and without annotations demonstrating a hypoechoic lesion in segment II of the liver. (c, d) Ultrasound of the left lobe of the liver with a biopsy needle (arrowheads) in the target lesion with and without annotations.

automatic needle has been shown to improve the diagnostic yield by increasing core length and reducing crush artefact [10]. The biopsy yield must be counterbalanced by safety considerations when the deep margin is threatened by a large vessel, duct or diaphragm.

Aspiration or Suction-Type Needles

Use of aspiration needles such as Jamshidi™ (Becton, Dickinson, Franklin Lakes, NJ, USA), Klatskin, and Menghini is declining, but was reserved for non-targeted parenchymal biopsies. The needles are an open core with either an internal or external bevel, which is passed into liver tissue and then withdrawn while steady suction is applied to a connected syringe. The specimen is separated distally from the liver by the power of suction. The technique is associated with a reduced risk of haemorrhage but variable core quality [11].

Coaxial Technique

A coaxial technique may be used for biopsy of a focal lesion. This entails image-guided positioning of an outer guide needle (Figure 14.2; at least one gauge larger than the actual biopsy needle), within or adjacent to the lesion. A second

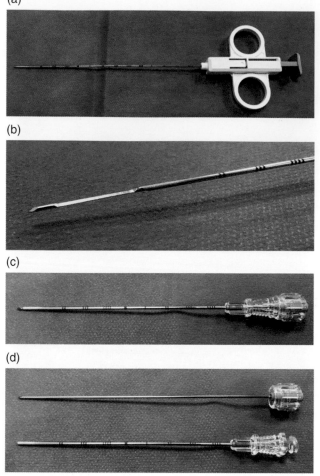

Figure 14.2 (a) Semi-automatic Tru-Cut–style biopsy needle. (b) Biopsy needle with the specimen obturator fully advanced prior to clicking the plunger and deploying the cutting cannula (note the specimen notch). (c, d) Coaxial introducer needle before and after removal of the stylet.

biopsy needle is then placed through the guide needle to obtain samples. The method allows multiple samples to be obtained without having to repeatedly reaccess the lesion, or indeed puncture the liver capsule. The theoretical impact on safety, however, has not been proven [12].

The authors therefore advocate the use of both coaxial and non-coaxial techniques, reserving the former for lesions high/deep within the liver where access is likely to be challenging, potentially increasing the requirement of multiple capsule punctures.

Needle Calibre and Number of Cores

Calibres used for liver biopsy vary among institutional protocols and purpose of the biopsy, with commonly used calibres being 16G, 18G, and 20G. In non-targeted biopsies assessing liver parenchymal disease, adequacy is determined by the number of complete portal tracts obtained, and there is good evidence to suggest that a larger needle has a greater yield, regularly exceeding the commonly accepted threshold of 11 tracts. A single 2–3 cm core with a 16G needle is therefore favoured by the authors in this context.

By contrast, biopsy to assess focal liver lesions does not require surmounting of such a threshold. In this instance, several cores to vary the sampling from a potentially heterogeneous or necrotic lesion are usually of greater diagnostic value. Core calibre is less correlated to diagnostic yield than number of passes. At least two cores with an 18G needle are usually sufficient in this instance.

Again, literature on the specific impact of core number on complication rate is varied. Recent evidence suggests that multiple biopsy passes are not on their own associated with an increase in severe complications, whereas infiltrative malignancy or deranged clotting had a greater impact [13].

Plugging the Tract

Plugged liver biopsy was first described in the mid-1980s. It has been advocated as an alternative method for obtaining liver tissue in patients with impaired coagulation or fibrotic liver disease. It has been adopted as standard practice by many operators in an effort to reduce haemorrhage risk. This requires the use of a coaxial technique. Following biopsy, the coaxial needle is left within the liver substance. Gelfoam pledgets or slurry are inserted/injected as the coaxial needle is withdrawn. The technique has been shown to reduce bleeding risk, but may be associated with increased pain, presumed secondary to liver capsular stretch, which deters many operators from using it.

Contrast-Enhanced Ultrasound in Hepatobiliary Intervention

Microbubble contrast assessment of liver lesions can be a useful adjunct in instances where the target lesion has been well demonstrated on cross-sectional imaging, but is poorly delineated on B-mode ultrasound against background liver parenchyma (Figure 14.3). This is most poignant in cirrhotic liver disease when the liver appears, as seen here, very heterogeneous and can easily mask small lesions.

Once the lesion has been confidently identified using microbubbles, the corresponding B-mode image can be reassessed and more accurately biopsied. The technique is fast and inexpensive and may allow biopsy of occult lesions.

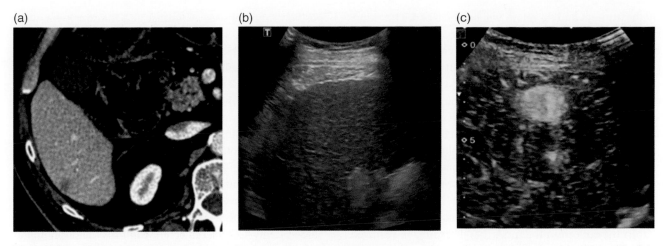

Figure 14.3 (a) Contrast-enhanced computed tomography demonstrating portal venous wash-out of the lesion in segment VI of the liver. (b) B-mode ultrasound of segment VI. The liver lesion is difficult to visualise, precluding precise ultrasound-guided biopsy. (c) Contrast-enhanced ultrasound demonstrating avid arterial enhancement of the lesion.

Ultrasound-Guided Drainage (Liver and Gallbladder)

Ultrasound-guided drainage or aspiration of liver collections has become the accepted treatment over surgery. The spectrum of diseases where image-guided treatments can be offered is wide-ranging, and includes infective causes in the case of pyogenic and amoebic liver abscess, inherited disorders such as polycystic liver disease that may result in symptomatic liver cysts, and emergent surgical presentations such as acute cholecystitis, where a percutaneous cholecystostomy may be offered to patients in specific circumstances.

Liver Abscess

Historically, surgery was the only therapeutic option in patients with liver abscess (Figure 14.4), but it has now been largely superseded by image-guided percutaneous drainage and aspiration. Advances in antibiotics have also improved outcomes in this patient group. Hepatic abscesses may occur through different routes, such as haematogenous spread from abdominal sepsis, biliary spread, and direct inoculation in the setting of penetrating liver injury [14].

Technique

There are two basic approaches to inserting a drain: Seldinger and trocar. The Seldinger approach is preferred

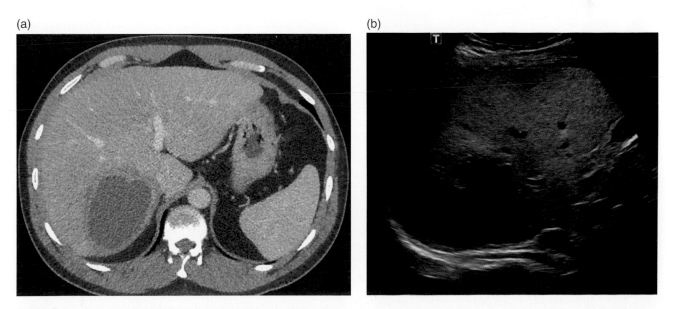

Figure 14.4 (a) Axial computed tomography demonstrating a thick-walled liver abscess in the right lobe of the liver. (b) Pre-drainage ultrasound showing the anechoic content of the liver abscess.

by the authors and therefore will be described. The skin is cleaned, draped, and local anaesthetic instilled, followed by making a skin nick at the planned entry point (see the section on liver biopsy technique). A 21G Chiba needle is usually used, but an 18G needle may sometimes be more appropriate. The ultrasound probe is positioned such that the target lesion and the needle are both visible. The needle is advanced in the pre-planned trajectory under ultrasound guidance. Only the needle or the ultrasound probe is adjusted at any one time to allow adequate needle visualisation. There is often a loss of resistance once the tip of the needle enters the abscess cavity.

In the case of a 21G Chiba needle, once the needle tip is within the collection the inner metal cannula is removed. Contrast is then used to opacify the abscess cavity and guide the remainder of the procedure with the aid of fluoroscopy. A 0.018 in. Mandril wire is advanced into the cavity, ensuring a proportion of the stiffer shaft of the wire is sited within the abscess. The wire position may also be checked with ultrasound. The needle is removed and a 4-French stiffener-dilator-sheath system is inserted (Figure 14.5). The stiffener and dilator as well as the 0.018 in. wire are removed, allowing a 0.035 in. J-tipped wire to then be inserted. If an 18G trocar needle is used, once within the abscess, the metal cannula is removed, and a syringe used to aspirate a sample confirming needle

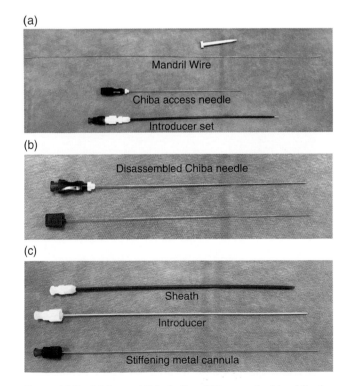

Figure 14.5 (a) Access kit including Chiba needle, Mandril wire, and introducer set. (b) Disassembled Chiba needle. (c) Disassembled introducer set (sheath, introducer, and stiffening metal cannula).

position in the abscess. Contrast and fluoroscopy may be used if required, and may reduce the risk of kinking the guidewire. A 0.035 in. J-tipped wire can be inserted directly through the needle shaft. For deeper, difficult to access abscesses, a 21G needle and fluoroscopy are preferred, while for more superficial abscesses, an 18G needle may be used under ultrasound guidance only.

The size of drain chosen is dependent on the contents of the abscess. If serous in consistency, an 8-French drain is sufficient, whereas if the contents are thick, a larger 10-French or 12-French drain is more appropriate. The tract is gently serially dilated over the wire. The selected drain is then advanced over the wire and the pigtail formed within the abscess cavity. Contrast injection confirms the position and demonstrates any potential communication with the biliary tree, which may alter further management. The drain is then connected to a drainage bag via a three-way tap and the contents aspirated and flushed into the drainage bag. The drain can be secured in place by means of an anchor suture. To ensure adequate drainage, the catheter should be flushed regularly with normal saline. Aspiration alone may be beneficial for smaller collections, but percutaneous drainage is more effective in achieving maximal cavity collapse [15–17].

Complications

Ultrasound-guided liver abscess drainage comes with small risks. The liver is a vascular organ and therefore there is an inherent risk of bleeding with any liver intervention. Inadvertent vessel laceration, pseudoaneurysm, and arteriovenous fistula formation are uncommon [18]. Bleeding from small vessels is usually self-limiting and can be managed conservatively; however, persistent bleeding from a pseudoaneurysm may require angiography and embolisation.

Although a low risk, spread of abscess contents into the peritoneal space or blood stream is a risk in percutaneous liver abscess drainage. This can be mitigated by ensuring the time between dilating the tract and inserting the drainage catheter is as short as possible. Given that the walls of liver abscesses are usually hypervascular, transient sepsis as a result of transfer of abscess contents into the blood stream occurs in up to 5% of cases [18].

The risk of injury to adjacent structures is small when the needle is visualised in real time and cross-sectional imaging used to plan entry route. Nevertheless, puncture of bowel and spleen has been reported. If the puncture is technically difficult, a 21G Chiba should be used.

Echinococcal Cysts

Echinococcal cysts are caused by the larval stage of the parasite *Echinococcus granulosus sensu lato* and occur most commonly in the liver. These wall-limited cysts, may be uni-or multilocular. For uncomplicated cysts, medical therapy with albendazole is the treatment of choice, but is less effective for more complex cysts (CE2 and CE3b). Percutaneous ultrasound-guided drainage is a treatment option for unilocular (CE1 and CE3a) cysts, but is ineffective for multiloculated ones (CE2 and CE3b), where surgery or modified percutaneous procedures may be necessary [19, 20] (See chapter 7).

Congenital Liver Cyst

Liver cysts in the context of polycystic kidney disease are usually innumerable. The dominant cysts may occasionally cause mass effect and sometimes pain. These dominant cysts may be treated with aspiration and injection of a sclerosant such as sodium tetradecyl sulphate (STS). It is advisable to assess for communication with the biliary tree by injecting contrast prior to sclerosing hepatic cysts. Recurrence is frequent in cases of aspiration alone.

Cholecystostomy

Although laparoscopic cholecystectomy is the gold-standard treatment for calculus gallbladder disease, there are two scenarios where percutaneous cholecystostomy should be considered. First, in patients with acute cholecystitis caused by an obstructing calculus who are poor surgical candidates (Figure 14.6), percutaneous cholecystectomy

can provide temporary drainage of the gallbladder. Second, cholecystostomy is beneficial in critically ill patients with sepsis and radiological evidence of cholecystitis refractory to antibiotic treatment.

The technique of cholecystostomy insertion is identical to liver abscess drainage described above, but the gallbladder is the target. Most interventional radiologists will also opt for fluoroscopic guidance; however, this is not essential, and cholecystostomy may be performed solely under ultrasound guidance on the intensive care unit in the critically ill patient. The operator has the option of a transhepatic or transperitoneal approach and should choose the route that appears safer and less technically challenging, as there is no significant difference in complications or morbidity between the two approaches [21].

Thermal Ablation

The liver is a site of both primary hepatic malignancy and secondary metastatic deposits, most frequently from colorectal cancer. Traditionally surgical resection, or in the case of hepatocellular carcinoma (HCC) liver transplantation, was the mainstay of treatment. However, in recent years percutaneous, ablative techniques have evolved, and now play a major role in treating malignant liver lesions with a curative intent. Ablative techniques include RFA, microwave, cryoablation, and irreversible electroporation. RFA will be described, given it is the most commonly used modality.

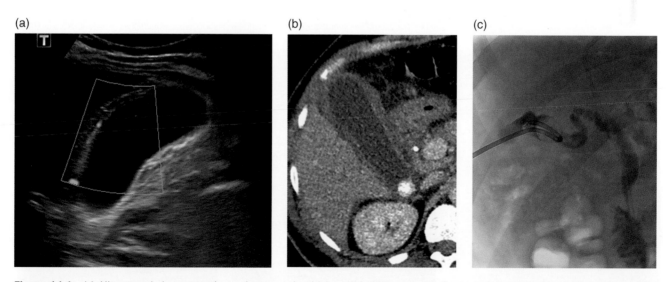

(a)   **(b)**   **(c)**

Figure 14.6 (a) Ultrasound demonstrating a hyperaemic, thick gallbladder wall. (b) Computed tomography of the same patient confirming acute cholecystitis and a gallstone at the gallbladder neck. The patient went on to have cholecystostomy, as he became increasingly unwell despite intravenous antibiotics. (c): A cholecystogram several weeks following cholecystostomy insertion demonstrating a plastic stent in the common bile duct (CBD), no CBD calculi, and a gallstone in the neck of the gallbladder. The patient eventually had an uncomplicated cholecystectomy following recovery from the acute event.

Technique

RFA utilises an alternating current (200–1200 Hz) passed through a closed-loop circuit consisting of a radiofrequency generator, electrode, grounding pads, and the patient [22]. Ionic agitation at the tip of the RFA probe, which is placed under ultrasound, CT, or MRI guidance, creates friction, heat (target 60–100 °C), and resultant cell death as the result of coagulative necrosis [23]. Similar to a surgical margin, the goal is to achieve a 1 cm ablation margin around the tumour to minimise the risk of tumour recurrence; therefore, a planned ablation diameter 2 cm greater than the tumour diameter is selected based on prior cross-sectional imaging (Figure 14.7).

The procedure is usually performed under heavy conscious sedation or general anaesthesia. Antibiotics are recommended to minimise the risk of developing hepatic abscess [24]. If the lesion is seen well on ultrasound, this is used to guide needle placement. CT is then used to confirm needle position.

Patient Selection

There is substantial evidence for the use of thermal ablation for HCCs smaller than 3 cm in patients who are not eligible for resection or transplantation [25, 26]. There is also mounting evidence for its use in the treatment of colorectal cancer liver metastases. In tumours adjacent to high-flow vessels larger than 3 mm, the heat-sink effect caused by thermal energy being dissipated away from the tumour and thereby impeding treatment efficacy must be considered during the patient selection phase as well as during follow-up.

Follow-Up

Imaging follow-up is essential to monitor treatment response. A commonly used imaging follow-up regime is using contrast-enhanced CT (pre-contrast/arterial and portal venous phase examinations) or liver MRI at 1, 3, 6, and 12 months after treatment. CEUS may also play a role during follow-up. A smooth, concentric, and symmetrical enhancing rim on follow-up imaging is typically seen and should be differentiated from irregular and nodular peripheral enhancement, which is suggestive of residual tumour.

Complications

Complications arising from RFA of liver lesions are infrequent. The largest study of 16 346 treated lesions in 13 283 patients performed by Koda et al. found a 3.5% complication rate and 0.04% mortality rate [27]. In the study, direct liver injury was caused in 1.69% of cases, including hepatic infarcts, liver abscess, bile duct injuries, and bile leaks. Extrahepatic injury as a result of RFA was also found to be uncommon (0.69%), including pleural effusion, pneumothorax, gastrointestinal injury, diaphragmatic injury, and gallbladder injury. The risk of extrahepatic injury can be reduced using hydro-dissection, which involves injecting 5% dextrose solution under image guidance between the target lesion and adjacent organ, separating them and thereby minimising the risk of injury.

(a)   (b)   (c)

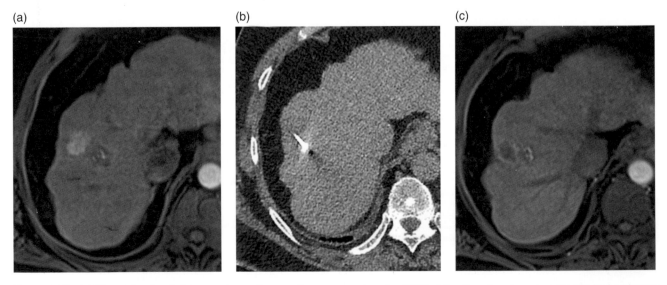

Figure 14.7 (a) T1-weighted gadolinium-enhanced magnetic resonance imaging (MRI) of the liver showing a hepatocellular carcinoma (HCC) in segment VIII. (b) Computed tomography image confirming the position of the microwave ablation needle in the HCC following insertion under ultrasound guidance. (c) Follow-up MRI at three months showing appropriate post-ablation appearances.

Biliary, Portal Venous Access

Biliary Access

Percutaneous transhepatic cholangiography was initially introduced as a diagnostic tool for imaging the biliary tree. It has been replaced by non-invasive modalities such as ultrasound, CT, and magnetic resonance cholangiopancreatography (MRCP). Over the years, however, percutaneous transhepatic biliary drainage (PTBD) has evolved into an effective therapeutic option to treat biliary obstruction, with a complementary role to endoscopic retrograde cholangiopancreatography (ERCP).

PTBD involves the percutaneous insertion of an internal/external biliary drainage catheter through the liver, biliary tree, and into the duodenum in the first instance. This allows internal as well as external biliary drainage as a temporary measure to decompress the biliary tree and eventually allows for further intervention, including transbiliary biopsy, stone clearance, as well as plastic and metal stent insertion.

Indications	Contraindications
Biliary obstruction and failed ERCP	Uncorrected coagulopathy
Biliary obstruction and impossible ERCP (e.g. gastric bypass surgery)	Undrained ascites
Hilar biliary obstruction with ≥first-order ductal separation	
Post-surgical bile leak to divert bile away from the site of leak	

Technique

A full discussion of biliary intervention is beyond the scope of this chapter. Instead, we will describe the use of ultrasound for initial biliary access. The lobe/segment to be drained is determined on cross-sectional imaging. In cases of a distal biliary obstruction, the authors' preferred approach is drainage via a peripheral segment III duct; this is because segment III is relatively superficial, with the ducts being easily visualised on ultrasound. Segment III ducts also allow for favourable angles for subsequent navigation through the biliary tree. This approach is more comfortable for patients compared with an intercostal approach. PTBD is usually tolerated with moderate conscious sedation, but some patients may require general anaesthesia.

Pre-procedural ultrasound is performed to identify a dilated peripheral segment III duct. The planned access point is marked on the skin. Following skin preparation and local anaesthesia, a 2 mm skin nick is made. The ultrasound probe is aligned along the long axis of the duct, which is then accessed using a 21G Chiba needle

(Figures 14.8 and 14.9). The inner stylet is removed and a pre-flushed extension tube with a 20 mL contrast syringe is attached to the hub of the needle, ensuring the needle is not displaced. An attempt should be made to aspirate bile, but this is not essential, particularly in cases of minimal biliary dilatation. Contrast is then injected gently under fluoroscopy guidance confirming biliary access (contrast flows slowly towards the liver hilum, in the biliary tree, in a dripping candle wax fashion). This is followed by the introduction of an 0.018 in. guidewire into the biliary tree, allowing subsequent insertion of a 4-French dilator-stiffener-sheath system. Once the dilator and stiffener are removed, the sheath allows the insertion of an 0.038 in. guidewire and subsequently a catheter. Care must be taken not to traverse the liver capsule too many times in attempts to cannulate the ducts, as this increases the risk of bleeding. The needle may be retracted and the trajectory adjusted without retracting it completely beyond the liver capsule. The puncture should be as peripheral as possible to reduce the risk of major vascular injury.

Portal Venous Access

Portal venous access is used in some instances of portal venous intervention, such as portal vein embolisation, portal venous stenting, and embolisation of parastomal varices. The access procedure is similar to biliary access described above, except for targeting a peripheral portal vein. Colour Doppler is useful to help identify a peripheral portal vein branch. Once a Chiba needle is used to puncture a peripheral portal vein, blood is aspirated confirming venous puncture. Contrast injection under fluoroscopy guidance should demonstrate flow towards the periphery of the liver.

Use of Ultrasound to Aid Transjugular Intrahepatic Portosystemic Shunt Creation

Transjugular intrahepatic portosystemic shunt (TIPS) is an effective treatment for some sequalae of portal hypertension, namely refractory variceal bleeding, ascites and hepatic hydrothorax as well as in the secondary prevention of variceal haemorrhage. TIPS is also indicated in patients with Budd-Chiari syndrome, where other less invasive management strategies have failed. There is also increasing evidence that TIPS may play a role in select patients with portal/mesenteric vein thrombosis. The aim of the technique is to create a communication between the portal circulation and the hepatic veins in order to reduce portal pressure. Portal venous puncture is often the most

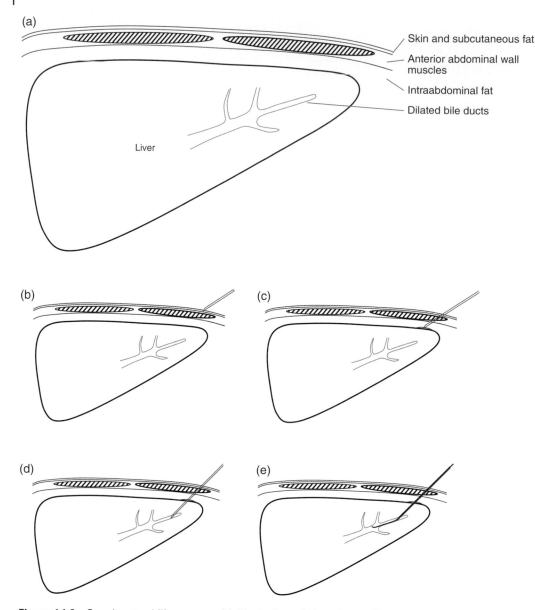

Figure 14.8 Step-by-step biliary access. (a) Illustration of the relevant liver anatomy on ultrasound. (b) Skin infiltration with local anaesthesia. (c) Infiltration of the liver capsule with local anaesthesia. (d) Peripheral bile duct access. (e) Introduction of an 0.018 in. guidewire to the biliary tree following aspiration of bile and contrast injection confirming biliary access.

challenging step of the procedure, with associated potential complications including haemorrhage. Numerous techniques have been described to aid portal venous puncture, with varying levels of success. Transabdominal ultrasound needle guidance is a cost-effective technique that remains underutilised.

Once the liver access kit is introduced into the right or middle hepatic vein via an internal jugular venous approach, a sonographer stands on the patient's right-hand side and images the liver with ultrasound via an intercostal approach.

The operator introduces the needle via the liver access kit, through the hepatic vein wall, as the sonographer visualises it using ultrasound as it courses towards the right portal vein. The sonographer guides the operator by stating the direction they have to move the ultrasound probe in order to visualise the right portal vein as they move it away from the needle tip. The operator then changes torque on the access sheath in order to alter the dirction of the needle accordingly. Continuous feedback is given until the portal vein is accessed. Care must be taken by the operator not to

(a) (b)

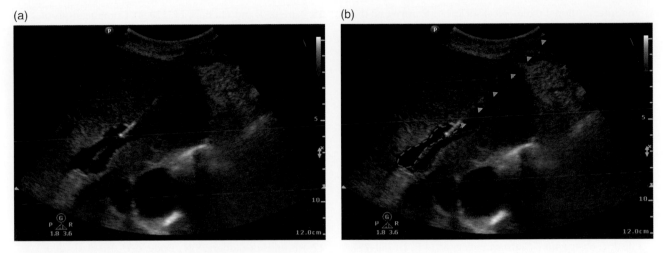

Figure 14.9 (a, b) Ultrasound images with and without annotations demonstrating biliary access using a Chiba needle. Yellow arrowheads: needle; blue dotted line: local anaesthetic near the liver capsule; green dotted line: dilated, peripheral segment VI bile duct; red dotted line: segment VI peripheral portal vein.

introduce air into the system, as this reduces the sonographer's ability to visualise the needle tip. The technique is associated with high levels of technical success while minimising radiation exposure [28].

TIPS Follow-Up

Most institutions will perform an ultrasound examination 24 hours following TIPS creation and prior to patient discharge. These serve as a baseline for subsequent ultrasound examinations. Follow-up varies between institutions. An example of routine TIPS follow-up is with ultrasound at three months, six months, and six monthly thereafter, with earlier follow-up if symptomatic. Klinger et al. suggested that routine follow-up in the absence of dysfunction after 24 months may not be necessary, as the incidence of TIPS stenosis is low in those who had no stenosis within two years and no other intervention [29]. Those who required intervention within the first two years of shunt creation remain at high risk of TIPS dysfunction and require ongoing routine imaging follow-up.

Shunt velocity measurements should be 1–2 m/s and should be consistent throughout the shunt. A variety of ultrasound parameters have been described in the assessment of TIPS dysfunction [30]. These include:

- Maximum velocity in the shunt of <60 cm/s along the length of the stent graft.
- A change in shunt velocity of >50 cm/s compared to baseline at the same site.
- Lack of flow through the TIPS stent.
- Change in direction of flow in the main portal vein, left, and right portal vein branches from the baseline ultrasound.
- Return of the main portal vein flow to hepatofugal.
- Worsening ascites or increase in spleen size.

Such abnormal parameters should prompt invasive venography and intervention.

References

1 Patel, I.J., Davidson, J.C., Nikolic, B. et al. (2012). Consensus guidelines for periprocedural management of coagulation status and hemostasis risk in percutaneous image-guided interventions. *J. Vasc. Interv. Radiol.* 23 (6): 727–736.

2 Haynes, A.B., Weiser, T.G., Berry, W.R. et al. (2009). A surgical safety checklist to reduce morbidity and mortality in a global population. *N. Engl. J. Med.* 360 (5): 491–499.

3 Royal College of Radiologists (2019). *Guidance on Implementing Safety Checklists for Radiological Procedures*, 2e. London: Royal College of Radiologists www.rcr.ac.uk/system/files/publication/field_publication_files/bfcr191_checklists-radiological-procedures.pdf.

4 Chehab, M.A., Thakor, A.S., Tulin-Silver, S. et al. (2018). Adult and pediatric antibiotic prophylaxis during vascular and IR procedures: a society of interventional radiology practice parameter update endorsed by the cardiovascular

and interventional radiological society of Europe and the Canadian association for interventional radiology. *J. Vasc. Interv. Radiol.* 29 (11): 1483–501.e2.

5 Al Knawy, B. and Shiffman, M. (2007). Percutaneous liver biopsy in clinical practice. *Liver Int.* 27 (9): 1166–1173.

6 Murphy, F.B., Barefield, K.P., Steinberg, H.V., and Bernardino, M.E. (1988). CT- or sonography-guided biopsy of the liver in the presence of ascites: frequency of complications. *Am. J. Roentgenol.* 151 (3): 485–486.

7 Grant, A. and Neuberger, J. (1999). Guidelines on the use of liver biopsy in clinical practice. *Gut* 45 (Suppl 4): IV1.

8 Morris, J.S., Gallo, G.A., Scheuer, P.J., and Sherlock, S. (1975). Percutaneous liver biopsy in patients with large bile duct obstruction. *Gastroenterology* 68 (4 Pt 1): 750–754.

9 Fohlen, A., Bazille, C., Menahem, B. et al. (2019). Transhepatic forceps biopsy combined with biliary drainage in obstructive jaundice: safety and accuracy. *Eur. Radiol.* 29 (5): 2426–2435.

10 Hall, T.C., Deakin, C., Atwal, G.S., and Singh, R.K. (2017). Adequacy of percutaneous non-targeted liver biopsy under real-time ultrasound guidance when comparing the Biopince and Achieve biopsy needle. *Br. J. Radiol.* 90 (1080): 20170397.

11 Karavaş, E., Karakeçili, F., and Balcı, M.G. (2019). A comparison of needle types and biopsy techniques used in liver biopsies of chronic hepatitis B patients. *Viral Hepat. J.* 25: 1–5.

12 Hatfield, M.K., Beres, R.A., Sane, S.S., and Zaleski, G.X. (2008). Percutaneous imaging-guided solid organ core needle biopsy: coaxial versus noncoaxial method. *Am. J. Roentgenol.* 190 (2): 413–417.

13 Chi, H., Hansen, B.E., Tang, W.Y. et al. (2017). Multiple biopsy passes and the risk of complications of percutaneous liver biopsy. *Eur. J. Gastroenterol. Hepatol.* 29 (1): 36–41.

14 Joshi, G., Crawford, K.A., Hanna, T.N. et al. (2018). US of right upper quadrant pain in the emergency department: diagnosing beyond gallbladder and biliary disease. *Radiographics* 38 (3): 766–793.

15 Dulku, G., Mohan, G., Samuelson, S. et al. (2015). Percutaneous aspiration versus catheter drainage of liver abscess: a retrospective review. *Australas. Med. J.* 8 (1): 7–18.

16 Zerem, E. and Hadzic, A. (2007). Sonographically guided percutaneous catheter drainage versus needle aspiration in the management of pyogenic liver abscess. *Am. J. Roentgenol.* 189 (3): W138–W142.

17 Cai, Y.L., Xiong, X.Z., Lu, J. et al. (2015). Percutaneous needle aspiration versus catheter drainage in the management of liver abscess: a systematic review and meta-analysis. *HPB* 17 (3): 195–201.

18 Lorenz, J. and Thomas, J.L. (2006). Complications of percutaneous fluid drainage. *Semin. Intervent. Radiol.* 23 (2): 194–204.

19 Brunetti, E., Kern, P., Vuitton, D.A. (2010). Writing Panel for the WHO-IWGE. Expert consensus for the diagnosis and treatment of cystic and alveolar echinococcosis in humans. *Acta Trop.* 114 (1): 1–16.

20 Stojković, M., Weber, T.F., Junghanss, T. (2018). Clinical management of cystic echinococcosis: state of the art and perspectives. *Curr Opin Infect Dis.* 31 (5): 383–392.

21 Loberant, N., Notes, Y., Eitan, A. et al. (2010). Comparison of early outcome from transperitoneal versus transhepatic percutaneous cholecystostomy. *Hepato-Gastroenterology* 57 (97): 12–17.

22 Rhim, H., Goldberg, S.N., Dodd, G.D. 3rd et al. (2001). Essential techniques for successful radio-frequency thermal ablation of malignant hepatic tumors. *Radiographics* 21(special issue): S17–S35.

23 Lencioni, R., Crocetti, L., Cioni, D. et al. (2004). Percutaneous radiofrequency ablation of hepatic colorectal metastases: technique, indications, results, and new promises. *Invest. Radiol.* 39 (11): 689–697.

24 Sutcliffe, J.A., Briggs, J.H., Little, M.W. et al. (2015). Antibiotics in interventional radiology. *Clin. Radiol.* 70 (3): 223–234.

25 Tateishi, R., Shiina, S., Teratani, T. et al. (2005). Percutaneous radiofrequency ablation for hepatocellular carcinoma. An analysis of 1000 cases. *Cancer* 103 (6): 1201–1209.

26 Lencioni, R., Cioni, D., Crocetti, L. et al. (2005). Early-stage hepatocellular carcinoma in patients with cirrhosis: long-term results of percutaneous image-guided radiofrequency ablation. *Radiology* 234 (3): 961–967.

27 Koda, M., Murawaki, Y., Hirooka, Y. et al. (2012). Complications of radiofrequency ablation for hepatocellular carcinoma in a multicenter study: an analysis of 16 346 treated nodules in 13 283 patients. *Hepatol. Res.* 42 (11): 1058–1064.

28 Tavare, A.N., Wigham, A., Hadjivassilou, A. et al. (2017). Use of transabdominal ultrasound-guided transjugular portal vein puncture on radiation dose in transjugular intrahepatic portosystemic shunt formation. *Diagn. Interv. Radiol.* 23 (3): 206–210.

29 Klinger, C., Riecken, B., Muller, J. et al. (2018). Doppler ultrasound surveillance of TIPS-patency in the era of covered stents - retrospective analysis of a large single-center cohort. *Z. Gastroenterol.* 56 (9): 1053–1062.

30 Maleux, G., Nevens, F., Wilmer, A. et al. (2004). Early and long-term clinical and radiological follow-up results of expanded-polytetrafluoroethylene-covered stent-grafts for transjugular intrahepatic portosystemic shunt procedures. *Eur. Radiol.* 14 (10): 1842–1850.

15

Advancing Ultrasound Technologies

Adrian K.P. Lim[1,2], James P.F. Burn[1], and Caroline Ewertsen[3]

[1] Department of Imaging, Imperial College Healthcare NHS Trust, London, UK
[2] Department of Metabolism, Digestion and Reproduction, Imperial College London, UK
[3] Department of Radiology, Riyshospitalet, Copenhagen, Denmark

Ultrasound technology continually improves in leaps and bounds and when first introduced, it was primarily to assess anatomical structures and detect focal lesions. The development of Doppler and subsequently contrast ultrasound added yet another dimension to ultrasonic assessment of the liver, and the current state-of-the-art technologies also employ texture analysis and elastography, with a multiparametric approach to non-invasive liver assessment in chronic hepatic disease. This chapter is a summary of current available technologies (accurate at time of publication), some of which are still undergoing trials to evaluate their efficacy.

Ultrasound B-Mode/Greyscale Imaging

Optimum image resolution has been the paramount goal of ultrasound manufacturers, where the detection of focal liver lesions and also texture appreciation rival those of other imaging modalities, namely computed tomography (CT) and magnetic resonance imaging (MRI), where sub-centimetre lesions can be better characterised with ultrasound. The spatial and temporal resolution is improved with better probe technologies, where the penumbra of the frequency range of the probe is increased, covering ranges between 2 and 9 mHz rather than 1–5 mHz previously. The ability to generate thinner ultrasound beams also provides improved image homogeneity and image processing algorithms remove noise and artefact, giving a 'cleaner' image.

One constant limiting factor has also been body habitus, where an increase in body mass index (BMI) significantly reduces ultrasound penetration and resolution. There are now lower-frequency probes allowing visualisation up to a 30 cm depth, but of course with a trade-off of poorer image quality than with more conventional probes. However, some imaging is better than none, particularly in populations where obesity is becoming an ever-increasing problem.

Doppler Technologies

Microvascular flow imaging (MFI) is the general terminology to encompass the more sensitive Doppler offerings, where clever algorithms allow the depiction of slow-flowing vessels separate from noise. The common acronyms include superb microvascular imaging (SMI, Canon Medical Systems, Tochigi, Japan), micro-flow imaging (MFI, Philips Medical Systems, Eindhoven, Netherlands), or just microvascular imaging (MVI, Samsung Medical Systems, Kyonggi, South Korea). GE Healthcare (Chicago, IL, USA) has in addition to microvascular flow Doppler technology, a version that utilises B-mode rather than Doppler technology and is termed B-flow.

MFI applies an advanced Doppler algorithm and unique wall filters to identify, isolate, and eliminate clutter. The result is preservation of low-velocity flow signals, allowing representation of microvessel blood flow to be depicted. This is achieved at low mechanical index, high frame rates (enabled with plane wave imaging), and without the need for contrast agents. The end result is a Doppler technique that has significantly improved sensitivity and spatial resolution, in comparison to standard colour Doppler/power Doppler ultrasound [1–4].

The visualisation is much refined (Figure 15.1), but is technically not seen down to micrometres and the vessels depicted are in the range of 1 mm or so. Nonetheless, this adds to the diagnostic capability and can sometimes obviate the need for contrast enhancement, particularly in the correct clinical setting (Figures 15.2 and 15.3).

Liver Ultrasound: From Basics to Advanced Applications, First Edition. Edited by Adrian K.P. Lim and Matteo Rosselli.
© 2024 John Wiley & Sons Ltd. Published 2024 by John Wiley & Sons Ltd.
Companion website: www.wiley.com/go/LiverUltrasound

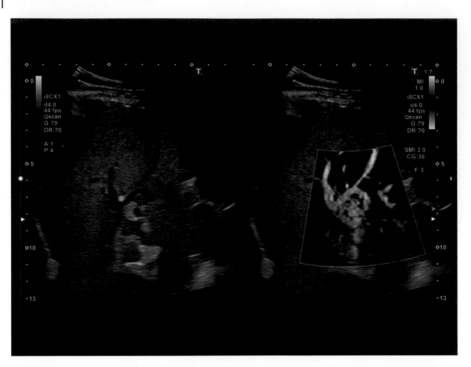

Figure 15.1 (Video 15.1) This shows a thrombosed portal vein with numerous collaterals. The right-hand image is the monochrome version of superb microvascular imaging (SMI), Canon Medical Systems' version of microvascular flow imaging. Note the superb resolution of the small vessels and collaterals, which are typically not shown with colour Doppler. *Credit:* A. Wilson, A.K.P. Lim., (2022), ELSEVIER , Licenced under CC BY 4.0.

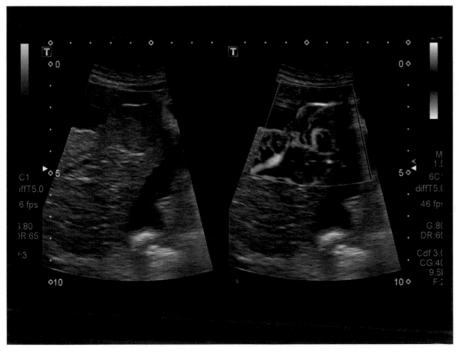

Figure 15.2 (Video 15.2) There is an exophytic focal lesion on a background of liver cirrhosis. Note the nodular edge and ascites within segment VI of this liver. The right-hand image is with superb microvascular imaging (SMI) turned on. Note how clearly the abnormal haphazard neoangiogenic vessels are displayed without the use of contrast. This microvascular pattern clearly denotes a hepatocellular carcinoma. *Credit:* A. Wilson, A.K.P. Lim., (2022), ELSEVIER , Licenced under CC BY 4.0.

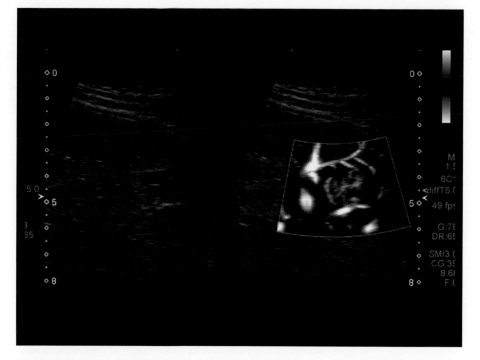

Figure 15.3 (Video 15.3) This was an incidental finding in a young female patient with no medical history of note. There was suggestion of a subtle hypoechoic lesion in the liver and on turning on monochrome superb microvascular imaging (SMI; right-hand image), the stellate, spoke–wheel pattern of this vascular lesion is clearly depicted. There has been no injection of contrast and, given the lack of a history of malignancy or chronic liver disease, it can safely be diagnosed as focal nodular hyperplasia (FNH), warranting no further imaging. The greyscale isoechoic appearance would also be compatible with FNH.

The changing vascular pattern of the liver parenchyma with significant chronic liver disease can be appreciated and, while still in the research realms, an attempt at quantifying this change is promising at staging disease and may provide a cancer risk stratification. These methods, however, are still work in progress, although artificial intelligence algorithms have significantly enhanced this process [5].

Contrast-Enhanced Ultrasound

The sensitivity and resolution of contrast images continually improve, but, more importantly, this technology is available even on portable and lower-end scanners, which will benefit more remote areas and developing countries, where the cost of premium-end ultrasound scanners can be difficult to justify and priority is given to more basic medical necessities.

The software to combine MFI and fusion technology with contrast-enhanced ultrasound (CEUS) also keeps improving and can be clinically useful, particularly with intervention.

Time–intensity curves for evaluation of tumour response remain under research, as it can be difficult to follow or evaluate the entirety of a tumour within the liver ultrasonically. It may be that developing artificial intelligence algorithms provide an evaluation of the patterns of disease within the liver that cannot be perceived by the human eye.

Shear Wave Elastography

Shear wave elastography (SWE) is an innovative application enabling indirect assessment of liver stiffness and thus fibrosis. It has seen much development over the years and validation studies are ongoing, but its utility in many guidelines as an adjunct or even instead of a liver biopsy is becoming more frequent. These have been discussed in detail in Chapter 11.

Manufacturers and scientists are still looking into increasing the volume of the liver being sampled in the form of 3D-SWE, which has been shown to be efficacious in other organs (e.g. breast tumours) and has been promising on some studies with 3D magnetic resonance elastography (MRE) [6, 7].

This technology remains under evaluation for liver applications where the equipment and technique are more challenging compared with 2D-SWE, but the advantages over the latter are not clear.

The SWE community has also managed to tackle the problem of different SWE systems giving slightly different values. The cut-offs to 'rule in' or 'rule out' compensated advanced chronic liver disease may prove clinically more useful than trying to correlate SWE values and histological levels of fibrosis [8].

Viscosity

SWE has been shown to be an effective method of assessing liver stiffness and thus indirectly liver fibrosis, although this can be erroneous in patients with inflammation or steatosis. When liver inflammation occurs, viscosity is also increased leading to an increase in shear wave propagation speed and thus stiffness values. In acute hepatitis of different aetiologies and non-alcoholic steatohepatitis (NASH) where the viscosity is increased, so is liver stiffness. This is in turn, misinterpreted as fibrosis, and probably explains the inaccuracies and mis-classifications of SWE. The main reason for these discrepancies is that viscosity properties are neglected in current algorithms for quantifying liver elasticity.

Shear wave dispersion (SWD) imaging is a new technology developed by ultrasound manufacturers. In viscoelastic tissue, shear wave speed experiences frequency dispersion; that is, the change of shear wave speed is dependent on the shear wave frequency. There is a positive correlation between dispersion and viscosity, and thus SWD technology that measures the dispersion slope, indirectly provides a handle on the viscosity of the tissue sampled. This is typically expressed in m/s/kHz and is additional information while performing a 2D-SWE measurement (Figure 15.4). Recent clinical studies have shown that this measurement of the dispersion slope (SWD) is better correlated with necroinflammation within the liver than is 2D-SWE [9, 10].

Attenuation Imaging/Parameter

The degree of attenuation of the ultrasound beam varies depending on the type of tissue, and a measurement of the attenuation coefficient (dB/cm/MHz) in a given sample indirectly provides the 'make-up' of the tissue. In the

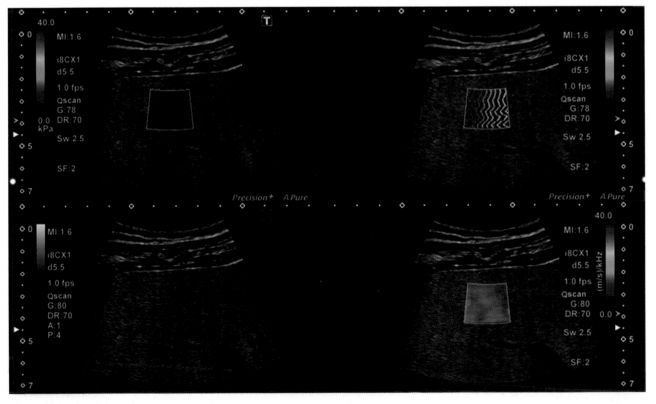

Figure 15.4 The quad view function on the Aplio i-series (Canon Medical Systems), where the top left colour map is 2D shear wave elastography (note the scale in kPa), the top right line image is the propagation map denoting a good study where all the lines are nicely parallel, and the bottom right image is the colour map for dispersion slope/viscosity (note the scale in m/s/kHz). Lastly, the bottom left image is the localising greyscale image showing the segment assessed, depth, and that the liver capsule is parallel with the probe.

(a)

(b)

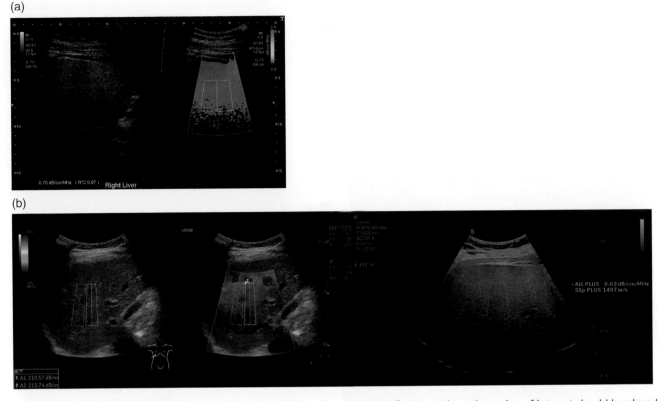

Figure 15.5 (a) A map showing attenuation imaging (ATI) from Canon Medical Systems, where the region of interest should be placed below the liver capsule (orange bar) and the attenuation coefficient is given in the numbers below. Note that the R^2 value denotes the reliability of the study: the closer to 1.0, the more accurate the acquisition. (b) Examples of the different offerings of attenuation imaging on premium-end scanners by GE (left) and Supersonic (right), respectively. Note that the scale and values will differ among manufacturers between what is considered to be normal versus the varying degrees of hepatic steatosis severity. *Source:* Courtesy of Prof Ioan Sporea.

liver, the commonest attenuating factor is fatty infiltration, and therefore this parameter has been utilised to estimate fatty change of a liver. This concept was first introduced in FibroScan, known as the controlled attenuation parameter (CAP) score, and many of the ultrasound manufacturers have now followed suit, combining it with their 2D-SWE, commonly termed as attenuation imaging or variations of that terminology. The latter, unlike FibroScan, also provides visualisation of the liver that has been sampled (Figure 15.5). There have been many studies now that have shown this parameter can be correlated with hepatic steatosis and also has a similar performance when compared with MRI proton density fat fraction (MR-PDFF), which is an accepted non-invasive method for assessing steatosis [11–13].

Fusion

The technology to fuse ultrasound imaging with CT or MRI volume datasets has been available for many years. This technology has been cumbersome, but is now fast and easy to use, with the number of steps to set it up significantly reduced. Many systems now also utilise a generated magnetic field and a probe sensor rather than an optical sensor to detect the 'position in space' of the ultrasound probe (Figure 15.6). This allows the scanner to manipulate the CT/MRI images to move in a similar and synchronised fashion with the real-time ultrasound scan and images (Figure 15.7).

The synchronisation algorithms have continually improved and while this technology is predominantly utilised for interventional purposes, such as in ablation procedures, it can also be helpful in diagnosis. This is highlighted in Figure 15.6, where frequently indeterminate tiny (<5 mm) lesions in the liver seen on CT can be difficult to find with cognitive fusion; the ability to fuse the CT images with ultrasound allows more accurate characterisation of these lesions. The method can also be used to keep track of lesions in patients with multiple lesions, for instance in the liver. Here it can be used to count and mark lesions, so they will not be counted twice.

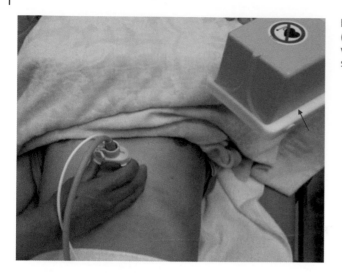

Figure 15.6 The typical set-up for ultrasound fusion, with the box (arrow) showing the magnetic field generator. Note the additional wiring attached to the probe, which is the sensor to enable the scanner to detect the 'position in space' of the probe.

(a)

(b)

(c)

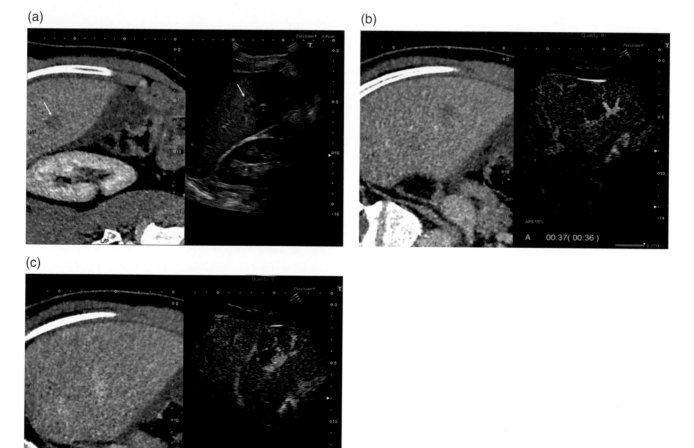

Figure 15.7 (Video 15.4) (a) The left-hand image shows the subtle low-density lesion (arrow) in the liver in a patient with a known malignancy. Note that on the synchronised ultrasound image there is only a suggestion of a subtle hypoechoic lesion (arrow). (b, c) Contrast-enhanced ultrasound can also be used. This delineates more clearly where there is peripheral nodular enhancement and gradual centrifugal infilling, clearly denoting a haemangioma.

Conclusion

Ultrasound technologies can now provide a multiparametric assessment of the liver and not only information on anatomical structure and vascular flow. Many of these advancing technologies are continually being evaluated and refined against more traditionally accepted forms of liver assessment, but are showing great promise. The cheap, easily accessible, and non-invasive nature of ultrasound when compared with the other imaging modalities makes it more attractive and a viable tool for the mass population.

References

1 Bae, J.S., Lee, J.M., Jeon, S.K., and Jang, S. (2020). Comparison of MicroFlow Imaging with color and power Doppler imaging for detecting and characterizing blood flow signals in hepatocellular carcinoma. *Ultrasonography* 39 (1): 85–93.

2 Lee, D.H., Lee, J.Y., and Han, J.K. (2016). Superb microvascular imaging technology for ultrasound examinations: initial experiences for hepatic tumors. *Eur. J. Radiol.* 85 (11): 2090–2095.

3 Lim, A.K. (2014). The clinical utility of superb microvascular imaging (SMI) for assessing musculoskeletal inflammation. White paper, Toshiba Medical Systems.

4 Hata, J. (2014). Seeing the unseen. New techniques in vascular imaging: superb microvascular imaging. *White paper, Toshiba Medical Systems.*.

5 Kuroda, H., Abe, T., Kakisaka, K. et al. (2016). Visualizing the hepatic vascular architecture using superb microvascular imaging in patients with hepatitis C virus: a novel technique. *World J. Gastroenterol.* 22 (26): 6057–6064.

6 Choi, H.Y., Sohn, Y.M., and Seo, M. (2017). Comparison of 3D and 2D shear-wave elastography for differentiating benign and malignant breast masses: focus on the diagnostic performance. *Clin. Radiol.* 72 (10): 878–886.

7 Loomba, R., Cui, J., Wolfson, T. et al. (2016). novel 3d magnetic resonance elastography for the noninvasive diagnosis of advanced fibrosis in NAFLD: a prospective study. *Am. J. Gastroenterol.* 111 (7): 986–994.

8 Barr, R.G., Wilson, S.R., Rubens, D. et al. (2020). Update to the Society of Radiologists in Ultrasound Liver Elastography Consensus Statement. *Radiology* 296 (2): 263–274.

9 Sugimoto, K., Moriyasu, F., Oshiro, H. et al. (2020). Clinical utilization of shear wave dispersion imaging in diffuse liver disease. *Ultrasonography* 39 (1): 3–10.

10 Sugimoto, K., Moriyasu, F., Oshiro, H. et al. (2020). the role of multiparametric us of the liver for the evaluation of nonalcoholic steatohepatitis. *Radiology* 296 (3): 532–540.

11 Karlas, T., Petroff, D., Sasso, M. et al. (2017). Individual patient data meta-analysis of controlled attenuation parameter (CAP) technology for assessing steatosis. *J. Hepatol.* 66 (5): 1022–1030.

12 Ferraioli, G., Maiocchi, L., Savietto, G. et al. (2021). Performance of the attenuation imaging technology in the detection of liver steatosis. *Ultrasound Med.* 40 (7): 1325–1332.

13 Ferraioli, G., Maiocchi, L., Raciti, M.V. et al. (2019). Detection of liver steatosis with a novel ultrasound-based technique: a pilot study using MRI-derived proton density fat fraction as the gold standard. *Clin. Transl. Gastroenterol.* 10 (10): e0008.

Index

Liver Ultrasound: From Basics to Advanced Applications, First Edition. Edited by Adrian K.P. Lim and Matteo Rosselli.
© 2024 John Wiley & Sons Ltd. Published 2024 by John Wiley & Sons Ltd.
Companion website: www.wiley.com/go/LiverUltrasound